**The Dartmouth
Institute for Better Health
The Dartmouth Medical School**

MEDICAL AND HEALTH GUIDE FOR PEOPLE OVER FIFTY

Eugene C. Nelson, D.Sc.
Ellen Roberts, M.P.H.
Jeannette Simmons, D.Sc.
William A. Tisdale, M.D.

**A Program for Managing
Your Health**

An AARP Book

published by

American Association of Retired Persons, Washington, D.C.
Scott, Foresman and Company, Lifelong Learning Division, Glenview, Illinois

19-25 The quizzes and scales of functional health were developed by the Rand Corporation and can be used without permission with the proper acknowledgment.

38-40 From CAN FRIENDS HELP YOU STAY WELL? Copyright © 1981 by California Department of Mental Health. Reprinted by permission.

54-55, 274-286 Adapted by permission of Scott, Foresman and Company from FITNESS FOR LIFE by Theodore Berland. Copyright © 1986 by Theodore Berland.

73 Reprinted from RECOMMENDED DIETARY ALLOWANCES, 9th edition, 1980, National Academy of Sciences, Washington, D.C.

82 From FEELING FIT: A GUIDE TO AN ACTIVE LIFESTYLE. Copyright © 1982 Pawtucket Heart Health Program, Pawtucket, Rhode Island. Reprinted by permission.

Library of Congress Cataloging-in-Publication Data
Main entry under title:

Medical and health guide for people over fifty.

  Includes bibliographies and index.
    1. Geriatrics—Popular works.   2. Aging.   3. Medicine,
Popular.   I. Nelson, Eugene C.   II. Dartmouth Institute
for Better Health.   III. American Association of
Retired Persons.   [DNLM: 1. Aging—popular works.
2. Geriatrics—popular works.   3. Hygiene—in old age—
popular works.   WT 120 M489]
RC952.M39 1986   613'.0438   85-22072
ISBN 0-673-24816-X (Scott, Foresman)

AARP Books is an educational and public service project of the American Association of Retired Persons, which, with a membership of 20 million, is the largest association of persons fifty and over in the world today. Founded in 1958, AARP provides older Americans with a wide range of membership programs and services, including legislative representation at both federal and state levels. For further information about additional association activities, write to AARP, 1909 K Street, N.W., Washington, DC 20049.

■■ PUBLISHERS' NOTE

Informed practice of medical self-care includes making appropriate use of the health care facilities in your community. If you know or suspect that you have a serious health problem, consult a professional health worker.

CONTENTS

PART ONE   PERSONAL HEALTH ASSESSMENT AND PERSONAL ACTION

PART TWO   ORGANIZING SELF-CARE

PART THREE   COMMON HEALTH PROBLEMS AND SELF-CARE TECHNIQUES

FOREWORD

What is health? Do we merely define it as "freedom from physical disease or pain"? Or does it transcend the physical realm and encompass the whole gamut of "well-being" including the social and emotional? Are we always as old as the calendar says we are? Or as young?

Actually, investigators are telling us that there is a lot of truth in the adage "You are only as old as you feel." More and more, we are learning that a positive attitude and a healthy, active lifestyle help forestall many of the traditional effects of aging.

No longer does increasing age necessarily mean years in a wheelchair or an institution. There are today 27 million people in the United States over the age of sixty-five. This number is projected to double by the year 2020. Contrary to the popular notion that old people cannot take care of themselves, only 5 percent of today's over-sixty-five population, and only about 23 percent of those over eighty-five, live in institutions. Without doubt older people are not only living longer and healthier lives but also doing so within the community.

It is important—indeed, vital—to understand the concept of "normal aging." What bodily changes are due to aging per se? What changes are caused by destructive lifestyles or treatable diseases? It has been carefully documented at the National Institute on Aging's Gerontology Research Center in Baltimore, Maryland, and in studies by other investigators as well, that an individual free of disease may have little if any decline in physical or mental functioning with age. It has been found that personality remains constant as well. Additional studies have yielded important findings. For example, research has shown that lung function improves after a person, at any age, stops smoking. These are all important concepts with which to grapple. For years we have been led to believe that transformations caused by advancing years rob a person of his or her special characteristics, leaving that individual to be considered simply one more of "the elderly." Now, for the first time, we understand that healthy aging means, for the most part, a continuation of one's individuality.

That is not to say that changes do not occur with age. We know that there are certain chronic conditions that become more prevalent with age. These conditions are, indeed, very real and cause a great deal of anguish to older people and their families in later years. We know, for example, that there are definite changes in hearing and vision and in the way drugs react in the body. We are aware, too, of the great toll arthritis, heart conditions, and Alzheimer's disease place on many older people. Such disabilities may require the aid of another person in order to carry out some daily functions.

There is a lot we still need to know and understand about aging. With continued research and an adequate number of trained professionals in the field, the future is a hopeful one.

We also recognize that aging people have many concerns, not only about themselves but also about their loved ones. People want to know more about proper nutrition and exercise, about insomnia and depression, about forgetfulness and headaches. These concerns are not trivial and need to be addressed. Herein lies the purpose for this book: to address issues, discuss causes and symptoms, and then suggest possible ways the problem might be solved or prevented. *Medical and Health Guide for People Over Fifty* by no means is meant as a substitute for medical care. It is, however, a way to promote awareness, encourage a healthier lifestyle, and offer constructive suggestions to an individual responsible for his or her own health management. It is meant as a guide that should help people become knowledgeable about the body in the hope of avoiding some detrimental habits and adopting some that may be beneficial toward a healthy old age. It provides the reader with an opportunity to become actively involved in health maintenance.

I began with a question, What is health? It is, in my opinion, the ability to remain functional throughout one's lifetime with a minimum amount of disease and chronic ailment. This is the goal, and this book should help you achieve it.

T. Franklin Williams, M.D.
Director
National Institute on Aging
Bethesda, Maryland

PREFACE

People can improve the quality of their lives by taking more responsibility for their own health. Recognition of this fact led some members of the Dartmouth Medical School faculty to form the Dartmouth Institute for Better Health for the purpose of developing community health-education programs. The first program developed by the institute was called Self-Care for Senior Citizens and began in 1977. Within a few years, the authors of this book shaped the program into a twenty-six-hour course held in communities in various parts of the United States.

The success of the program—in helping hundreds of older people learn how to take more responsibility for staying healthy—prompted the W. K. Kellogg Foundation to award a grant to the Dartmouth Institute for Better Health, the American Association of Retired Persons, and the American Red Cross. The grant gives these three organizations the opportunity to work together to offer an updated version of the original course, now called "Staying Healthy After 50," in communities throughout the nation, using this book as the basic text.

ACKNOWLEDGMENTS

Many people contributed generously to the development of this guidebook. The authors are especially grateful to the following individuals and organizations:

To John E. Ware, Jr., Ph.D., and his colleagues at the Rand Corporation—Allyson Ross Davies, Ph.D.; Cathy Sherbourne, M.A.; and Anita L. Stewart, Ph.D.—for their guidance in how to measure health status.

To the Henry J. Kaiser Family Foundation, for allowing us to reprint the results of its research on national norm scores for people aged fifty and older.

To Elaine Shamos for her major contribution to the writing of chapters 3 and 4, which focus on self-improvement and adjusting to stress.

To Nancy Mason, who, through her involvement in the Health Promotion for Older Americans Program at the Dartmouth Institute for Better Health, gave guidance to the development and testing of concepts in Part One, "Personal Health Assessment and Personal Action."

To Anne Harvey at AARP, who supported the concept of this book from the beginning, and to editors Gloria Mosesson and Elaine Goldberg, who provided valuable guidance and advice along the way.

Finally, to Linda J. McLean for the skill and energy she gave to preparing Part Three, "Common Health Problems and Self-Care Techniques," and to Lynda MacElman, who worked diligently and tirelessly on the preparation, typing, and revising of the manuscript.

INTRODUCTION

If you are like most people, you want to be as healthy as possible for as long as possible—to get the most out of life. Health is not just a matter of inherited genes and luck. It can be shaped by those who care about it at any age. What you do to and for yourself *will* make a difference in the level of health you enjoy.

Learning how to get better control of your health is an active process. Once you kow the basics of good health, as described in this book, you can confidently take charge of your health, deal with medical problems if they arise, and, if necessary, work effectively with your doctor and other health professionals.

Medical and Health Guide for People Over Fifty is an important book for you if want to do more to take care of your own health, need information on how to go about doing this, and want to know when to get help from a health professional. It is not meant to replace common sense or professional advice.

The book is divided into three parts.

PART ONE: Personal Health Assessment and Personal Action

This part of the book helps you assess your own health from three perspectives—physical, emotional, and social (chapter 1, 2, and 3). It will help you adopt a healthier lifestyle by coping with the troubling feelings that loneliness and stress cause (chapter 4), becoming more physically fit (chapter 5), following a well-balanced diet (chapter 6), and improving your social relationships, if you wish.

PART TWO: Organizing Self-Care

Chapters in this part of the book help you learn what is important in forming a positive partnership with your doctor (chapter 7), how to keep good medical records (chapter 8) and handle medications (chapter 9), and how to locate community resources when you need help (chapter 10).

PART THREE: Common Health Problems and Self-Care Techniques

Here you will find information on almost sixty health ailments common to older people that lend themselves to self-care techniques. Each ailment is described, and causes and symptoms are given. Specific sections alert you to symptoms potentially severe enough that you should consult your doctor instead of treating yourself. Your doctor may refer you to another health professional, but your first stop should be with your own doctor or at a health facility where you are known. The ailments described were selected because associated problems can be dealt with fairly simply, and early attention and care can prevent serious consequences. Major illnesses that might require hospitalization for treatment are not included, such as some forms of cancer and heart disease.

No textbook or educational program can fully cover your unique health habits and needs. But you can get personal insights into techniques that lead to fewer worries and more enjoyment—and, therefore, a healthier life. This book was written to give you a good start.

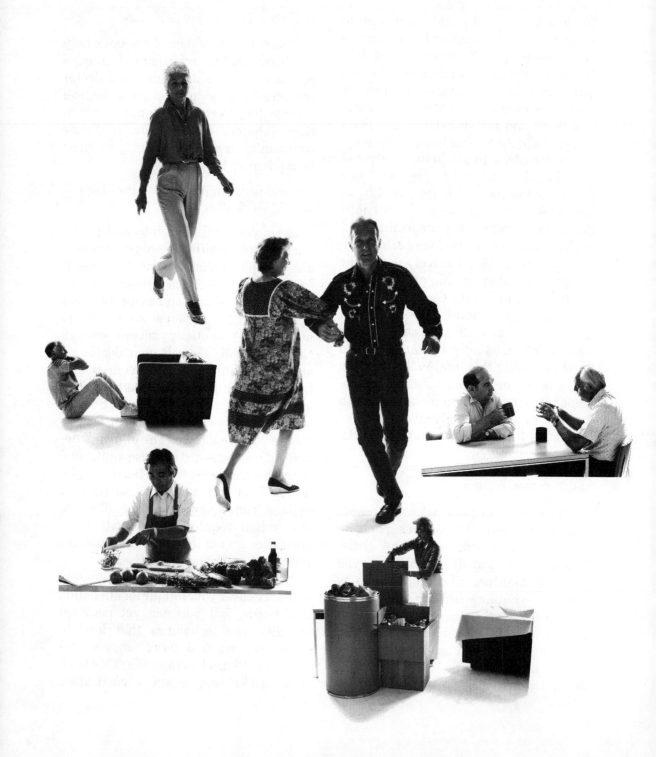

PART ONE

PERSONAL HEALTH ASSESSMENT AND PERSONAL ACTION

Chapter 1

Health: It Depends on You

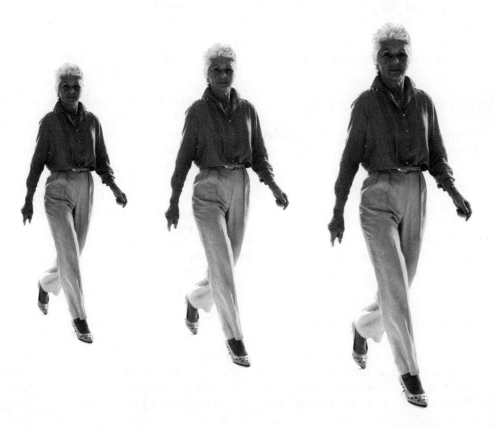

This part of *Medical and Health Guide for People Over Fifty* will give you information on ways to take charge of your health. You will be provided tools to assess your own level of health and your health-related daily behaviors (for example, emotional responses, physical activity, and eating). You will be introduced to specific things you can do to feel better.

You will be challenged to take stock of what you *know* and *believe* about good health and to compare it to what you *do* about your health. When you spot gaps or inconsistencies, you can take charge and make changes.

Before taking some tests to assess your health (chapter 2) and finding out the steps you can take to feel better than you may be feeling now (chapters 3 to 6), you need first to explore what health really is and how aging ties into health.

HEALTH AND FUNCTION

When you've got your health, you've got everything, the saying goes. But what is good health? More important, is good health a matter of luck, or is it something you can work for?

A quick look at a day in the lives of two women, Susan S. and Barbara C., both of whom are in their sixties, may help answer these questions.

Susan's Day: Susan begins her day by rising early and doing a few stretching exercises. After stretching, she dresses, has a glass of juice, and meets her neighbor Elsie for their two-mile morning walk. After their walk, Susan comes home and fixes herself a good breakfast—a half of a grapefruit, a bowl of bran cereal with banana slices and low-fat milk, and coffee. Since Susan is diabetic, she has to adhere to her diet strictly and eat properly. After breakfast, Susan washes the dishes, dusts the furniture in the apartment, and vacuums the living room. She then showers and dresses for her afternoon work as a volunteer at a local nursing home, where she has her lunch with some of the other volunteers. At three-thirty, Susan returns home to rest and relax for a little while before going to her daughter's home for dinner. She leaves her apartment at 6:30 P.M. to drive to her daughter's home.

Barbara's Day: Barbara rises at 10:30 A.M. She had trouble getting to sleep the previous night and was up most of the time. Upon arising, Barbara goes into the kitchen, turns on the TV, and fixes herself coffee and toast. She spends the next hour watching television, drinking coffee, and smoking cigarettes. Barbara is still tired, however, because she did not sleep well, and after breakfast she goes back to bed for a little nap. Upon awaking, Barbara gets up and goes into the kitchen for a snack of cookies and hot tea. She then proceeds to do her ironing while watching the TV soap operas. Later in the afternoon, Barbara's niece phones and invites her for dinner that evening. Barbara thanks her niece but declines the invitation by saying that she did not sleep well the previous night and thus is too tired to go out.

Everyone knows people like Susan and Barbara. Susan is busy and productive, enjoying pleasant experiences each day. Barbara, on the other hand, is often lonely and tired and feels unproductive.

Of the two, Susan appears healthier than Barbara.

From a biomedical point of view, however, Barbara could be considered the healthier one. Susan has a chronic disease, diabetes, while Barbara has no major chronic disease. Yet Susan is healthier from a *functional* point of view. Functional health is the capacity to perform the normal activities of daily living in a natural home environment and the ability to enjoy life.

Susan understands her health problem and has made the decision to take positive action to manage and improve her condition and make the most of her life. She takes responsibility for herself and creates a daily pattern of living that is rewarding and satisfying to her. *Good health is more than simply not having an obvious disease.* It is realizing your physical, emotional, and social potential as an individual. It is being able to participate in your community and being able to enjoy life. It is an active effort to cut down your chances of suffering from disease. It is your own strong belief that, for your age, your health is excellent.

DIMENSIONS OF HEALTH

The World Health Organization views health as complete physical, emotional, and social well-being. Good health is a combination of good genetics, a healthy body, a sound mind, and positive social relationships. Thus these dimensions of health—physical, emotional and social— add up to an overall health status.

Having "complete" or totally good health in every dimension is rare. Therefore, thankfully, it is not essential to have perfect health in all dimensions in order to gain a full measure of life satisfaction. This is because strength in one dimension—for example, emotional health—can more than make up for weakness in another dimension, such as physical health.

Thus, in the cases of Susan and Barbara, Susan would score high on physical, emotional, and social dimensions. She does her best, by working with her doctor, to maintain her well-being and to control her problem of diabetes. The result is an overall health status rating that is highly positive. Barbara, in contrast, would score higher on physical dimension, since she is free from a chronic disease. But the high mark on physical dimension would be counterbalanced by a low score on emotional and social dimensions. The outcome is an overall health status rating for Barbara that is more negative than Susan's.

A person's health status can move in either direction, positive or negative, as time passes. Getting older does not guarantee a negative shift on any of the health dimensions. Most people at any age can improve their health status by a bit of work and self-study.

DETERMINANTS OF HEALTH STATUS

What determines a person's health status? Most medical experts now agree that five factors—heredity, environment, health outlook, health care, and lifestyle—are the prime determinants of health (see figure 1).

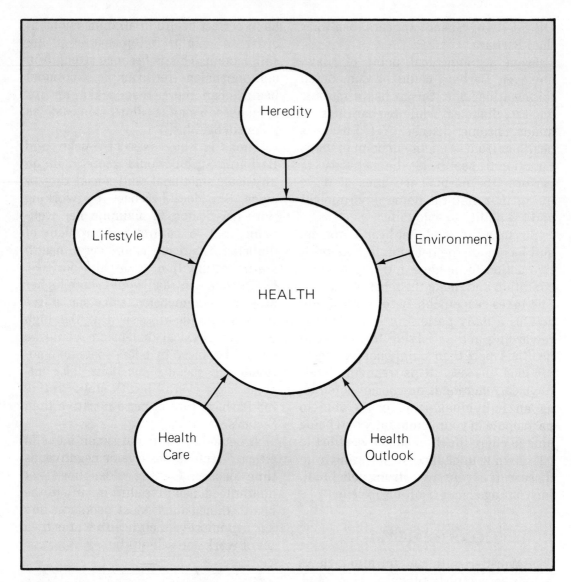

Figure 1. Determinants of Health

This is what is meant by these five terms:

- **Heredity** refers to your individual biological inheritance. This determines your body build and the way your body responds to wear and tear throughout life.

- **Environment** has two aspects: the physical environment in which you live (air, water, earth, noise) and the social environment (friendly or hostile, safe or dangerous, fast pace or slow pace).

- **Health outlook** refers to your feelings,

thoughts, beliefs, and images about your own level of health and well-being.

■ **Health care** is the action that you take on your own, through self-care, or on the recommendations you receive from physicians, nurses, and other health professionals to prevent or treat disease or to promote health.

■ **Lifestyle** is the unique pattern of your daily life. It is the food you eat, the exercise you get, the alcohol you drink, the cigarettes you smoke, and the way you react to stress. Lifestyle is related to your philosophy of life. It is knowing when to take care of things on your own and when to seek help. Lifestyle is also expressed by the way you handle difficult situations and loneliness.

Today the average person is still likely to believe that keeping healthy simply means visiting a doctor regularly for a general physical examination and evaluation. Many people put their health in their doctors' hands because they feel that good health stems first and foremost from good medical care. This can be thought of as the "good health equals good medical care" equation.

In today's world, however, medical care may very well *not* be an important determinant of health. Consider this startling fact: At the turn of the century, the leading causes of death were infectious diseases such as tuberculosis, scarlet fever, and smallpox. These were all caused by microorganisms, or germs. Today, by contrast, the three leading causes of death are all noninfectious chronic diseases. They are, in rank order, heart disease, cancer, and stroke.

What this change means is that the major factors that cause most disability and that may ultimately cause death have turned around completely over the past eighty years. The causes of today's major diseases are not microorganisms, but, in a sense, ourselves. This is because the development of chronic disease is often associated with lifestyle. In addition, chronic disease, at times, is caused by human-made problems in the environment such as air pollution and water pollution. Therefore, both the lifestyle that you choose for yourself and the places where you live and work, your environment, can make positive or negative contributions to your health.

CONTROL OVER DETERMINANTS OF HEALTH

When you review the five main determinants of health, you can quickly see that factor one, heredity, is beyond personal control. Sometimes a person can influence the second factor, environment, for example, by moving to a warmer climate or by becoming more actively involved with community groups. But often people are forced to accept the environment "as is."

With the three remaining factors—health outlook, health care, and lifestyle—you can see a tremendous opportunity to take charge, to be the captain of your own fate. Health outlook is almost completely under your own control. It is simply your personal view of your overall health status and sense of well-being. A small proportion of people do not have a personal physician and have great difficulty gaining access to health care. The majority, however, have two options: (1) to be active, knowledgeable practitioners of self-care and responsible users of medical care or (2) to be passive patients who do only "what the doctor says," invest little personal energy in health maintenance, and hope for the best. Finally, while recognizing that lifestyle is largely imposed on people when young and is subsequently shaped by the environment, the bottom line is that it is up to the individual to choose his or her lifestyle.

It is obvious that the person who believes that his or her health is potentially top-notch, learns and practices safe and medically assisted self-care, is a knowledgeable and responsible user of professional medical care, and develops a positive lifestyle stands the best chance of optimizing his or her own health status.

SCIENTIFIC EVIDENCE ON LIFESTYLE AND HEALTH CARE

While it is recognized that on occasion medical care backfires (for example, by producing severe drug side effects), scientific evidence confirms the fact that health care is a determinant of good health. In addition, there is also increasing scientific evidence that lifestyle has a dramatic effect on health and that health care works best when it includes the active involvement of the person through medically assisted self-care. Here are the findings of some recent studies.

■ In a study of 7,000 people aged forty-five and over, researchers found that

chances for a long and vigorous life were much better for those who had positive lifestyles that included these seven features.

1. three meals a day
2. breakfast every day
3. moderate exercise several times per week
4. adequate sleep
5. no smoking
6. moderate weight
7. no alcohol or moderate use of alcohol

(Belloc and Breslow, 1972)

■ A study of deaths resulting from cirrhosis of the liver and lung cancer concluded that the death rates for these diseases are lifestyle-related. Study participants were residents of Utah and Nevada, states with similar socioeconomic and climatic characteristics. Researchers found that the Nevadans were more likely to die from these two diseases than were their neighbors in Utah. Thus, the study results served to reinforce earlier findings that death from cirrhosis of the liver is related to drinking and death from lung cancer is related to smoking. Researchers credited the difference in death rates to the following:

1. the tendency of Utah residents to avoid alcohol and tobacco due to the influence of Mormonism
2. the tendency of Nevada residents to lead a more hard-driving, rough-and-ready way of life, including the use of alcohol and tobacco

(Fuchs, 1974)

■ Several studies into trends in life expectancy since the turn of the century have been conducted recently.

Researchers discovered that a new trend became apparent between 1975 and 1980: life expectancy among individuals who reached age fifty has increased dramatically since the turn of the century. Men have gained five years and women more than ten. That means that a man who turned fifty in 1981 can expect to reach age seventy-five, and a woman who turned fifty in the same year can look forward to her eighty-first birthday. Most of the gain in years of life was attributed to a decrease in deaths due to cardiovascular problems such as heart attack and stroke. The studies concluded that the decrease in the number of deaths, and thus the increase in life expectancy, was due to more moderate lifestyles. This measurable moderation included the following features.

1. People smoked less.
2. People consumed less fats.
3. People exercised more.
4. People practiced better weight control.
5. People formed more active partnerships with their doctors to control high blood pressure.

(NEJM, 1985)

■ Studies dealing with self-care for minor problems such as colds and sore throats reached the following conclusions.

1. Self-care is safe for these minor problems.
2. Self-care can save the doctor's time.
3. Self-care can save the individual's money.

(Zapka and Averill, 1979; Kemper, 1982; Vickery et al, 1983)

■ In a study evaluating the value of self-care for people with chronic diseases such as hypertension, emphysema, arthritis, and diabetes, researchers came to several conclusions:

1. Self-care practiced along with on-going professional supervision can improve the physical and mental health of the individual.
2. Self-care can help people avoid unnecessary expense.

(Butler, Gertman, Oberlander, and Schlinder, 1979–80)

In short, it makes sense that a positive lifestyle along with prudent self-care and adequate medical care can improve your health and, at the same time, save you money. The scientific evidence is mounting in support of this position.

SCIENTIFIC EVIDENCE ON POSITIVE HEALTH OUTLOOK

It has been shown that a person's health outlook—how he or she perceives his or her own health level—can also help the person feel better and live longer.

A large study involving more than 3,000 Canadians aged sixty-five and older was done to determine whether a person's perception of his or her own health predicted death. All the people in this study were asked a single simple question, For your age would you say, in general, your health is excellent, good, fair, poor, or bad? These 3,000 Canadians were then "tracked" for seven years to establish who lived and who died, what their medical problems were, how much medical care they used, and what their actual clinical status was, based on objective measures.

The results were amazing. First, persons who had rated their own health as "poor" in 1971 proved almost three times more likely to die than people who said their health was excellent. Second, the person's self-rating of health status predicted risk of death much better than did a clinical rating of health status based on the physician's medical diagnosis and the use of medical care.

This study, and others like it, strongly suggest that what an older person *believes* about his or her own health level—the person's thoughts, feelings, and images—is more important than the individual's actual physical level of health. It is not known for sure that if a person thinks positively about his or her own health, it will actually improve that person's health. It could be that many people who believe they are very healthy are in fact already healthy. However, it may well be true that a person can also help "will" himself or herself into good health. (Read chapter 4, "Coping with Stress.")

AGING—THE BASICS

Aging, the complex process of growing older, is a universal fact of life. Although most people realize that stepwise changes in appearance and behavior are inevitable, many persons tend to ignore or resist them. Some of this denial results from misplaced fear. Many people are frightened by their own ignorance of the nature of aging. While it is true that certain aspects of old age are still poorly explained, other aspects are now well understood and understandable.

As noted earlier, one vital dimension of health is *physical*. That is, quality living—and aging—depends on your having strong, well-functioning organs and body tissues. This physical part of living and aging has been shown to follow a certain pattern, or set, of timed stages: (1) intrauterine, or prenatal, development, which ends at the time of birth; (2) growth and maturation, which ends with full adult physical and sexual development; and (3) older adulthood, the stage that ends with death.

Unlike chronological aging, or aging as measured by clock and calendar, true physical aging begins subtly in humans as they reach their twenty-fifth to thirtieth year. This complex process, once under way, seems to proceed slowly and rather steadily. Physical changes in various parts of the body may not take place at the same rate (for example, gray hair arrives before bifocals are needed), and individuals differ considerably in the speed and pattern of aging.

Four general types of physical change characterize human aging:

1. **Changes in body composition**. On the average, height and weight decrease as persons move from age fifty to seventy-five and beyond. Much more important, from a physical point of view, are changes in the makeup, or composition, of the body parts. After age thirty, the percentage of body water declines, body fat increases dramatically, muscle bulk tapers off, and the bony skeleton shrinks in size and strength. These physical facts have important implications for health and survival. Potent sleeping medications (for example, Valium and its derivatives) are "trapped" in this

larger fat compartment and may cause dangerous morning drowsiness, and minor falls in elderly women are likely to result in crippling fractures of weakened hips.

2. ***Changes in body reserve capacities.*** An individual rarely draws upon the ultimate reserve powers of his or her body—even a marathon run by a young athlete will not exhaust the extra "safety valve" power built into his or her heart and lungs. Careful studies have shown that in healthy older persons who do not have chronic disease conditions, heart, brain, and kidney functions may be maintained well into the very late years. However, there is considerable variability among individuals; in addition, the frequent presence of one or more chronic disease conditions—heart disease, high blood pressure, diabetes, and so on—may lead to reduced functional reserves. It has been shown that regular exercise of muscles and most body systems may go far toward preserving their vital functions throughout the years.

3. ***Changes in the body's capacity to repair injury.*** For most of life, injuries to body tissues are followed promptly by a stepwise growth of new tissues and repair of the local damage. Thus a fractured wrist "knits" within weeks, and the lung damage caused by pneumonia is healed completely within ten to twelve days. Compared with young adults, older persons repair or restore injured tissues more slowly. The ultimate repair is complete and effective, but the process involved is slower.

4. ***Changes in response to stress.*** With advancing age, many people respond less efficiently to all sorts of stress. The important lesson to remember is that although aging can slow and dampen the reactions to physical and other types of stress, older persons *do* respond effectively, given time and support.

These four physical patterns observed among older people are generalizations that describe average tendencies. *Individuals age uniquely and distinctively.*

Aging processes in various organs proceed at different rates within a particular person—hence the eighty-year-old woman who is blessed with a sharp, creative intellect but cursed by "old age" arthritis of the hips.

Dramatic differences in levels of body function may be found within a group of people of similar age and background. Scientists have shown, for example, that heart and circulatory performances vary widely within a group of seventy-five-year-old male volunteers—more widely, in fact, than when some seventy-five-year-olds are compared with thirty-five-year-olds. Diversity or uniqueness tends to increase with age.

Both physical and emotional functions tend to change gradually with advancing age, but there is no real evidence to suggest that losses accelerate or snowball. Although loss of many body reserves may begin by age thirty, no one risks "running out of sand" by living to be a hundred.

Much is known about aging in humans, but much more is still either unknown or unclear. Some physical changes, such as loss of muscle tone and bone strength, may be preventable or partly reversible by exercise and proper diet. Others, such as age-related thickening of the heart wall, may be inevitable elements of old age. Research into aging, its basic causes and critical effects, is still a new enterprise, but one fact is known for sure: Physical aging is not simple!

No one pretends that scientists can describe complex human events adequately in simple physical terms. Consideration of older adulthood demands, therefore, that scientists also take into account the emotional and social dimensions of health as well. Fortunately, temporary or even permanent deficiencies in one dimension may be counterbalanced by strength in the others. Thus, the elderly woman who is temporarily handicapped following cataract surgery can rely on guardrails, supportive friends, and an optimistic outlook until she recovers. Equally important, one may lose some physical capabilities without a major change in critical personal *functions*. Osteoarthritis (see pages 255–257) may render a hip lame and stiff, for example, but physical therapy and judicious use of a cane may ensure good functional health.

Few aspects of total health are more important than level of intelligence, or mental functioning. Basic intellectual powers change very little in the course of normal aging. These powers—which include the abilities to learn, remember, use language, and reason, among others—seem to decline very little, if at all, between the ages of twenty-five and seventy-five. Some experts feel that very intelligent people live longer. Others doubt this relationship, pointing out that intelligence probably contributes to longevity by providing ample income, safe housing, and greater life satisfaction. At any rate, although many specific types of mental functions are difficult to measure, some psychologists report that older persons tend to perform mental tasks less efficiently. At worst, they simply take longer to carry out certain test exercises. Still others suggest that forgetfulness and confusion—often misnamed "senility"—characterize the very old. Careful testing indicates that this perception is incorrect and that the intellectual difficulty is simply slowness of recent recall (see pages 147–149). The really essential intellectual skills remain intact in normal older people, so active learning, creativity, critical reasoning, and sound judgment should be sustained throughout later life.

Many older people cite distinct advantages to advanced age: lessened family responsibilities, new freedoms, unique personal opportunities, and fewer social pressures. The intelligent and thoughtful older person capitalizes on these advantages and enjoys the ultimate intellectual reward—wisdom.

PRESCRIPTION FOR SUCCESSFUL AGING

Dr. Robert N. Butler, a Pulitzer Prize winner and the first director of the National Institute on Aging, has issued a general prescription for healthful aging. Dr. Butler's prescription stresses three types of action: physical, mental, and social.

■ ***Physical***. Watch nutrition, keep fat under 30 percent in your daily diet, don't smoke, limit alcohol use, and get plenty of exercise (for example, a brisk walk several times each week).

■ ***Mental***. Keep your mind active! Build up your interest in sports, reading, the arts, hobbies, current events, civic activities, or whatever captures your imagination. People who have goals, ambitions, and some organized pattern of daily activities are likely to live longer and enjoy life more.

■ ***Social***. Cultivate strong bonds with people. Having good social networks—close friends and relatives—and sharing activities with people you know and trust not only make life more fun but also lead to better health outcomes. It is especially important to have friends and relatives available to help out in hard times, such as with sickness or the death of a loved one.

Your health depends on you. You are the doctor, and you can write your own prescription for *successful* aging.

Chapter 2

How Healthy
Are You?

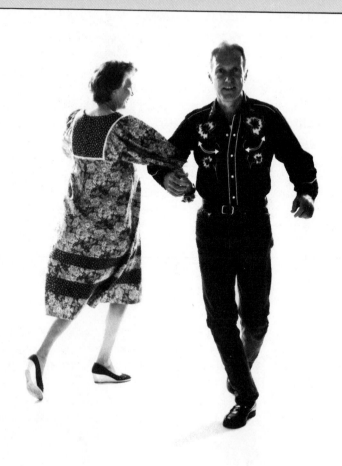

The purpose of assessing your own health is to help you become better acquainted with your health strengths and to identify any health weaknesses. You then can use this information to plan more effectively ways to maintain and/or improve your health—both on your own and with the aid of your physician. The main question to be answered in this chapter is, How can I evaluate my own health status?

FUNCTIONAL VIEW OF HEALTH

There are many different ways to view health and to measure it. Doctors, on the one hand, traditionally have learned to view health almost totally from a *physical* perspective. They learn to evaluate their patients' health in terms of disease or lack of it. Any changes from a normal physical state are assessed to confirm the absence or presence of disease and, if a disease is present, its severity. This physical view of health is now being recognized by leading physicians as being too narrow.

Lay people, on the other hand, often look at health more broadly and from a different vantage point than doctors. They usually think in terms of *illness* rather than disease and in terms of *function* rather than physical status. Illness, from the lay perspective, is the individual's view of how a disease disrupts important activities essential for daily functioning or how a disease undermines the individual's ability to do things that add zest and happiness to life, such as socializing with friends, engaging in hobbies, or working on enjoyable projects. For example, you may think of illness in terms of how severely it interferes with your ability to do work around the house, walk around town, go shopping, or participate in activities like golf, dancing, and fishing.

Most people are concerned with maintaining an active and pleasurable daily lifestyle, pursuing whatever they consider their normal activities without being held back by health problems. This functional view of health is a very practical one and is gaining acceptance among doctors and other health professionals. The functional approach is especially useful in assessing the health of older persons. As individuals age, they become increasingly concerned with finding the best way to stay active and live normal, happy, independent lives. For these reasons, it is best for the individual to evaluate his or her health primarily from a functional perspective, which includes physical, emotional, and social considerations. It is also helpful to document the general perceptions of the individual's current health. This is very important because scientific studies show that people's perceptions of their own health predict how well they function, both physically and emotionally, and are even associated with longevity (see chapter 1).

HEALTH MAINTENANCE AND IMPROVEMENT

Whether a medical visit is for a specific problem or a routine health examination, the doctor customarily goes through a four-step process, shown in figure 1. First, the doctor collects information about you by taking a medical history, performing a physical examination, and ordering laboratory and other diagnostic tests. Next, the doctor makes an assessment of your condition that takes into account all the information about you that has been collected; if indicated, he or she makes a diagnosis regarding any abnormal conditions found. Third, the doctor works with you to establish a plan of treatment or a routine for health improvement if either is indicated. Fourth, the physician follows your progress in carrying out your plan and monitors your health status. As the need arises, adjustments are made in your treatment plan.

As figure 1 indicates, the health maintenance and improvement process begins with the collection of information about you and your health. The four self-assessment quizzes on pages 19, 20, 21, and 23 can assist you with your own data collection. These quizzes on your health perceptions, physical health, emotional health, and social health are based on health measures developed by John E. Ware, Jr., Ph.D., and his colleagues at the Rand Corporation. These health measures have been shown to be valid and reliable indicators of a person's health. They were used in the National Health Insurance Study to find out whether people who got more medical care enjoyed better health.

It is important to take the quizzes. First, you'll probably find them easy to complete and quite enjoyable. Second, you may see that you are in better health than you thought. Third, you can compare your health score with the national average score for people aged fifty and older. So find a quiet place where you

can write comfortably, and give yourself a free health evaluation!

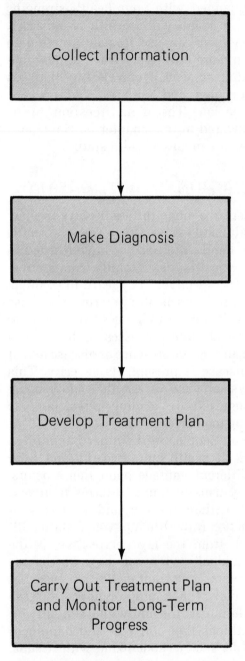

Figure 1. Health Maintenance and Improvement Process

QUIZ: *Health Perceptions*

This quiz measures your views about your overall health. There are no right or wrong answers.

Read each statement at the left. Then read the headings at the right. Circle the number in each row that tells whether the statement is definitely true, mostly true, mostly false, or definitely false—*for you,* or circle the number that tells that you are not sure about the statement.

Statement	Definitely True	Mostly True	Mostly False	Definitely False	Not Sure
1. I am somewhat ill.	1	2	4	5	3
2. I'm as healthy as anybody I know.	5	4	2	1	3
3. I have been feeling bad lately.	1	2	4	5	3
4. My health is excellent.	5	4	2	1	3

To determine your score on the health perceptions quiz, add all the circled numbers.

Put an X on the health perceptions scale, shown on page 25 at the place that corresponds to your score.

You can see how you stand compared with other persons aged fifty to sixty-five by noting where your score is relative to the ⊙ on the health perception scale. The ⊙ marks the average score of a sample of people aged fifty to sixty-five living in the United States.

- A high rank on the health perceptions scale shows that you have a very good view of your health.
- A middle rank on the health perceptions scale suggests that you may view your health as something that could be improved.
- A low rank on the health perceptions scale means that you are far more likely to have one or more chronic diseases, and this may give you an even more negative outlook.

Most people rate their own health as pretty good. If you did not score as well as you would have liked to on this quiz, start to ask yourself these questions.

- What keeps me from feeling better?
- Are there physical, emotional, and/or social reasons for my not feeling better?
- Am I bothered by pain or chronic disease?
- What can I do to make myself feel better?

QUIZ: *Physical Health*

This health quiz will help you quickly size up your physical functioning in activities that are usually essential for daily living.

Answer each question about your general physical capabilities as realistically as possible by circling either 0 or 1 for the answer.

Question	Your Answer	
1. Does your health limit the kinds or amounts of vigorous activities you can do such as running, lifting heavy objects, or participating in strenuous sports?	Yes—limits. 0	No—does not limit. 1
2. Do you have trouble bending, lifting, or stooping because of your health?	Yes—have trouble. 0	No—do not have trouble. 1
3. Does your health limit the kinds or amounts of moderate activities you can do such as moving a table, carrying groceries, or bowling?	Yes—limits. 0	No—does not limit. 1
4. Do you have any trouble either walking uphill or climbing a few flights of stairs because of your health?	Yes—have trouble. 0	No—do not have trouble. 1
5. Do you have any trouble walking one block because of your health?	Yes—have trouble. 0	No—do not have trouble. 1
6. Do you have any trouble eating, dressing, bathing, or using the toilet because of your health?	Yes—have trouble. 0	No—do not have trouble. 1

To figure out your physical health score, follow these steps.

1. For questions 1 and 2, give yourself 1 point if you answered no to both questions. Give yourself 0 if you answered yes to *either* question.

2. Add all the circled numbers for questions 3 to 6.

3. Now, add the points from steps 1 and 2 to get your total score.

Put an X on the physical health scale on page 25 at the place that corresponds to your score.

You can see how your score on the physical health scale compares with the scores of other people aged fifty to sixty-five by noting where the bull's-eye ⊙ appears on the scale.

- A high rank on the physical health scale signifies a very good level of physical function. There are few, if any, physical activities that you cannot do.

- A middle rank on the physical health scale suggests that you can do many physical activities but are not able to do the more strenuous ones.

■ A low rank on the physical health scale means that your physical health prevents you from carrying out many physical activities associated with daily living—in both work and leisure.

Congratulations if you scored near the top of the physical health scale. Although most people do score quite high on this measure, often there may be room for improvement.

If you scored on the Very Poor end of the scale, do not be upset or become too discouraged; you still have to check several other dimensions of health.

If you wish to improve your physical health, keep this in mind for a goal when designing your health improvement plan in chapter 3. There are ways to meet this goal that can be incorporated in your prescription for successful aging. (See chapter 5).

QUIZ: *Emotional Health*

This quiz will help you evaluate your emotional health. It asks about different feelings you may have experienced during the past month.

Read each question at the left. Then read the answer choices at the right. Circle the number in each row that tells whether the answer is All of the time, Most of the time, A good bit of the time, Some of the time, A little bit of the time, or None of the time during the past month.

Question	All of the time.	Most of the time.	A good bit of the time.	Some of the time.	A little bit of the time.	None of the time.
1. How much of the time have you been a very nervous person during the past month?	1	2	3	4	5	6
2. How much of the time have you felt calm and peaceful during the past month?	6	5	4	3	2	1
3. How much of the time have you felt downhearted and blue during the past month?	1	2	3	4	5	6
4. During the past month, how much of the time were you a happy person?	6	5	4	3	2	1
5. During the past month, how often have you felt so down in the dumps that nothing could cheer you up?	1	2	3	4	5	6

To determine your score on the emotional health quiz, add all the circled numbers.

Put an X on the emotional health scale on page 25 at the place that corresponds to your score.

You can see how your emotional health score compares with the scores of other persons in the fifty to sixty-five age bracket by noting where the bull's-eye ⊙ appears on the emotional health scale.

- A high rank on the scale signifies that your emotional health is top-notch; however, there still might be room for improvement.

- A low rank means that your emotional health is likely to be bothersome.

Many people score on the high end of the emotional health scale. A large number, however, fall in the middle or on the low end. If you scored on the Very Poor end of the scale, keep in mind that you assessed your emotional health for only the past month. For various reasons (for example, the loss of a friend, a move to a new location, or a physical health problem), this past month may have been a difficult one for you and thus not a true indicator of your emotional well-being. If, however, you feel that last month was fairly typical for you, you may be truly suffering from poor emotional health. Ask yourself what may be bothering you.

- Am I sad and lonely? Why?

- Am I anxious and worried? Why?

- Do I want to feel better emotionally?

- What might I do to help myself?

If your emotional health ranking was low, there are many ways to improve the situation and thus enable you to feel better and move toward the positive end of the emotional health scale. (See chapter 4.)

QUIZ: *Social Health*

This quiz will help you assess your social health—your relationships with family, friends, and the community.

Read each question at the left. Then read the answer choices at the right and circle the number after the correct answer.

Questions	Your Answer
1. Over *a year's time*, about how often do you get together with friends or relatives, like going out together or visiting in one another's homes?	Several times a week .... 6 About once a week .... 5 Two or 3 times a month .... 4 About once a month .... 3 Five to 10 times a year .... 2 Less than 5 times a year 1
2. During the *past month*, about how often have you had friends over to your home? (Do not count relatives.)	Every day .... 6 Several times a week .... 5 About once a week .... 4 Two or 3 times in past month .... 3 Once in past month .... 2 Not at all in past month 1
3. About how often have you visited with friends at *their* homes during the *past month?* (Do not count relatives.)	Every day .... 6 Several days a week .... 5 About once a week .... 4 Two or 3 times in past month .... 3 Once in past month .... 2 Not at all in past month 1
4. About how often were you on the telephone with close friends or relatives during the *past month?*	Every day .... 6 Several days a week .... 5 About once a week .... 4 Two or 3 times in past month .... 3 Once in past month .... 2 Not at all in past month 1
5. How often have you attended a religious service during the *past month?*	Every day .... 6 More than once a week .... 5 Once a week .... 4 Two or 3 times in past month .... 3 Once in past month .... 2 Not at all in past month 1
6. In general, how well are you getting along with other people these days—would you say better than usual, about the same, or not as well as usual?	Better than usual .... 3 About the same .... 2 Not as well as usual 1

To determine your score on the social health quiz, add all the circled numbers.

Put an X on the social health scale on page 25 at the place that corresponds to your score.

As before, you can see how your social health score compares with the scores of other persons in the fifty to sixty-five age bracket by noting where the bull's-eye ⊙ appears on the scale.

- A high rank on the social health scale signifies that you enjoy a very active social life.

- A middle rank on the social health scale suggests that your social life is relatively active.

- A low rank on the social health scale indicates that you are not mixing much socially with friends or relatives.

By and large, people are happier when they have ample opportunity to mix socially. If you scored on the Very Poor end of the scale, however, you need not be too disturbed. Some people are quite content with a low level of social activity, and you may be that kind of person. Remember, you are in the process of collecting information on your social health. Besides, you may have scored quite well on your health perceptions, physical health, and emotional health quizzes.

If, however, you want to improve your social health, there are many ways to do so. Keep this goal in mind when designing your health improvement plan. (See chapter 3.)

THE FOUR SCALES OF FUNCTIONAL HEALTH

Use the scales on the next page to plot your results on the quizzes on pages 19, 20, 21, and 23. The bull's-eye ⊙ shows the average score of people aged fifty to sixty-five on that quiz.

The whole of health is much greater than the sum of these four parts. This means it is impossible to add up your scores to summarize your total health in any precise way.

The physical, emotional, and social dimensions of health are all fairly separate and distinct. Each dimension contributes to a person's overall health. Each person will have his or her unique pattern of health and will value that pattern in a personal way.

Keep in mind that the different aspects of health can interact with one another, thereby multiplying their effects on you. For instance, think back to a time when you were feeling physically on top of the world—full of energy, sleeping well, and so on. How were your emotional outlook and social activities? A problem in one area or another can change how one handles other aspects of living. However, when you know this, you can take positive steps to compensate.

PUTTING THE PIECES TOGETHER

You have just taken the first step in writing your own successful prescription for healthy living. You have acquired some new information about your health and functioning. You have increased your own knowledge base by learning a bit more about yourself and perhaps by

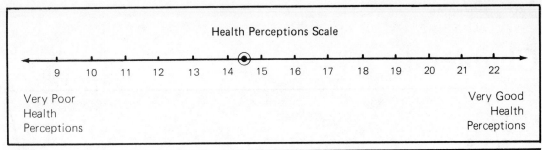

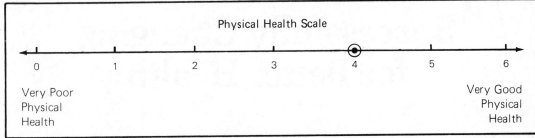

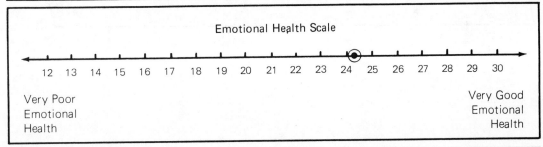

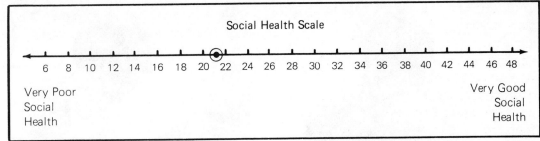

seeing yourself from a slightly different angle. When you look at your standing on the quizzes, there are two important things to remember:

1. *Your score in each area*—health perceptions, physical health, emotional health, and social health—*can change by chance or can be changed* by effort.

2. *An area of outstanding health strength can make up for areas of weakness.*

People have no control over chance events. However, many people do have the capabilities to apply themselves to a task and thereby improve themselves. If, for example, you want to be more physically fit or more socially active, chances are you can!

Chapter 3

Successfully Changing for Better Health

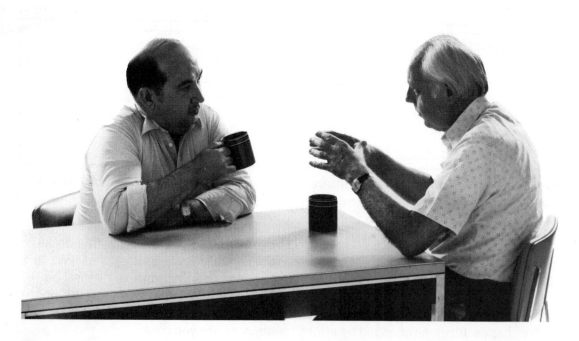

Lifestyle is the unique pattern of your daily life: the food you eat, the medications you take, the cigarettes you smoke, the exercise you get or don't get. Establishing and maintaining a healthy lifestyle is an important goal, and achieving this goal is a lifelong process. But what is a healthy lifestyle?

■ A healthy lifestyle is knowing when to take care of things on your own, and doing what is needed, as well as knowing when to seek help, and getting it.

■ A healthy lifestyle is pursuing a hobby or helping others. It is doing something enjoyable and not allowing yourself to be bored.

■ A healthy lifestyle is knowing how to handle difficult situations and loneliness. It is dealing with yourself, your life, your family, and your friends in a positive manner. It is changing some things in your life but living with those things you cannot change.

Your lifestyle, at this moment, whether good or bad, is distinctly your own and indicates, with some accuracy, your future health status.

You must continually strive to create the kind of life you want to keep up with constantly changing needs and the changing environment. If you don't make the effort, you become the victim of impulse, circumstance, and simple chance.

All people have habits that they automatically follow as part of daily living. At times they make conscious personal decisions to change some of those habits to improve their health.

Oftentimes, however, they choose certain goals, such as losing weight or quitting smoking, because someone has urged them to, such as a family member or a doctor. Think carefully. How well have you succeeded in your past efforts to carry out a decision that was designed to please *others*? It may take some time to make the decision to change something in your life, and it may take even more time to act upon that decision. Therefore, it is much easier to carry out a decision that you have chosen freely because you truly feel that it will help *you*. You are the best judge of your habits, priorities, and weak spots, and you alone experience the rewards or discomforts. You must decide!

Part of the decision-making process involves gathering as much advance information as possible and weighing the pros and cons of making a particular decision. What, for example, are the pros and cons of your losing weight? If, after considering all the possibilities, you decide to lose weight, the decision has now become your choice, not someone else's. Then it is important that your behavior be consistent with your decision. For example, if you decide to lose weight, your eating habits should reflect that decision. One inconsistent move or wrong behavior, however, does not negate the decision or mean that you are a failure. It may simply be the result of inadequate knowledge or a routine habit.

Generally, if you feel good about your decision to make a change in your behavior, the chances are good that you will be able to make the change. The formula on the next page can help you

---

FORMULA FOR ATTAINING BETTER HEALTH

Task 1.   Assess your lifestyle and determine your goals.

Task 2.   Choose one specific behavior in a lifestyle area where you desire some self-change.

Task 3.   Observe yourself and gather information about your behavior patterns in this area.

Task 4.   Identify and evaluate any thoughts, feelings, and attitudes that may either aid or hinder your efforts to change your lifestyle.

Task 5.   Pinpoint the skills and tasks required to change your behavior and practice them.

Task 6.   Constantly monitor the results of your self-change efforts and revise your behavior as needed.

■ CASE STUDY

Sally L. is a seventy-two-year-old woman who had lived in a cold climate for the last forty years. Within the past year, she and her husband moved to Florida because of his failing health. Sally is suffering at present from osteoarthritis and hypertension. Several factors contribute to her medical condition: a smoking habit of two packs of cigarettes per day, an overweight condition of twenty pounds, and a diet high in salt and saturated fats. Most of all, however, she is bothered by the absence of a new social circle.

What has recently motivated Sally to assess her lifestyle is the fact of her husband's recent heart attack, which has left her as his primary caregiver. Her increased responsibility has made her more aware of her own health, and she wants to feel better in her new role.

TASK 1. ASSESS YOUR LIFESTYLE AND DETERMINE YOUR GOALS

Before Sally, or anyone, can start a self-change process, she must assess her entire lifestyle. In chapter 2, you began the process by completing the quizzes. Another way to assess your lifestyle might be to sit down with a pencil and paper and list all the areas in which you have the desire to change or improve yourself. Think of the areas as falling into these categories: physical, emotional, and social well-being. For example, consider Sally.

As with most people, Sally has several lifestyle areas in which improvement is desired. In the area of physical health, she realizes that losing twenty pounds, decreasing her salt intake, eating less fatty foods, and exercising regularly would improve her osteoarthritis and hypertension. Her smoking habit is also detrimental to good health, but Sally finds it difficult to deal with at this time. In the area of emotional well-being, she wants to decrease her anxiety as a primary caregiver by becoming more knowledgeable and competent in caring for her frail husband. She also recognizes that her social well-being would benefit from developing a strong circle of friends in her new community.

TASK 2. CHOOSE ONE SPECIFIC BEHAVIOR IN A LIFESTYLE AREA WHERE YOU DESIRE SOME SELF-CHANGE

Before selecting one specific behavior, you first need to *identify the lifestyle area* where self-change is most desired, for example, the area of physical health. Second, you need to *determine what the problem actually is*—in Sally's case, perhaps not exercising enough. Finally, you need to *pinpoint one specific behavior that is measurable* and to which you can make a commitment to change— in this instance, resolving to get regular exercise by walking twenty minutes per day.

Factors influencing the selection of priorities should include *your personal desire* to change and *your ability to succeed realistically* at change. Ask yourself honestly whether the change you are contemplating is physically possible and economically feasible for you.

In Sally's situation, there are many areas in which she can make efforts at self-change. Sally's social well-being is of top priority to her, and through her assessment she has decided that loneliness and lack of close friends are her major problems. Because of recent relocation and her time-consuming role as caregiver, Sally is now realizing that she must make the effort to meet new people and make new friends. One specific behavior that she has decided to undertake is to initiate conversations with the neighbors in her apartment complex. Sally is highly committed to this behavior change because her husband is now less able to provide emotional support for her. This targeted behavior is both physically possible and economically feasible in her new apartment complex and is a small-enough step to assure her success.

TASK 3. OBSERVE YOURSELF AND GATHER INFORMATION ABOUT YOUR BEHAVIOR PATTERNS IN THIS AREA

Accurate self-observation is the foundation of a successful self-change process. By observing yourself, you become more *aware* of your behavior patterns, especially your established habits. In *analyzing* these behavior patterns, you can understand better the *internal cues* (thoughts or feelings) that trigger your behavior and also learn to recognize the *social and environmental cues* that influence your actions.

To make accurate self-observation easier, it is extremely helpful to record your observations on paper. This will help you describe behaviors that you wish to eliminate and behaviors that you want to continue. (See Appendix E for a full-sized, blank copy of a self-observation chart.)

Sally has decided to record some positive behavior: Get to Know My New Neighbors. Not having made any new friends for a while, Sally has become less confident with this skill. In an effort to make friends in her new location, she is interested in learning more about her behavior patterns as she attempts to begin conversations with her neighbors. Below is a sample of one of her records.

	Self-Observation		
Behavior:			
Date	**Situation** (Briefly describe where you were and whom you were with.)	**Thoughts and Feelings in This Situation** (Briefly describe how you were feeling and what you were thinking.)	**Actions** (Describe how you responded to the situation.)
Wed. 3/20	In the elevator with neighbor from the apartment next door.	Felt silly and nervous. Thought I wouldn't know what to say.	Got off at the next floor.
Thurs. 3/21	In the laundry room with Mrs. J.	Felt excited. Thought she was someone I'd like to get to know.	Mrs. J. started to talk. Had a nice chat with her.
Sat. 3/23	Heard from Mrs. N. that Mrs. Brown downstairs was sick—with 3 kids!	Felt sorry for the family. Thought maybe I could help.	Left a note under door with a get-well card and offered to help with laundry or shopping if they wanted it.

TASK 4. IDENTIFY AND EVALUATE ANY THOUGHTS, FEELINGS, AND ATTITUDES THAT MAY EITHER AID OR HINDER YOUR EFFORTS TO CHANGE YOUR LIFESTYLE

To be successful with your self-change efforts, you must be aware of the thoughts, feelings, and attitudes that affect your behavior. Through record keeping, you will note things you say to yourself. The thoughts, feelings, and attitudes that hinder self-change can be classified as those that happen before making a desired behavior change ("I'm too old to start exercising now") and those that occur while attempting a behavior change ("I should have exercised twice this week; I'll never be able to catch up"). Becoming aware of the things you say to yourself is the first step toward modifying these thoughts.

Let's refer to Sally's record keeping. The thought that hindered her ability to begin a conversation with her neighbor in the elevator was, "What if I don't know what to say?" Thus, her fear of being unable to communicate appropriately kept her from even attempting to meet a new person. In the laundry room, however, Sally had different thoughts when Mrs. J. started a conversation: "This is someone I'd like to get to know." Sally felt excited and enjoyed her chat. Thus, the likelihood of future behavior change was enhanced. Lack of confidence and self-doubts are acquired habits. However, with continued effort and new skills, better attitudes can be learned, thus improving your self-esteem and helping you succeed with a self-change plan.

TASK 5. PINPOINT THE SKILLS AND TASKS REQUIRED TO CHANGE YOUR BEHAVIOR AND PRACTICE THEM

Now that you have monitored your behavior patterns and analyzed your thought processes, you are ready to *determine those specific skills that you will need* to implement your self-change plan. You may need to gain new skills from various sources or recall old ones. But in any case, *practice is essential* for success. A key to any change process is the ability to set small, manageable goals; to think positively; and to communicate effectively. For many people, the commitment to change behavior is made easier by sharing those plans with others who can be supportive by making a written contract with or an oral statement to family and friends.

In Sally's case, the new skills she needs to acquire and practice involve communication and relaxation. Sally needs to practice setting small manageable goals: "Today I will sign up for an art class at the adult center." She needs to practice thinking positively: "I had a group of close friends before; I can make new friends again." She needs to communicate her plan to someone supportive, such as her husband.

TASK 6. CONSTANTLY MONITOR THE RESULTS OF YOUR SELF-CHANGE EFFORTS AND REVISE YOUR BEHAVIOR AS NEEDED

Completing a chart such as the one that follows may prove helpful when you wish to review your self-change process. This chart reviews Sally L.'s total self-

Self-Change Plan			
Self-Change Goal	Specific Behavioral Change	Self-Observation	
Build a good social support network in my neighborhood.	Get to know my neighbors.	Keep records of attempts I made to start talking with my new neighbors.	

change process, focusing in particular on the area she has given top priority, that of improving her social well-being by making new friends.

After Sally felt she could accomplish and maintain that first step, to begin conversations with her neighbors, her next step would be to *select increasingly more difficult, yet attainable, behavioral changes* (joining a social group, perhaps, or inviting guests in) in order to accom-plish her overall goal of developing a strong social support network. Once she had achieved this goal, she could con-tinue with her total self-change process by *selecting another lifestyle area*, such as becoming a more knowledgeable care-giver. (See Appendix E for a blank self-change plan chart).

Lifestyle is an important factor that can influence an individual's health. It is clear that individuals must accept re-

Patterns that Aid or Hinder Self-Change Efforts	Skills and Tasks Required for Self-Change	Plan Summary
Feeling silly and nervous in talking to strangers. Feeling excited about good responses. Having doubts about my ability to chat with strangers. Can't get out to social functions because of John's illness.	To relax more. Remember the good experiences. Keep trying to learn to talk easily with people. Invite people to my home.	Continue to begin talking with neighbors for two more weeks.

sponsibility for maintaining their health. No doctor or team of health professionals can influence a person's health in the way that the individual's lifestyle can. The way you live your daily life either enhances your health or diminishes it. Certain lifestyle behaviors become risk factors related to physical and emotional illness. It is important to note that *these risk factors accumulate* (for example, inactivity, smoking, and high blood pressure together increase the risk of a heart attack far above any of the three factors separately) and that *these risk factors are interactive* (for example, people under stress are more likely to overeat, smoke, and have a high blood cholesterol level). The fact that risk factors accumulate and are interactive makes it possible for you to address many potential risk factors by making changes in individual lifestyle behaviors.

The Formula for Succeeding at Self-Change can help you maintain a healthier lifestyle. It can further be used to help develop more understanding and gain more control in the areas of stress, physical fitness, and nutrition.

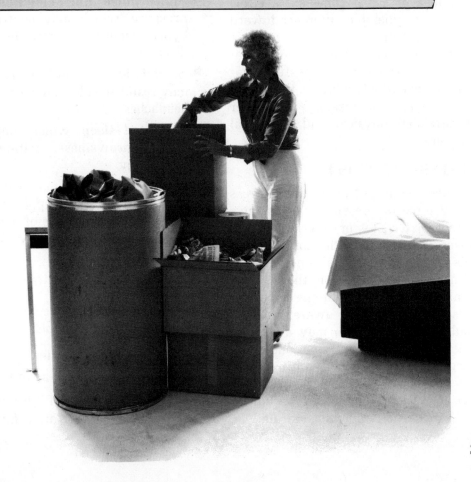

Chapter 4

Coping with Stress

All people throughout the ages have experienced stress. Stress is a major factor in an individual's personal and professional life, affecting the person positively or negatively. Managing stress can make the difference between facing the stresses and strains of day-to-day living as a challenge and an opportunity for growth or allowing those stresses and strains to adversely affect one's physical and emotional well-being. By learning how to relax, solve problems, and communicate more effectively, an individual can teach himself or herself to both minimize distress and maximize the positive aspects of stress, such as when that little extra pressure triggers a great idea or when some extra effort makes a considerable difference toward a desired outcome.

Strong medical evidence shows that the strain derived from stressful situations can eventually increase the risk of heart disease, depression, and other stress-related physical and emotional disorders.

STRESS—WHAT IS IT?

Consider a concept from physics. *Stress* is any force or pressure exerted on a system (externally or internally) that causes a change from the normal state. This change from normal functioning is defined as the *strain* on the system. What this means is that the aspect of stress you need to be aware of is the resulting strain, which may adversely affect your physical and emotional well-being. Strain is a frequent but unnecessary result of stress. Since stress is a part of everyday life, it is important to be aware of the symptoms of strain.

Symptoms of Strain

In stressful situations, symptoms of strain include the following:

- *increased muscle tension and tightness*, especially in the face, neck, and back, which may result in headaches, backaches, or teeth grinding
- *upset stomach and dysfunction of the gastrointestinal tract*, which may cause heartburn, ulcers, diarrhea, or constipation
- *automatic troubling thoughts, feelings, and images*, which may lead to worry, anxiety, inner tension, or poor self-esteem
- *rapid pulse and elevated blood pressure*, which may contribute to hypertension or other cardiovascular diseases
- *constriction of blood vessels*, which may result in cold hands or migraine headaches
- *disrupted sleep*, which may cause fatigue, drowsiness, irritability, or low energy
- *depression*, which may cause poor concentration, loss of appetite or compulsive eating, feelings of irritability, mood swings, or loss of sexual interest

Sources of Stress

Older adults face many common stressful situations. For example:

- a move to a new location
- a change in role, such as retirement
- changes in physical appearance
- a change in social relationships

- a change in financial situation
- taking vacations or holidays

These situations can be viewed as challenging and lead to growth or can be viewed negatively and lead to strain.

Other situations commonly produce strain and necessitate the use of adaptive coping skills. These situations include the following:

- loss of spouse, family members, or friends through death
- loss of immediate contact with family members or friends because of relocation
- declining health

- decreasing independence
- loss of finances

STRESS LEVELS AND STRENGTH OF SUPPORT NETWORK

Studies have shown that when a person is faced with stressful situations, the presence of a strong social support network (family, friends, and community) helps decrease the strain the individual experiences. Below are self-tests that you can take to help you identify your personal stress level and the strength of your support network.

Stress Level

Read each stress-related event at the left. If you have experienced that event within the last twelve months, circle the corresponding number at the right. Add the numbers circled for your stress level score.

	Score
Personal Life	
Serious injury or illness	6
Alcohol, drug, or emotional problem	6
Marriage	4
Death of close friend	4
Trouble with friends or neighbors	2
Beginning or ending of school or training program	2
Work and Finances	
Loss of job, retirement	6
Selling or buying of home	4
Change of jobs, promotion	2
Trouble with boss	2
Family	
Death of spouse or immediate family member	10
Divorce	8
Reconciliation or separation	6
Serious illness or injury of family member	4
Family arguments	4
Child's entering or leaving home	4
Moving of relative into household	2
Move to new residence	2

Stress Total:

Support Network Strength

Read each question at the left. Then circle the number of your response at the right. Add the numbers circled for your score on support network strength.

		Score	
1. At work, how many persons do you talk to about a job hassle?		0 3 4 5	None (or not employed) One or two Two or three Four or more
2. How many neighbors do you trade favors with (loan tools or household items; share rides, baby-sitting, and so on)?		0 1 2 3	None One Two or three Four or more
3. Do you have a spouse or partner?		0 2 6 10	No Yes, several different partners Yes, one steady partner Yes, married or living with someone
4. How often do friends and close family members visit you at home?		0 1 4 8	Rarely About once a month Several times a month About once a week or more
5. How many friends or family members do you talk to about personal matters?		0 6 8 10	None One or two Three to five Six or more
6. How often do you participate in a social, community, or sports group?		0 1 2 4	Rarely About once a month Several times a month Once a week

Support Total: ☐

On each barometer on the next page draw a line to show where your respective score falls

If your Stress Level score is

—less than 10

You have a **low stress level**, and your life has been stable in most areas for the past twelve months.

—10 to 15

You have a **moderate stress level**, and there has been a lot of change in your life this past year.

—16 or more

You have a **high stress level**, and there have been major adjustments in your life this past year.

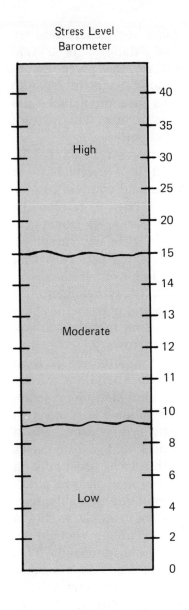

Stress Level
Barometer

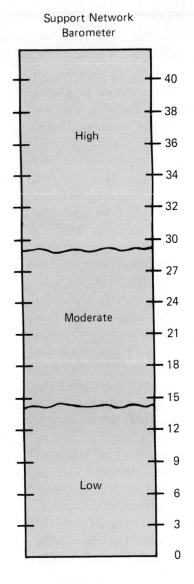

Support Network
Barometer

If your Support Network Strength score is

—less than 15

Your support network has **low strength** and probably does not provide much support. You need to consider making more social contacts.

—15 to 29

Your support network has **moderate strength** and likely provides enough support except perhaps during periods of high stress.

—30 or more

Your support network has **high strength** and will likely maintain your well-being even during periods of high stress.

THE STRESS PATTERN AND HOW TO COPE—THE "FIGHT OR FLIGHT" RESPONSE

Despite the differences in sources of stress, the resulting strain produces predictable changes in the body that are often referred to as the *"fight or flight"* response. This is an age-old response that at one time in early evolution was the body's way of adapting to real physical dangers. The response includes the following major physical changes: increase in heart rate, constriction of blood vessels, perspiration, muscle spasm, and a brief shutdown of the stomach's digestive actions. For example, a cave dweller in response to the sight of a tiger may have experienced this "fight or flight" response. The physical changes were necessary adaptive responses in preparing to either fight or flee the tiger. Today humans continue to react with this physical response under strain, but these reactions are no longer appropriate for most of today's problems.

The majority of stresses that confront people are not physical dangers, such as that experienced by the cave dweller, but rather everyday troublesome situations such as being the primary caregiver for a loved one who is ill, dealing with retirement, or managing financial problems. It is neither adaptive nor appropriate to fight or flee these situations. However, the body has prepared itself to do so. Furthermore, perceptions of danger, such as the fear of not being able to provide care for an ill spouse, can and often do produce the physical "fight or flight" response. That is, *thoughts* of perceived danger can trigger such symptoms as rapid pulse, blood vessel constriction, and upset stomach. Regardless of whether the "danger" is a real physical threat or one perceived in the mind, the body tends to react to sources of stress in a predictable and often uncomfortable way. This pattern is called the *stress pattern*.

On page 41 is an arrow diagram of the stress pattern. It is a useful way to understand stress, and you will be able to use it to show how to resolve the resulting strain. Take, as an example, a person who is a primary caregiver, someone who is taking care of a frail spouse or person in his or her home.

The way to read the arrow diagram is to start at the top and to trace the chain of events down, going from box to box as directed by the arrows.

The stress in this situation is from caring for a loved one who has a fever and a rash, a mild but alarming reaction to prescribed medication. *Physically*, this caregiver experienced tension, which produced tight neck and scalp muscles and a tension headache. *Mentally*, a common response to an unpleasant situation is to have troubling thoughts, feelings, and images. For example, as shown in figure 1, the troubling thought is, "What if he has to be hospitalized?" This worrisome thought leads to a further increase in the caregiver's stress level, making it even more difficult to deal with her responsibilities.

Another common reaction to a stressful situation is *avoidance*. For example, in this situation the caregiver had a drink and put off calling the doctor. Drinking alcoholic beverages, using medications inappropriately, and a combination of the two are common ways

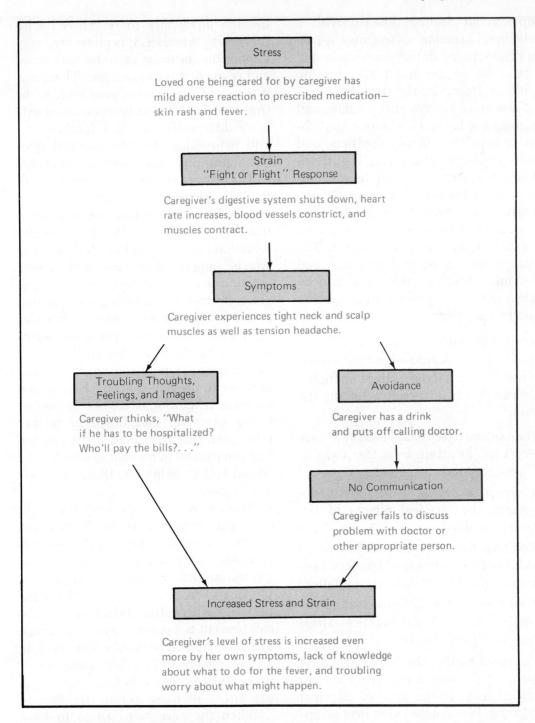

Figure 1. How the Stress Pattern Works

people avoid dealing directly with a problem or situation. Oftentimes, a person drinks to try to feel good again and to take his or her mind off pressing problems. However, the stressful situation is almost always still present, and the drinking becomes a major contributor to accidents, family conflicts, and health problems. By avoiding the stressful situation and continuing to *not communicate or interact* (see figure 1), the caregiver puts herself under still more stress, only making the situation worse. This can become a vicious cycle. The unhappy results are both physical and emotional. However, this cycle can be broken with the introduction of specific coping mechanisms.

Coping Techniques

Here are some techniques an individual can use to help handle a "fight or flight" response that is adversely affecting the person.

- **Relaxation exercises.** These exercises decrease the strain from the "fight or flight" response.
- **Physical exercise.** This activity decreases the physical effects of the stress involved.
- **Positive thinking.** The ability to do this fosters constructive thoughts, feelings, and energies about the situation.
- **Communication.** Effectively and assertively expressing thoughts and feelings decreases the strain.

As noted earlier, the body's response to prolonged stress is strain, which can manifest itself in the form of physical symptoms. In response to the first symptoms of tension (in this example, tight neck muscles), you can teach yourself to become physically more relaxed with *relaxation exercises*. It is physiologically impossible for muscles to be both tense and relaxed at the same time. Therefore, if you can learn to relax your body at the first signs of tension (tension manifests itself differently for all individuals), it will help eliminate your harmful emotional and physical responses to stress.

The stress pattern can be broken with the introduction of relaxation. (See Appendix B for instructions on relaxation training.) For example, the stressful situation in figure 1 is that the loved one who is being cared for has a mild adverse reaction to a new medication. The caregiver notices her loved one's reaction and feels her own neck and scalp muscles tightening. She knows this is the beginning of a headache for her. At this point, the caregiver is aware of the tension and in order to prevent a headache, she can do some relaxation exercises. However, if the caregiver had failed to do her relaxation just then, and if the tension had progressed to a slight headache, she would still be able to do these exercises at this point.

Another way to cope with the "fight or flight" response is to do *physical exercise*, thus minimizing the physical response to the stress. These two coping techniques, relaxation exercises and physical exercise, used early in the stress pattern—where strain is first apparent—can prevent the onset of symptoms such as headache and backache. However, in an emergency or a crisis situation, it may not be practical to take time out to use either of these coping techniques.

When the caregiver begins to have troubling thoughts (in this example, "What if he has to be hospitalized?"), her ability to cope is diminished. This part of the pattern can be broken by another technique—positive, or constructive thinking. For example, "Before worrying, let me get the medical facts by calling the doctor. I'll feel better if I know." Such self-talk, in conjunction with relaxation, can help the individual regain the composure needed to handle the situation more appropriately.

The fourth coping technique is effective, or assertive, communication. Communicating about thoughts and feelings, *even if no direct change occurs*, reduces the physical impact that strain has on an individual. The goal here is to relieve the feeling of distress and/or frustration. In the example above, the stress pattern continues when the caregiver has a drink and avoids calling the doctor. This part of the stress pattern can be broken by effectively communicating (in this example, by calling and speaking to the doctor).

Below are the most common reasons people don't communicate effectively.

- They fear to sound aggressive, since firmness is often confused with anger.

- Assertiveness is considered improper in some families and cultures.

- Some people overreact to situations, which prevents them from communicating appropriately.

- Some people simply lack communication skills.

These are the most common errors people make in dealing with stress.

- They approach the stressful situation with a skeptical attitude.

- They avoid the use of appropriate coping techniques that will help them succeed in reducing strain.

- They do not communicate effectively thoughts and feelings that need to be expressed.

The Formula for Attaining Better Health (introduced in chapter 3) can be used to begin your own stress-management program. This formula gives you a systematic approach to behavioral change.

FORMULA FOR ATTAINING BETTER HEALTH

Task 1. Assess your lifestyle and determine your goals.

Task 2. Choose one specific behavior in a lifestyle area where you desire some self-change.

Task 3. Observe yourself and gather information about your behavior patterns in this area.

Task 4. Identify and evaluate any thoughts, feelings, and attitudes that may either aid or hinder your efforts to change your lifestyle.

Task 5. Pinpoint the skills and tasks required to change your behavior and practice them.

Task 6. Constantly monitor the results of your self-change efforts and revise your behavior as needed.

■ *CASE STUDY*

Bill M. retired four months ago at age sixty-six from his job as an accountant for an automobile dealer. Over the past four months, he has been suffering from insomnia, feelings of nervousness (feelings that his heart is racing), increased irritability, and difficulty in concentrating. Bill's fear of experiencing these symptoms, sometimes called panic attacks, has made him increasingly more anxious about leaving home, and thus he has been avoiding social events. His family became aware of these changes because he has been absent from weekly family dinners with his grandchildren. Because of their concern, family members recently approached him about his health. His family's concerns, along with his own fears that he may have a serious illness, have prompted Bill to assess his lifestyle. In addition, he has asked his physician to evaluate and monitor his health with periodic examinations.

toms of fatigue, poor sleep, and occasional rapid heartbeat. Bill's wife has become aware of her husband's irritability and depressed mood. Bill is the first to admit he has avoided seeing people and going places for fear of having a panic attack. Bill wants to concentrate in the social area with the goal of eliminating his panic attacks.

Task 2. Choose One Specific Behavior in a Lifestyle Area Where You Desire Some Self-Change

Of all areas, Bill is most concerned about his panic attacks and wants to get them under control. His recent medical exam assured him that he has no serious illness. When Bill has a panic attack, his symptoms include a "racing" heart, shortness of breath, feelings of nervousness, and an overwhelming desire to be safe at home. These panic attacks are specific, measurable episodes that he has resolved to control.

Task 1. Assess Your Lifestyle and Determine Your Goals

With the aid of his family, Bill decides to sit down with pencil and paper and make a list of the major changes that have occurred in his life during the past four months. He groups these changes under the headings of lifestyle areas—physical, emotional, and social. He then checks only the lifestyle area that *he* would like to improve. Bill has not felt "just right" for a while; he notes symp-

Task 3. Observe Yourself and Gather Information About Your Behavior Patterns in This Area

By using the following record-keeping format, Bill is able to keep a diary of episodes of panic attacks for two weeks in order to understand better the conditions under which these attacks occur. (See Appendix E for a blank copy of this self-observation chart.) Here's what some of the entries on Bill's record looked like.

Self-Observation

Behavior: *Panic Attacks*

Date	Situation (Briefly describe where you were and whom you were with.)	Thoughts and Feelings in This Situation (Briefly describe how you were feeling and what you were thinking.)	Actions (Describe how you responded to the situation.)
Tues. 12/10	In the supermarket, alone.	Felt nervous — short of breath. Thought I might pass out. I wanted to be home.	Quickly left the store. Went home and to bed.
Thurs. 12/12	At George and Judy's home for dinner. Elaine with me.	Began to feel nervous and afraid of a panic attack. I thought about doctor saying I'm in good shape; that I just need to relax.	Stepped outside for some fresh air for a few minutes.

Task 4. Identify and Evaluate Any Thoughts, Feelings, and Attitudes That May Either Aid or Hinder Your Efforts to Change Your Lifestyle

Bill has realized from having kept records of his panic attacks that his behavior in two different situations created different outcomes. In the first situation, certain troubling thoughts and images—for example, anticipating a panic attack and predicting that the physical symptoms would get worse—clearly made his anxiety worse. In the second situation, constructive thoughts and feelings—for example, reassuring thoughts about his medical examination and, in turn, understanding his need to relax—made his anxiety less. Furthermore, he has realized that these attacks are more likely to occur when he is with people outside his family, especially old friends and colleagues from work. Bill's analysis of what is going on in these situations leads him to conclude that he is uncomfortable with what he is doing in his retirement and often feels useless and somehow unfulfilled.

Task 5. Pinpoint the Skills and Tasks Required to Change Your Behavior and Practice Them

Having analyzed his behavior, Bill is ready to determine the specific skills he needs to implement his self-change plan. The primary skill he needs to acquire and practice is the use of relaxation techniques in order to decrease the strain of the "fight or flight" response leading to his panic attacks. He should first practice these techniques under nonthreatening conditions. After mastering the skill of relaxation, he should then apply the relaxation techniques at the first sign of panic. Thus, he will be able to lessen the severity of these attacks and possibly prevent future ones. (See Appendix B for relaxation instructions.) The second skill that applies to Bill's case is mastering *positive thinking*, or self-talk, in order to keep him from anticipating panic attacks and making his condition worse.

Bill acknowledges that, along with setting concrete plans for his retirement, communicating with relatives and friends who have gone through this life change would be helpful. Effectively *communicating* at appropriate times then becomes another skill he will practice. Bill will record his success.

Task 6. Constantly Monitor the Results of Your Self-Change Efforts and Revise Your Behavior As Needed

Bill's stress-management self-change plan as he hopes to follow it through toward his six-months goal of controlling his panic attacks is on pages 48–49. (See Appendix E for a blank self-change plan chart.)

After Bill can maintain the first steps of his plan, learning and applying relaxation and positive thinking skills to control his panic attacks, his next step will be to select another skill. A second skill may be developing and communicating with a support network of other retirees and/or consulting with a psychiatrist or other counseling professional.

He must, of course, note the results of his behavioral changes and review his specific behaviors from time to time so that his self-change goal can be met.

Understanding the various sources and symptoms of stress in one's life and learning how to cope effectively by using techniques of relaxation exercises, physical exercise, positive thinking, and effective communication may decrease the health risks of stress-related medical and emotional problems. Thinking of problems in the context of the stress pattern and using the Formula for Attaining Better Health, you can begin to make positive changes toward a healthier emotional state. While skilled professionals should be sought out for more severe symptoms of strain, these self-care strategies can be applied effectively to cope with the daily stresses and strains faced by everyone.

Self-Change Plan

Self-Change Goal	Specific Behavioral Change	Self-Observation	
Enjoy retirement more.	Cut down number of panic attacks.	Keep record of panic attacks for one month.	

	Patterns that Aid or Hinder Self-Change Efforts	Skills and Tasks Required for Self-Change	Plan Summary
	Episodes of fear feelings — spasms, sweating, heart racing, etc.	Relaxation exercises.	Practice exercises over next 4 to 6 weeks and write what happens.
	Having negative thoughts and feelings. Easily get mad.	More positive thinking.	Practice over next 4 to 6 weeks and record progress.
	Having doubts about ability to be happy in retirement — don't like what I do.	Decide on specific plan to do something more important with my time.	Begin something over next 6 months.
		Get along better with others — Talk with family more. — Talk with retirees. — Talk with counselor or doctor.	 —Do over next 2 weeks. —Do over next 2 months. —See if need this after 6 months.

Chapter 5

Physical Fitness

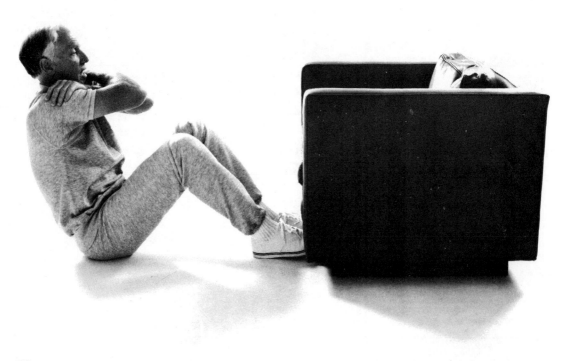

The ability to carry out important daily tasks and activities with vigor, comfort, and alertness is known as physical fitness. Physical fitness can also be interpreted as maintaining optimum physical activity and/or stimulating circulation. It does not necessarily mean calisthenics, running, or jumping rope.

Physical fitness is not a cure-all, but being physically fit does contribute to improved breathing, better circulation, and improved muscle tone, which, in turn, aid with such body functions as digestion, bowel regularity, and sleep. In addition, calcium loss from bone may be decreased with exercise. No one standard of fitness is suitable for all persons, but some level of physical fitness is an achievable goal for almost everyone.

THE BENEFITS OF BEING FIT

Your functional health status depends on good physical fitness. (See the physical health quiz in chapter 2, page 20.) Physical activity and physical fitness will help with the following:

- Increasing joint flexibility.
- Enhancing agility and mobility.
- Improving heart, arteries, and lungs.
- Controlling body weight.
- Feeling more energetic.
- Feeling stronger.
- Feeling more relaxed.
- Sleeping better.
- Developing new social contacts.
- Having fun.
- Improving morale and confidence by feeling and looking younger.
- Maintaining an independent lifestyle.

Medical experts agree that many of the physical changes that people attribute to normal aging actually are a result of inactivity and could be diminished by a continuing program of physical exercise. However, only about one-third of older adults engage in regular exercise. What are your thoughts and feelings about exercise? Check them against the following myths and facts.

MYTHS AND FACTS ABOUT EXERCISE

Myth 1: Exercising makes you feel tired.

Fact: A gradual buildup to and continuation of regular exercise will improve your circulation and give you more energy, helping you resist fatigue and stress. Regular exercise can also improve the strength and efficiency of your body, making daily tasks much easier and less tiring. It can also help you sleep better at night and wake up refreshed.

Myth 2: The older you are, the less exercise you need.

Fact: Much physical frailty attributed to aging is actually a result of inactivity. At any age, an exercise program needs to be tailored to the person's physical condition and his or her pattern of daily living. Regardless of age, all parts of the body need to be used regularly.

Myth 3: You have to be athletic to exercise.

Fact: Studies show that individuals

who have been sedentary for many years achieve significant improvement in cardiovascular endurance, muscle strength, and body flexibility when they actively engage in a fitness program.

Myth 4: When an illness or accident weakens the body, it's too late to exercise.

Fact: It is rarely too late. The initial step is to plan a gradual but steady return to regular physical activity. Exercise can improve how you feel physically as well as emotionally and help you gain strength. However, if you are ill or have a chronic medical problem, you should talk with your doctor about the kinds of exercises you should do and how you should go about building up to your desired level of activity.

Self-Test Before Beginning a Physical Activity Program

Below is a self-test you can take to help you determine whether you should consult your doctor before embarking on a program of physical activity. Put a check after each statement that is true for you.

1. You have been told you have heart trouble, or you have had a heart attack. ____
2. You frequently have pains in the left-chest or mid-chest area, left neck, left shoulder, or left arm during or immediately after exercise, after meals, or when out in the cold. ____
3. You often feel faint or dizzy. ____
4. You experience bothersome breathlessness or wheezing after mild exertion. ____
5. Your doctor has said that your blood pressure is too high and that it is not under control. ____
6. Your doctor has said that you have bone or joint problems such as arthritis. ____
7. You are over sixty and not accustomed to vigorous exercise. ____
8. Your father, mother, brother, or sister had a heart attack before age fifty. ____
9. You have a medical condition not mentioned here that might need special attention. ____
10. You take one or more prescription medicines. ____

If you checked any of the above statements, consult your doctor before starting a program of physical activity. A positive answer does not exclude you from all fitness programs, but rather indicates that you need to select an appropriate one with your physician's advice. In addition, if you have been inactive or if you wish to begin a more vigorous exercise program, it is essential that you first consult your doctor.

If you did not check any of the statements, you can feel *reasonably* confident of your suitability to engage in measured physical activity. However, if you are worried about any specific exercises or if you intend to engage in very strenuous activities, you should first consult your physician. Your doctor may want to give you a physical examination and/or stress test to determine your fitness level. He or she can then recommend an exercise or physical activity program tailored to your capability.

With any physical activity program it is important to begin gradually, progress slowly, and not exercise to the point of pain or excessive fatigue.

ACHIEVING AND MAINTAINING FITNESS

Descriptions and examples of different types of exercises for body conditioning follow. A systematic program to attain fitness includes stretching muscles, strengthening weak muscles, relaxing tight muscles, and building up one's physical endurance.

There are four basic types of exercises:

1. *Flexibility exercises,* which stretch muscles.
2. *Strengthening exercises,* which firm and strengthen muscles.
3. *Relaxation exercises,* which help release physical tension from the muscles and reduce emotional stress.
4. *Endurance exercises,* which increase vitality, energy, and stamina.

Flexibility Exercises

As persons get older, they tend to lose flexibility (range of motion), and movements can become slow and painful. Inactivity adds to this problem. By stretching their muscles, individuals become more flexible, and it becomes much easier for them to accomplish daily activities. Stretching often improves posture and relieves the pain associated with arthritis, tension, and sore backs.

Stretching can be done in a sitting, lying, or standing position. It can be done while doing other things, such as watching TV or talking on the phone.

On the following page are examples of flexibility exercises.

Turn to Appendix A for photographs and explanations of additional flexibility exercises for the older adult.

Strengthening Exercises

Strengthening exercises firm up the muscles and help maintain or improve muscle condition. Although there comes a time when muscles can only be maintained but not expanded, the rate of decline of muscle condition can be slowed through regular exercise. Unused muscles become weak, flabby, and tired, whereas strong muscles make it easier to perform daily chores and activities.

Strong back and stomach muscles improve posture and relieve back pain. Strong leg muscles make walking, climbing stairs, lifting, and housework easier.

One form of strengthening exercises, isometric exercises, "holds" a contraction. People tend to hold their breath while doing isometric exercises, with a resultant increase in blood pressure. Therefore, this type of exercise is not recommended. *Remember to keep breathing regularly during any type of activity.*

On page 55 are some photographs and explanations of strengthening exercises for the older adult.

Turn to Appendix A for additional strengthening exercises for the older adult.

Flexibility Exercises

Main Street Stroll and Twist.   Simply walk around briskly for six minutes on a level surface. Indoors is OK, but outdoors is even better. Breathe deeply. The first two minutes, walk with an exaggerated swing in your arms, forward and backward. The third and fourth minutes, raise your arms as you walk, and put them through swimming-the-crawl motions. The fifth and sixth minutes, clasp your hands behind your head, and walk with an exaggerated twist of the shoulders—left and then right, and so on. Keep your hips stable in this warm-up exercise that limbers most of your body. It is best if done daily.

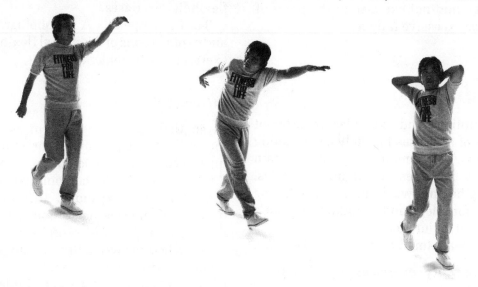

Raised-Knee Crossover.   Lie on your back, arms spread-eagle. Raise both knees together until your thighs are vertical; then swing them to the left as far as you can, trying to touch your knees to the floor. Then swing back to the center, and twist to the right as far as you can. Exhale deeply as you twist to the side; inhale as you return to the center position. The exercise should be done daily: five times the first week, ten times the second week, fifteen times thereafter, to increase trunk, hip, and knee flexibility and to strengthen abdominal muscles.

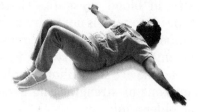
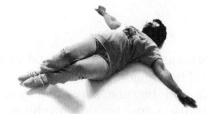

Strengthening Exercises

Half Knee Bend. Standing, legs apart, place your hands on your hips. This is a two-count exercise: (1) lower your body halfway on bent knees as your arms extend forward, palms down; (2) rise, and return to the starting position. Move smoothly, keep your back straight, and breathe deeply. Exhale as you lower your body; inhale as you raise it. Do six bends every other day the first week, nine every other day the second week, and twelve every other day the third week, to strengthen your thigh muscles.

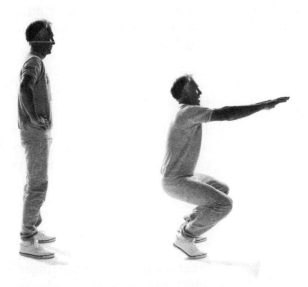

Knee Push-up. Lying on your tummy, legs together, place your hands under your shoulders, palms on the floor. Bend your knees so that you raise your feet off the floor. Now, keeping your back straight, push against the floor until your arms are fully extended and your body, from the knees up, is off the floor. Slowly lower yourself to the floor, keeping your knees bent. Repeat five times. On the third week, increase to eight. On the fifth week, increase to twelve. Done every other day, this exercise strengthens arm, shoulder, chest, and abdominal muscles.

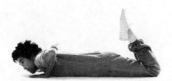 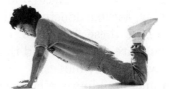

Relaxation Exercises

Relaxation exercises are systematic activities designed to take the tension out of muscles. These activities can help prevent headaches and fatigue, as well as contribute to better sleep. An individual needs to learn what the difference in feeling is between tightening up muscles and relaxing them. Several techniques are available to relax your muscles and your mind. Total well-being includes both the ability to be active and the ability to relax. Examples of relaxation exercises can be found in Appendix B.

Other relaxation techniques include the following:

- lying on the floor, bending the legs at the knees, and resting the lower legs on a sofa or bed
- yoga
- meditation
- T'ai Chi
- massage

Endurance Exercises

To improve energy and stamina, an individual must participate in activities that elevate the heart rate for sustained periods of time and thus supply the body muscles with extra oxygen and nutrients. Such activities are endurance exercises, and examples include brisk walking, swimming, cross-country skiing, jogging, aerobic dancing, hiking, and bicycling. In these forms of exercise, movements are repetitive and rhythmic, and the whole body moves.

Endurance-building exercises improve the function of the heart, lungs, and blood vessels when the following characteristics are present.

- The exercises are *brisk*; the person must move fast enough to raise his or her heart and breathing rates.
- The exercises are *sustained*; they must be done at least fifteen to twenty minutes without interruption.
- The exercises are *regular*; they must be repeated at least three times per week, preferably with no more than a forty-eight-hour lapse of time in between.

A RESTING AND AN EXERCISE HEART RATE

To control and self-monitor your heart rate before, during, and after exercising, you need to learn how to take your pulse and how to determine your maximum heart rate and "target zone."

Taking Your Pulse

Press the index (second) finger and third finger of one hand firmly against the wrist just below the thumb side of the other hand (see figure 1). Count the beats

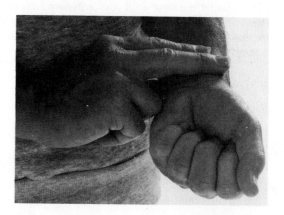

Figure 1. Taking a Pulse

(pulse) for fifteen seconds, multiply by four, and you have the number of beats per minute.

Calculating Your Heart Rate and Target Zone

The heart is one of the best indicators of your body's reaction to physical activity. During exercise, the heart beats faster than its normal sixty to eighty beats per minute. When you take your pulse during exercise, you should count for only fifteen seconds to identify the fastest heartbeat rate attained. To improve stamina and increase energy, it is important to exercise hard enough to elevate the heart rate to what is called the heart rate "target zone." The target zone has upper and lower limits that are based on your age.

To determine the heart rate you need to sustain during endurance exercises, locate your target zone in figure 2. Look for the age category closest to your own age on the chart, and read the line across. For example, if you are fifty-two years of age, the closest age on the chart is 50; the target zone is 102 to 127 beats per minute. This is 60 percent to 75 percent of your maximum heart rate, which is the fastest that your heart should beat. This maximum heart rate is usually determined for an individual by subtracting the person's age from 220. The figures in the chart are averages and should be used as general guidelines. If you are taking medication for high blood pressure, consult your physician to find out whether the heartbeat target zone for your exercise program needs to be adjusted.

During the first few months of an exercise program, you should aim for the lower (60 percent) level in the target zone. As you build up your fitness, gradually move up to the higher (75 percent) level.

STEPS TO FOLLOW WHEN ENGAGING IN ANY ENDURANCE-BUILDING ACTIVITY

Before making any major changes in the amount of physical activity you perform, take the *self-test* on page 52.

- Select an endurance-building activity to follow, such as walking, bicycling, swimming, or cross-country skiing.
- Start all endurance exercises with a warm-up period; after five to ten

Age	Target Zone 60 percent to 75 percent	Average Maximum Heart Rate 100 percent
50 years	102–127 beats per minute	170
55 years	99–124 beats per minute	165
60 years	96–120 beats per minute	160
65 years	93–116 beats per minute	155
70 years	90–113 beats per minute	150

Figure 2. Heart Rate for Target Zone

minutes of stretching exercises, gradually increase your breathing and heart rate with slow, rhythmic movements.

■ Add time and intensity to your endurance activity over four to six months, progressing from 60 percent of your maximum heart rate for ten minutes of continuous exercise, three times a week, to 75 percent for twenty minutes, three to five times per week. Do not exercise to the point of pain or excessive fatigue.

■ Always cool down for five to ten minutes with the same slow, rhythmic movements and stretching you did in the warm-up period.

■ Supplement your fitness program with light physical activity in your everyday lifestyle. For instance, use stairs instead of elevators; walk short distances rather than drive; and do lawn, garden, and household chores when possible.

You should not get out of breath with any of the endurance exercises you perform. If you do, rest a few minutes. Remember to go at your own pace—not your neighbor's. If you have been inactive, take it easy. If you have been told by your doctor not to do certain endurance exercises, stay with the ones allowed.

If you have been sedentary and are not already in a physical fitness activity, you may want to consider the benefits of walking or swimming. Either of these physical activities can be developed to include all four types of exercise: flexibility, strengthening, relaxation, and endurance.

WALKING FOR FITNESS

Walking is one of the best all-around exercises. The massaging action the leg muscles exert on the veins improves the flow of blood back to the heart and strengthens the leg muscles.

There are several advantages to walking over other types of exercise: (1) it is a familiar activity, (2) it can be done alone or with someone, (3) it requires no equipment, (4) it requires no transportation, (5) it requires no travel or travel time, (6) it requires no lessons, (7) it can be done almost anywhere, (8) it can be done at any time of day or night, (9) it can be done in almost any kind of weather, (10) it can be done indoors or outdoors, (11) it costs nothing to do, and (12) the injury rate for walking is the lowest for any form of exercise— jogging included. Conditioning benefits are achieved through walking only a little less slowly than through more strenuous activities, but these benefits improve dramatically if you increase your pace to faster than three miles per hour (twenty minutes per mile).

For building cardiovascular endurance, walking must be maintained for twenty minutes, three times a week, preferably on alternate days. Several times during your walk, check your pulse to see whether you are in your heartbeat target zone, and decide if you need to speed up or slow down. At fifty years of age, your target zone pace will be about a mile in twenty minutes, or three miles per hour.

A suggested gradual buildup for an endurance walking program is shown in figure 3.

	Warm Up	**Target Zone Exercising**	**Cool Down**	**Total**
Weeks 1-2	Stretch and limber up 10 minutes.	Swim one length* and walk back. Continue this for 5–8 minutes.	Walk slowly and stretch 10 minutes.	25 minutes approximately
Weeks 3-4	Stretch and limber up 10 minutes.	Try two lengths before pausing. Continue for 8–10 minutes.	Walk slowly and stretch 10 minutes.	30 minutes
Weeks 5-6	Stretch and limber up 10 minutes.	Try three lengths before pausing. Continue for 10–12 minutes.	Walk slowly and stretch 10 minutes.	35 minutes
Weeks 7-8	Stretch and limber up 10 minutes.	Try four lengths without stopping. Continue for 12–15 minutes.	Walk slowly and stretch 10 minutes	35 minutes
Weeks 9-10	Stretch and limber up 10 minutes.	Try five lengths without stopping. Continue for 15–18 minutes.	Walk slowly and stretch 10 minutes.	35–40 minutes

Do At Least Three Exercise Sessions During Each Week of the Program!

After Week 10	Work up to a swimming distance that you can cover in twenty minutes and at a pace that enables you to achieve 60 percent of your maximum heartbeat rate. The buoyancy of the water and a lower rise in body temperature in the water create conditions where the heart beats ten to fifteen times less to produce the same amount of work as exercise done on land. Remember, your pace should be set by listening to your body. You should not swim at a pace that causes breathlessness or a pounding heart. Overexertion causes problems; it does not help you build physical fitness.

*The length of most standard pools is twenty to twenty-five yards.

Figure 4. A Sample Swimming Program

When you have built up to twenty minutes, you have met the criterion for an endurance exercise. You should maintain a pattern of endurance and sustain the pace of the swimming exercise three times per week, preferably on alternate days.

CAUTION ON OVEREXERTION

If you are enthusiastic about exercising, you may have a tendency to overdo. There are various ways to regulate yourself. It is normal to feel warm during exercise and for your heart rate to increase. Be aware, however, of other changes that may be signals from your body that you are overexerting.

These include the following:

- dizziness
- heavy breathing
- sore muscles or muscle cramps
- a heart rate higher than your target zone level
- nausea
- chest pains
- a feeling of being very hot
- pains in the lower abdomen
- extremely heavy perspiration

If you have any of these symptoms, walk slowly or sit down. If you are nauseated or light-headed, sit down and put your head between your knees.

To quote Dr. Herman Kanenetz,

Exercise and overexertion are two different things. Overexertion is bad for the young and even worse for the elderly. The purpose of exercise is to get rid of muscle pain, not to increase it; to create relaxation, not anxiety; to train the lungs, not exhaust them; to improve circulation, not to tax the heart.

SELECTING YOUR PHYSICAL ACTIVITY

Choose your physical activity on the basis of the following:

- **Time Needed.** How much time do you have? This estimate must include the time required to get to and return from the place where you will take part in the activity.

- **Season of the Year.** Will the weather restrict your doing the activity year-round? If so, what activity will you substitute?

- **Skills Needed.** Will you need to take lessons? What will the lessons cost, and where can you get them?

- **Access.** Is the place where this activity can be performed accessible?

- **Cost.** What fee is charged? Must you buy special clothing? Is there a charge for parking?

- **Partner or Partners Needed.** Do you like to be with others? Will doing an activity with other people help you maintain a regular schedule?

The Formula for Attaining Better Health can be used as a systematic approach to behavioral change as you begin your own physical fitness program.

■■ CASE STUDY

George R. is sixty-seven years old. He retired from a position with a textile company a few years ago. During a visit to his personal physician last week, the doctor told George he was concerned that George's blood pressure was up to 170/110 and that George was twenty pounds heavier than when he retired. The doctor discussed the kinds of action that George should take. He prescribed medication to help control George's blood pressure, but he also pointed out to George that some changes in George's lifestyle needed to be made. The doctor suggested that George begin an exercise program to condition his heart and lungs. However, he cautioned George not to undertake strenuous physical

---

FORMULA FOR ATTAINING BETTER HEALTH

Task 1.   Assess your lifestyle and determine your goals.

Task 2.   Choose one specific behavior in a lifestyle area where you desire some self-change.

Task 3.   Observe yourself and gather information about your behavior patterns in this area.

Task 4.   Identify and evaluate any thoughts, feelings, and attitudes that may either aid or hinder your efforts to change your lifestyle.

Task 5.   Pinpoint the skills and tasks required to change your behavior and practice them.

Task 6.   Constantly monitor the results of your self-change efforts and revise your behavior as needed.

---

activity until his weight came down a bit. The doctor also indicated that George needed to take off at least ten pounds over the next two to three months.

Task 1. Assess Your Lifestyle and Determine Your Goals

The doctor gave George a booklet about exercise and the heart, which explained the kinds of physical activity required to condition the heart and lungs. According to the booklet, George's target zone ranges from 93 to 116 beats per minute. He would have to exercise at a pace that puts his heart rate at the lower range of heartbeats for three to five minutes at a time and would need to check his pulse periodically. Over a three-month period, he should be able to build up to fifteen minutes of sustained activity. George needs to exercise at least three times per week and with no more than a forty-eight-hour break between exercise periods, or the buildup of benefits will not occur.

George looked over the list of activities in the booklet to determine which ones could fit into his weekly pattern of living. Twenty years ago, he played tennis in the summer and racquet ball in the winter, but he felt too out of shape to think of those, and his doctor had warned him about not doing too much until he lost ten pounds. However, the same list included walking, swimming, and bicycling, so he does have a choice!

Task 2. Choose One Specific Behavior in a Lifestyle Area Where You Desire Some Self-Change

George had been a good athlete in high school and one of the better weekend tennis players throughout his thirties and forties. However, he didn't want to be embarrassed by breathlessness and a flabby appearance on the tennis court or at the swimming pool. Only children rode bicycles in his neighborhood, so George figured that his best choice was to begin his exercising with walking. The booklet described a sample walking program.

Task 3. Observe Yourself and Gather Information About Your Behavior Patterns in This Area

George has always used his time well, so he doesn't want to *just* go walking. He analyzed what he usually does each day of the week, hoping to identify some activities in which he could walk rather than use the car.

Tuesday and Thursday are his golf days—days filled with exercise and fun with his foursome. What does he do on Monday, Wednesday, Friday, and Saturday? Monday includes an hour at the elementary school, where he volunteers to help fourth graders with their math problems. The school is three miles from his house—too far for an initial walk, but he could drive part of the way. That's one day. Now how about Wednesday? That is the day his wife, Dorothy, plays golf, so she takes the car. When she returns, he dashes off on personal business to the bank, hardware store, and so on, which are about five miles away. He could do these errands by bus if he walked a half-mile. How about Friday? He goes grocery shopping with Dorothy, and they need the car. He could start out, and she could pick him up along the way. What about Saturday? Well, Tim, his eight-year-old grandson, usually spends the day with him, and their activities vary with the season. They usually go off to a ball game, go fishing, or go bowling. The strategy of

parking the car and walking part of the way or walking to the bus stop could be used here.

George decides to keep a record of times he walked instead of rode in a car or bus. (See Appendix E for a full-sized, blank copy of the self-observation chart on the next page.)

Task 4. Identify and Evaluate Any Thoughts, Feelings, and Attitudes That May Either Aid or Hinder Your Efforts to Change Your Lifestyle

George discovered that he needs to plan ahead even for something as simple as walking. In his first week, he learned that he really had not believed the booklet's advice about how slowly you need to start an exercise program. A fifteen-minute walk didn't appear to be too long, but he found it more tiring when most of it was uphill. He needs to allow time to rest halfway until he gets in shape.

Task 5. Pinpoint the Skills and Tasks Required to Change Your Behavior and Practice Them

George needs to start taking his pulse regularly on his walks—at the beginning of the walk, in the middle of the walk, and at the end of the walk.

There must be a way to be subtle when you don't want to interrupt your exercise (even brisk walking) to talk to people along the way—perhaps more arm swinging and a quick "hi."

George needs to keep a record of how he is increasing his walking time and distance. He will get a notebook and jot down specific times and places.

Self-Observation

Behavior: *Walking Instead of Riding*

Date	Situation (Briefly describe where you were and whom you were with.)	Thoughts and Feelings in This Situation (Briefly describe how you were feeling and what you were thinking.)	Actions (Describe how you responded to the situation.)
Mon. 6/10	Dorothy drove me part way to school. Started to walk alone the last mile.	Felt exhausted in 6 blocks. The walk is all uphill. I didn't realize I was in such poor shape.	I accepted a ride with another school volunteer for the last 6 blocks.
Sat. 6/15	Drove to the football game with Tim.	Felt good. Decided to park at the shopping center and walk to the stadium.	Parked at the shopping center and walked to and from the stadium with Tim. Took about 15 minutes each way. Saved $1.50 on parking fee.

It's easy to find excuses to skip a day, then two, and so on. George should start thinking ahead to what he will do during the cold, snowy days before going south

Self-Change Plan			
Self-Change Goal	Specific Behavioral Change	Self-Observation	
A regular exercise program to condition heart and lungs.	Build up to 15 minutes of brisk walking a day, 3 days a week.	Analyze my activities so I can combine walking with other chores. Keep a pocket notebook record of where and when I walk. Write down my pulse rate during brisk walking.	

in January and then what he will do down there. Maybe his wife will want to join him in regular swimming.

George needs to pick up an exercise booklet with directions on how to maintain joint flexibility.

Patterns that Aid or Hinder Self-Change Efforts	Skills and Tasks Required for Self-Change	Plan Summary
Usually go too fast and then get tired and sweaty. Don't consider how my plans affect others involved. Makes me frustrated if problems come up.	Allow more time to walk with some rest stops. Learn to take my pulse daily. Talk over plans with others far in advance. Set routines where possible.	Develop plans for beginning and increasing distances to walk. Ideas —park farther from school. —take bus farther down the line. —ask Dorothy to pick me up farther from home on way to shopping. Use pulse-rate records to guide rate of increase in time and distance to walk.

Task 6. Constantly Monitor the Results of Your Self-Change Efforts and Revise Your Behavior As Needed

George filled in the chart above to track how he will work up to his heart rate target zone and increase his walking distance. (See Appendix E for a blank self-change plan chart.) George is also using a chart to monitor changes in his weight (see Appendix C, page 336). He wants to take off those ten extra pounds before he sees his doctor in three months. In addition to the increased walking, George has decided to reduce the amount of beer he drinks from two bottles a day to one bottle a day.

Finally, George reviews the booklet his doctor gave him to determine how much swimming he will need to do to replace one or more of his walking sessions. George needs to design a schedule for his exercise program that fits into his other activities; he becomes frustrated when activities don't "mesh."

George must, of course, note the results of his behavioral changes and revise his specific behaviors from time to time so that his self-change goals can be met.

HOW PHYSICALLY FIT ARE YOU?

You may not be overweight or flabby, but, in your honest judgment, how physically fit are you? Now is the time to assess your physical fitness. While the experts cannot state scientifically that being fit makes you live longer, they do point to studies that suggest that high and sustained levels of physical activity are associated with longevity and with decreased atherosclerosis and cardiovascular disease.

Physical fitness is an achievable goal. An exercise program begun at any age can produce many benefits, including emotional well-being. So evaluate your fitness level. If you need to improve your fitness, see the sample exercises in Appendix A. A complete exercise program can be found in *Fitness for Life: Exercises for People Over 50,* by Theodore Berland (AARP Books, 1986).

You can revise your choices and decisions about a physical activity program following the same procedures described in George's case. There is no one standard of fitness; you need to choose activities that fit conveniently into your daily schedule—activities that can be added easily and will not be forgotten. When you decide to switch some aspect of your routine, you need to be certain that you can build regular physical activity into the revised weekly plan. If you are best motivated exercising with others, you might consider joining a local exercise group for walking, bicycling, or swimming.

Chapter 6

Eating to Stay Healthy

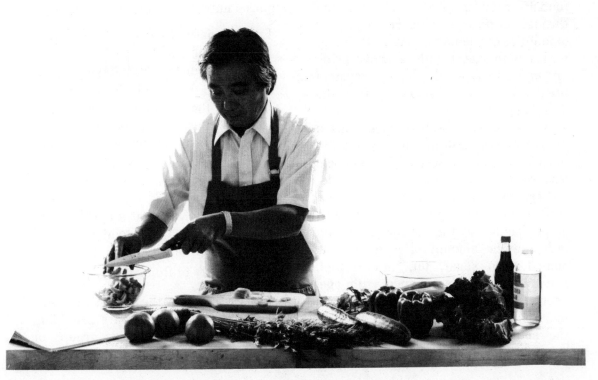

The media present an endless barrage of news and notions about cholesterol, food additives, saturated fat, natural foods, artificial sweeteners, sodium (salt), fiber, and so on. The scientists quoted do not agree, so the public receives mixed and confusing messages about the quantity and types of food people should eat. More research is needed on just what *are* the most nutritious eating practices for older people. In the meantime, how should an older person eat to stay healthy? Some simple basic rules about good nutrition should guide your decisions.

NUTRITIONAL NEEDS FOR OLDER ADULTS

All nutrients needed by the body for health and growth are available through food. Everyone needs the same nutrients throughout his or her life. However, the amount of nutrients needed by the body varies with age, health, activity level, and how effectively the digestive system breaks down and absorbs the food the individual eats.

As people age, the body composition tends to increase in fat and decrease in muscle mass and water. As physical activity and basic metabolic rate decrease, fewer calories are needed. These shifts require that individuals eat a greater percentage of their calories wisely, reducing the amount of calories consumed from sugar, fat, and alcohol. However, as bodies change with age, people must pay special attention to include adequate calcium and fiber in the diet. Balanced meals with adequate calories help achieve this.

BASIC CONCEPTS OF NUTRITION

The human body needs over fifty separate nutrients. Fortunately, a person does not have to check every day to see whether he or she is consuming all of them. These nutrients are contained in five plant and animal food sources. These five food groups are as follows:

- meat, poultry, fish, seafood, eggs, or meat alternatives such as dried beans, peas, nuts, peanut butter, and tofu
- milk, cheese, and yogurt
- fruits and vegetables
- whole-grain breads and cereals, pasta, and rice
- fats, sweets, and alcohol

To assure that you get your daily required nutrients, go by these four rules.

1. Eat a variety of each kind of food in the first four food groups. Select foods that have some fat each day.
2. Maintain a balanced diet among the first four food groups. Add sweets or alcohol, if used, to your diet if your total calorie allowance enables you to do so.
3. Practice moderation in the size and number of servings you eat each day. For overindulgence at a special celebration, reduce your food consumption the day before or the day after.)
4. Drink plenty of fluids daily.

When you follow these rules in selecting a balanced diet, you are providing your body with the major groups of essential nutrients scientists have identified. The main nutrients in food are as follows:

- proteins
- carbohydrates
- fats
- vitamins
- minerals

In addition, the body needs adequate amounts of water.

CELL GROWTH AND DEVELOPMENT (PROTEINS)

Humans need proteins in their diet to build and maintain all body cells. Proteins help form antibodies to fight infection and are responsible for regulating major body functions such as growth and digestion; they also supply calories.

Protein is found in three of the food groups:

- meat, poultry, fish, seafood, eggs, or meat alternatives such as dried beans, peas, nuts, peanut butter, and tofu
- milk, cheese, and yogurt
- whole-grain breads and cereals, pasta, and rice

Proteins are made from smaller units called amino acids. The body can manufacture some amino acids, but eight essential ones can be obtained only from food. Most proteins from meat and dairy products are "complete proteins," meaning they have all the essential amino acids. However, proteins from plants (grains, rice, legumes, and seeds) do not contain all the essential amino acids and are "incomplete proteins." Complete

proteins may be obtained in two ways:

- by mixing proteins from plant sources (grains, rice, legumes, and seeds) with a meat or dairy product or with milk (macaroni and cheese)
- by eating in the same meal a combination of the right proportions of complementary proteins from plant sources, such as legumes with grains (baked beans and brown bread, lima beans and corn, peanut butter on whole-grain bread, rice and beans, tortillas and beans, green beans and almonds)

PRIMARY SOURCES OF ENERGY (CARBOHYDRATES AND FATS)

All human energy is supplied by food, especially by foods in the whole-grain group, such as breads and cereals (carbohydrates), those in the milk group, and those in the fat and alcohol group. These foods provide sufficient energy (calories) to maintain vital body functions and to carry out daily chores such as cooking, house and yard work, or walking to the store. The carbohydrates also provide fiber, which adds bulk to the diet and serves as a natural laxative. Fats and oils have more than twice the calories, ounce for ounce, of carbohydrates. The higher the percentage of alcohol in a drink, the higher the calories.

The following foods are ready sources of carbohydrates.

starches: breads, cereals, rice, pasta, corn, potatoes, dried beans, and peas

sugars: sugar, honey, molasses, jams, syrups, soft drinks, candy, cakes, cookies, and puddings

These foods are sources of fats.

unsaturated fats:	cooking oil, margarine, salad dressings, and other oils
saturated fats:	fat in meat, whole milk, butter, cream, cheese, ice cream, avocados, chocolates, and solid hydrogenated vegetable shortenings

Some fat is visible, such as the "marble" in meat. Some fat is invisible, such as in cheese and avocados. Fats are classified as saturated or unsaturated. The saturated fats are usually animal in origin, coming from such sources as steak, bacon, butter, and cheese. Saturated fats are often used in nondairy creamers and cake mixes. This type of fat is solid at room temperature. The *unsaturated* fats come from plant sources, such as peanut oil and corn oil. They are liquid at room temperature. Margarine has been processed so it will be solid at room temperature and thus contains some saturated fat. Look at the label on the margarine package and select one that has twice as much polyunsaturated fat as saturated fat.

To maintain good nutrition, your body requires about one tablespoonful of fat per day. In the average U.S. diet, however, approximately 40 percent of the total calories are provided by fat. It is recommended that the fat you eat should be less than 30 percent of your daily calories. Whenever possible, saturated fats should be replaced with unsaturated fats. Excess saturated fat tends to raise blood cholesterol levels and predisposes the body to hardening of the arteries. Cholesterol is a waxy substance, related to fats, which is present in foods of animal origin and is manufactured by the body.

HEALTH MAINTENANCE (VITAMINS AND MINERALS)

To maintain health and prevent disease, you also need to eat foods that contain all fifty-plus nutrients, which include vitamins and minerals.

Vitamins and minerals cannot be produced by the body and must be obtained from food. Most vitamins and minerals work together with proteins to enable the body to obtain energy from food, build new tissue, and contribute to forming hormones, genetic material, and chemicals present in the nervous system. Nutritional surveys of older persons find as many as 50 percent of this population consuming less than the recommended amounts of the following vitamins and minerals.

vitamins:	A, C, and three of the B-complex—B_1 (thiamine), B_2 (riboflavin), and niacin
minerals:	calcium and iron

The Recommended Daily Allowance (RDA), as determined by professionals at the National Academy of Sciences, is the amount of essential nutrients required daily to meet the needs of a healthy person. The allowances differ by age, weight, sex, and physical condition (pregnancy and lactation).

Figure 1 lists the RDAs for men and women fifty-one and older. These persons are treated as a single group in this table; adequate studies have yet to be done on very old people. These

Recommended Daily Dietary Allowances, Designed for the Maintenance of Good Nutrition of Practically All Healthy People in the USA		
	Males	**Females**
Age (years)	51+	51+
Weight (kg/lb)	70/154	55/120
Height (cm/in)	178/70	163/64
Protein (g)	56	44
Fat-soluble vitamins		
Vitamin A (μg)	1000	800
Vitamin D (μg)	5	5
Vitamin E (mgα)	10	8
Water-soluble vitamins		
Vitamin C (mg)	60	60
Thiamin (mg)	1.2	1.0
Riboflavin (mg)	1.4	1.2
Niacin (mg)	16	13
Vitamin B_6 (mg)	2.2	2.0
Folacin (μg)	400	400
Vitamin B_{12} (μg)	3.0	3.0
Minerals		
Calcium (mg)	800	800
Phosphorus (mg)	800	800
Magnesium (mg)	350	300
Iron (mg)	10	10
Zinc (mg)	15	15
Iodine (μg)	150	150

Figure 1

RDAs, therefore, can only serve as general guides for later years. The requirements for vitamins and minerals are exceedingly small: milligrams (mg = one-thousandth of a gram) for some, micrograms (μg = one-millionth of a gram) for others. There are twenty-eight grams in an ounce.

The RDAs for vitamins are much greater than those actually required for disease prevention or treatment. There is still no convincing proof that large, or "mega," doses of any vitamin improve health or alter aging processes. If food intake is limited for any reason, a single multivitamin capsule will provide RDAs of the essential vitamins and minerals.

However, to obtain all the essential nutrients, an individual needs a balanced diet. When a variety of food is eaten, the body gets all the minerals, vitamins, and proteins it needs. Additional minerals should not be taken as supplements, since the margin between safe and toxic amounts is very small.

Vitamins

The process of aging may increase the need for some vitamins and minerals. Vitamins are found in fruits, vegetables, meats, dairy products, and cereals. One group of vitamins is classified as fat-soluble, the other as water-soluble.

Fat-soluble vitamins (A, D, E, and K) can be stored by the body and can build up to toxic levels if they are consumed in large doses (ten to twenty times the RDA) over a prolonged period of time. The absorption of these fat-soluble vitamins is inhibited if mineral oil is consumed in salad dressings or as a laxative.

Vitamin A is essential for good vision in dim light (it prevents night blindness), healthy skin, and protection against infection. Good sources of Vitamin A are dark green and deep yellow vegetables, liver, butter, and fortified milk.

Vitamin D (the sunshine vitamin) is necessary for the absorption and utilization of calcium in the body. A deficiency of this vitamin results in brittle, fragile bones (osteomalacia), muscle cramps, and nerve irritability. The best sources of vitamin D are fortified milk, yogurt, green vegetables, salmon, sardines, and liver.

Vitamin E helps transport oxygen to the cells and protects red blood cells. Studies have shown that vitamin E is rarely deficient in human beings. Good food sources of vitamin E are whole grains, seeds, nuts, eggs, sweet potatoes, and leafy vegetables.

Vitamin K is essential for normal blood clotting. It also helps maintain liver function and aids in the absorption of food in the intestines. The best food sources are dark green, leafy vegetables; cauliflower; soybeans; milk; yogurt; egg yolks; and safflower oil.

The water-soluble vitamins are vitamin C and the B-complex vitamins, which include those identified by the letter *B* with a number and/or a chemical name. The water-soluble vitamins are not stored well in the body, so foods containing these must be eaten daily. These vitamins can be destroyed by heat in cooking and also when exposed to air. Juices containing vitamin C should be kept in airtight containers and refrigerated when opened. The fruits and vegetables containing the water-soluble vitamins should be cooked in small amounts of water.

Vitamin C is essential for maintaining healthy cells in all parts of the body. A deficiency of vitamin C can result in bleeding gums, easy bruising, and the disease called scurvy. Citrus fruits are readily identified as a good source of vitamin C. However, if digestive problems or seasonal prices limit the use of citrus fruit, other good sources are green vegetables—especially broccoli, cabbage, and peppers—tomatoes, and baked potatoes (including the skins).

The vitamin B-complex group—B_1 (thiamine), B_2 (riboflavin), niacin, B_6 (pyridoxine), B_{12}, and folic acid—is essential for a healthy nervous system and for healthy eyes and skin. The B-complex group also aids the appetite and digestion. This group of vitamins is necessary for the production of energy in the cells of the body. Deficiencies among the B vitamins can result in exhaustion, depression, nervousness, poor appetite, constipation, skin disorders, and insomnia. To obtain all eight B-complex vitamins, an individual needs to eat such foods as poultry, liver, dairy products, eggs, oatmeal, rice, nuts, seeds, whole-grain breads, cereals, and vegetables.

Minerals

The body requires very small quantities of the thirty-one minerals that are used to build and maintain strong bones and teeth and to supply hemoglobin to red blood cells. The minerals of particular nutritional concern to older adults are calcium, iron, and sodium chloride (salt).

Calcium

Calcium helps blood clot and is needed for muscles to contract and relax and for nerves to respond to stimulation. Calcium is an essential mineral for maintaining bone strength. When an inadequate amount of calcium is consumed, the body takes calcium from the bones for other uses in the body. As part of the normal aging process, especially in women, the bones become more brittle and fragile due to a loss of calcium-containing minerals from the bones, and/or a reduction in the ability of the body to absorb calcium (see "Menopause," pages 261–262).

Thus, as you grow older, it is important to consume adequate amounts of calcium. Associated with loss of calcium in the bones (see pages 257–259) is a dramatic decrease in bone strength and a higher rate of hip fractures in older women—more than 120,000 per year in the United States. It is, therefore, important to consume adequate amounts of calcium and vitamin D. The recommended amount of calcium in the diet of older adults has been increased from 800 milligrams to 1,500 milligrams per day to minimize loss of bone calcium to other parts of the body.

Milk and milk products have a good ratio of calcium and phosphorus for the bones and contain vitamin D (if milk is fortified) which improves calcium absorption. In addition, nonfat powdered milk can be added to soups and stews for additional calcium in meals. Other sources of calcium are dark green, leafy vegetables; sardines; and salmon with bones. The use of mineral-oil laxatives blocks the absorption of vitamin D, and this in turn reduces the absorption of calcium.

Physical activity helps maintain strong bones and reduces the loss of calcium from them. Too much alcohol and antacids that contain aluminum will interfere with the body's ability to absorb calcium. If you have arthritis or kidney stones, consult your doctor about taking supplemental calcium such as bone meal.

Iron

Iron is an important mineral element found in all tissue cells of the body. It helps make hemoglobin, the red substance in blood that carries oxygen to the cells. Iron is stored in the liver and used over and over again. This efficient conservation of iron greatly reduces the amount a person needs to consume each day. Under normal conditions, the body absorbs an adequate amount of iron from a balanced diet. The advertisements that imply that older persons have iron-poor blood are misleading. When an older individual has an iron deficiency, it is of disease origin and not part of normal aging. The loss of blood in the intestinal tract from a peptic ulcer or tumor is an example. A doctor can decide how best to replace iron lost when there is a medical problem. A diet that includes red meat; whole grains; enriched flour; egg yolks; and dark green, leafy vegetables will adequately supply the need for iron.

Sodium Chloride (Salt)

Sodium has many important uses in the body. It maintains normal balance between the body fluids and cells, and it is needed for the transmission of nerve impulses and the relaxation of muscles. Medical research suggests that high sodium diets are associated with hypertension and abnormal fluid retention. The U.S. RDA recommends maximum intake of 2,000 milligrams of sodium per day—about the amount present in a teaspoonful of table salt. Most people eat too much—3,000 to 7,000 milligrams. One-third of this is from processed food, one-third is added in cooking or at the table, and the last third is present in foods in their natural form. If your doctor has advised you to reduce your intake of sodium (to help control hypertension or fluid retention), you need to take a close look at your food sources, not just the saltshaker. Salty foods include pretzels, potato chips, crackers, processed meats (bologna, bacon, sausage, frankfurters, and so on), canned meats, olives, pickles, canned and frozen vegetables, salted nuts, and soy sauce. Look for the sodium content on the label of the canned, frozen, and packaged foods you buy.

Ask your physician about the use of a salt substitute. Most salt substitutes contain a form of potassium salt; some are equal amounts of table salt and potassium chloride. Too much potassium can cause problems, especially for people with kidney disease.

You should check the label on the antacids you buy. You will see on the store shelves, along with the familiar packages of antacids, new packages of antacids that contain no sodium.

Newspapers and magazines feature a growing number of recipes that use spices and flavorings with ingredients instead of salt. Among the substitutes for salt as a seasoning are lemon or lime juice and herbs and spices such as garlic, dill, parsley, basil, and thyme.

WATER

One essential daily dietary component is not a food in terms of calories or vitamins—that component is water. The need to drink fluids is often overlooked. Drinking water or other fluids can aid your digestion and help prevent urinary tract problems. It is a good idea to start and end the day with a glass of water and add a glass at meals and with snacks. Fruits and vegetables are also important sources of water.

FIBER

Fiber is important all through life and especially in the later years, when constipation can be a problem. Fiber is a natural laxative; it promotes regularity. A daily intake of crude fiber will increase the water content of the stool and the softness of bowel movements.

Fiber is found naturally in fruits such as apples, in the bran portion of whole grains, and in vegetables. The bran portion of the grain is the covering around the kernel. Breads and cereals that are processed usually have the bran removed. Try to buy cereals or breads that are labeled "bran" or "whole grain." If you have difficulty chewing or digesting raw fruits and vegetables, you can still get a high fiber content from cooked and canned fruits and vegetables in your meals.

Eat a diet high in vegetable fiber, or roughage, to prevent the development of diverticulitis. A high-fiber diet helps protect against high blood cholesterol and certain types of tumors. For achieving regular bowel movements, the combination of fiber and adequate fluid is advocated over laxatives, which are costly and tend to cause a "lazy bowel." (See pages 211–214 for a discussion of constipation and pages 223–225 for information on diverticulitis.)

CAFFEINE

Caffeine is a stimulant and has a definite drug effect on the brain and heart. This stimulant is present in coffee, tea, cocoa, cola drinks, and some other soft drinks. Recent concern about the amount of caffeine people drink has led to the development of many new caffeine-free products. Check the labels on the beverages you buy.

DAILY FOOD REQUIREMENTS

You can stay healthy by selecting a variety of foods from the groups listed in figure 2. This chart provides a ready reference to check on the major nutrients you receive from each food group, how many servings you should select from each group, and the variety of food choices you have. It also reminds you of the importance of checking on the

amount of water you include each day through a variety of beverages.

YOUR DAILY FOOD INTAKE: A DIET LOG

Knowing the importance of essential nutrients and the cautions concerning fats, sugars, cholesterol, alcohol, salt, and caffeine, you may want to check your diet to determine whether it is reasonably balanced. Start with a diet log, or chart, on which you record everything you eat and when you eat it (see Appendix C, pages 338–339). Place the chart on the refrigerator or cupboard door so you will remember to record each and every nibble, snack, and meal.

The diet log lists the food groups from the balanced diet chart (figure 2) and has separate columns to enter the amounts of fats and oils, sweets, and alcohol you consume. Overconsumption of sweets and alcohol is likely to result in weight gain; in addition, calories derived from these sources have no nutritional benefits. You can check what you list in these columns for possible excess calories, caffeine, and alcohol, and the amount of fluid you drink each day. Use figure 2 as a guide in describing the food. Name the food so that you can check to see whether you are eating a variety from each group. The amount should be recorded to show whether it is one serving, one and one-half servings, or two servings. The total number of servings for each column should be checked with the balanced diet chart totals. Ask yourself these questions.

■ Does my meat group include a variety of fish, poultry, and legumes?

Food Groups	Amount per Day	Food Sources
I. Meat and Meat Substitute Group for protein, phosphorus, iron, vitamins B₆ and B₁₂, thiamine, and niacin	Two moderate servings	*One serving:* 2 oz. cooked lean meat, fish, or poultry; 2 slices (2 oz.) cheddar cheese; 2 eggs; 1 cup cooked dried peas, beans, or lentils; 1 cup cooked soybeans; 4 tablespoons peanut butter
II. Dairy Products for protein, calcium, phosphorus, vitamins A, B₆, and B₁₂, and riboflavin	Two servings	*One serving of low-fat dairy products:* 1 8-oz. glass milk; ½ cup cottage or ricotta cheese; 1 cup yogurt; 2 slices (2 oz.) cheddar cheese. Fortified milk adds vitamins A and D.
III. Fruits and Vegetables for carbohydrates, fiber, vitamins A, C, and K, riboflavin, folacin, iron, and calcium	Four or more servings	*One serving:* medium-sized apple, orange, banana, peach, or potato; 8-oz glass citrus fruit juice (orange, grapefruit); ½ cup cooked spinach, cabbage, carrots, or squash; 1 stalk broccoli; ½ green pepper
IV. Grains and Cereals for carbohydrates, iron, and B–complex vitamins, and fiber	Four or more servings	*One serving:* 1 slice whole-grain bread or muffin (enriched); 1 cup dry cereal; ½ cup cooked oatmeal, bran, rice, pasta, or barley
Fats, Sweets, and Alcohol for additional calories. Fats contribute vitamin E and an essential fatty acid.	Depends on your calorie needs	Includes butter, margarine, mayonnaise, fats and oils, and other salad dressings. Also canned or frozen fruits, jams, jellies, pastries, soft drinks, and alcoholic beverages. Approximately 9 calories per gram for fat, 4 calories per gram for sugar, and 7 calories per gram for alcohol.
Water for absorption of nutrients, regulation of body temperature, circulation, and excretion	Six to ten glasses	Includes all types of beverages and soups

Figure 2. A Balanced Diet

■ Does the fruit and vegetable group include a variety of yellow-orange and green, leafy vegetables and fruit?

■ Are the cereals and breads made from whole grains? If not, are they made from enriched flour?

When you look over your detailed record, you can quickly see whether you are eating enough from each of the food groups. You can also find the places where you may be getting extra calories and/or saturated fat. The Fats and Oils column should include the extra fat you get when you eat fried foods, add cream or whole milk to coffee or tea, or select whole-milk dairy products rather than low-fat products. The Sweets and Alcohol columns should tell you how many foods you are consuming that contain many calories but few nutrients.

FACTORS RELATED TO NUTRITIONAL INTAKE

As people age, medical, social, and environmental factors tend to influence their nutritional intake. These factors include gum disease, poor-fitting dentures, infection, medications, living alone, alcohol consumption, physical trauma, and stress. Over half the United States population fifty years of age and older no longer has their natural teeth. Painful gums and poor-fitting dentures decrease chewing effectiveness and create digestive problems. These problems can be reduced by slicing meat and fruit into small pieces, shredding vegetables, and cooking food until soft.

A number of medications affect appetite, absorption of foods, and utilization of nutrients. Diuretics increase the excretion of zinc and potassium. Some drugs produce side effects that include depressed appetite, nausea, vomiting, and diarrhea. On the other hand, some nutrients can decrease the action of drugs. When your doctor prescribes medicine for you, ask whether any of these side effects might occur and, if they should, what you can do to overcome them. The doctor may suggest changes in the times that you eat certain foods and/or an increase in the amount of vitamins you consume. When you take sulfa drugs and other antibiotics, the intestinal microorganisms that enable your body to use vitamins appropriately are affected. When the antibiotic tetracycline is taken, reduced absorption of both dietary fat and iron may occur. Your doctor needs to suggest a way you can protect your nutrition when you are taking a medication.

When you live alone, it is easy to lose interest in preparing meals or enjoying food. A positive approach is to plan regularly scheduled meals with family, friends, and neighbors. Eating out can include brown bag lunches and attending meal programs offered by nutrition centers, churches, and organizations.

Alcohol consumption can reduce nutrition in three ways:

1. It interferes with absorption of B_1, B_6, and folic acid.
2. It decreases appetite.
3. It often substitutes for the food needed in a well-balanced diet.

Stress that comes from infection or physical trauma (accidents or surgery) can alter the way the body uses nutrients. Under the stress of infection, body nitrogen and some vitamins and minerals are lost. If there is an acute or chronic infection in the digestive tract, the absorption of nutrients may be decreased. Intake of proteins, calories, vitamins, and minerals must be increased during the recovery period from infection or surgery.

A special word of caution. Older persons may have both decreased vision and a loss in sense of smell resulting in the inability to detect when foods are spoiled. Anyone with these losses should be especially careful to guard against food poisoning. If necessary, someone can check any questionable food.

TIPS TO SAVE FOOD DOLLARS

The commercial world encourages the consumer to buy many expensive foods and food substitutes, often in costly packages. A fixed and often limited income makes it very important to make economical as well as nutritional choices.

To make it possible for consumers to compare the nutrition in food products, the United States Food and Drug Administration has developed a nutrition label. Use of the nutrition label is voluntary unless a manufacturer adds nutrients to the product (for example, milk fortified with vitamins A and D) or makes a nutritional claim on the label or in advertising. Read the label to compare the percentage of Recommended Daily Allowances in food. A list of ingredients in a product appears on the label in order of the highest proportion first and the least last. In addition, the following information is provided.

- number of servings in package
- number of calories per serving
- amount of protein, carbohydrate, and fat (in grams) per serving (1 ounce = 28 grams)
- amount of vitamins and minerals as a percentage of the U.S. RDA
- information on fat, cholesterol, and sodium

Choose foods that provide the best nutritional value for the number of calories per serving. Skim milk provides major nutrients but fewer calories than whole milk. Whole-grain cereals without added sugar are nutritious and have fewer calories than sugared cereals.

Use unit pricing (displayed as price per ounce or pound or quart on the store shelf) to select the best buy. Bulk cheese or prepackaged sliced cheese is less expensive than individually sliced or shredded cheese. The largest size does not always have the lowest unit price. Individual packages of cereal may cost more than one large package; however, you should buy the size that you can use before it spoils. Check the date on perishable items. The balanced diet chart (figure 2) suggests a variety of choices for each food group, and these differ in cost as well as seasonal availability. Ignore the sales promotions for miracle pills, special diets, and exotic food products. Spend your dollars on a wide variety of foods at the grocery store. Intelligent consideration of the many options available from the nation's food supply means that everyone can be well nourished and enjoy eating, even on a limited budget.

IDEAL WEIGHT

A way of thinking about your ideal weight is to use the age twenty rule. If you were neither overweight nor underweight at twenty years of age, consider that your "ideal" weight at any age—allowing for a slow, modest gain. Judgments about your weight can best be made by looking in the mirror for changes in your body's fat distribution (roll around the waist? flabby thighs and arms?) and observing whether your clothes are tight or loose. It is helpful to use a scale once a week or at least once a month and to act on the five-pound weight changes as they occur rather than letting them accumulate to ten, fifteen, or twenty pounds. A sudden gain or loss of weight without a change in your activity level and/or your caloric intake is an "alert signal" of a change in the body's functioning, and should be brought to your doctor's attention (see "Unexplained Weight Loss," pages 153–154).

The major nutritional problem in the United States is overconsumption of fats and sugars, which results in obesity. It is associated with hypertension, atherosclerosis, heart attack, and diabetes.

BALANCING ENERGY NEEDS

The nutrients in food—proteins, fats, and carbohydrates—are the primary sources of energy to the body. The energy potential in food is expressed in calories. The body needs energy (calories) to keep it warm and to provide fuel so that all body systems can work. All foods contain calories. A calorie is a unit of measure just as a cup or tablespoon is a unit of measure. The caloric content of a food is calculated from the amount of protein, fat, and carbohydrate it contains. One gram of carbohydrate or protein contains four calories, whereas one gram of fat contains nine calories. This explains why fatty foods contain more calories than those low in fat content. When you eat and drink more calories than your body burns, you gain weight, since your body stores calories as fat. When you eat less, you lose weight because your body gets its extra fuel from stored body fat. A lowering of energy requirements can occur when changes are made in daily living patterns that require you to expend less energy. Examples are illness or injury that restricts your physical activity or a lack of motivation to keep physically active. With advancing age, the basic body composition changes, and the body's metabolic rate may decline, so the total caloric requirement also may decline.

If you consume 3,500 extra calories, you'll gain a pound. If you use up an extra 3,500 calories, you'll lose a pound. When trying to lose weight, experts agree that one to two pounds of weight loss per week is ideal. If you take the weight off slowly and gradually, you have a much better chance of keeping it off.

- To lose one pound per week: Reduce your total caloric intake by 3,500 calories per week, or 500 calories per day.
- To lose two pounds per week: Reduce your total calorie intake by 7,000 calories per week, or 1,000 calories per day.

The most efficient way to lose weight is to combine both diet and exercise and *not* depend on diet alone. Consider the example in figure 3. It shows that if you

Diet: 500 calories less	Calories saved	Exercise: 500 calories more	Calories used
Change from whole to skim milk.	(80)	Climb up and down stairs (5 minutes).	(55)
Have 2 less pats of butter.	(200)	Walk 2½ miles.	(250)
Have 1 less beer.	(150)	Do some gardening (1 hour).	(240)
Have diet cola instead of regular.	(106)		
Don't use cream in 2 cups of coffee.	(60)		
Total Calories:	496	Total Calories:	545

Figure 3. Combining Diet and Exercise to Lose Two Pounds per Week (1,000 calories per day)

add a little exercise to your day, you don't have to give up as much on the diet side.

FAD DIETS

Fad diets that promise *quick* and *easy* weight loss are not only misleading but oftentimes dangerous. The weight loss is usually temporary because it is often only a water loss. The fad diet does not change the dieter's general eating behavior, so when regular patterns of eating are resumed, the weight is gained back. Fad diets often emphasize eating foods from only one food group and excluding most other foods. This may result in malnutrition. The low-protein, low-fat "rice" type of diet may lead to potassium depletion and subsequent heart arrhythmia. The high-fat–low-carbohydrate or high-fat–no-carbohydrate diet creates a feeling of fullness; however, the immediate weight loss is because of partial dehydration, not loss of body fat. It can add fat deposits to the arteries.

Some people have developed kidney stones, disturbing psychological changes, and other complications while following fad diets. In addition, it is very difficult to obtain an adequate diet of all needed nutrients with less than 1,200 calories. Repeated loss and gain of weight puts stresses on the body that are injurious to health.

Consult your physician before going on a special weight-reduction diet. He or she will look for the cause of your weight gain (underlying disease, overeating, or reduced activity) and consider the proportion of fat to muscle on your body, your rate of metabolism, the desirable level of physical activity for you, and your eating habits. On the basis of all these factors, the doctor can make intelligent recommendations to reduce your weight to a desirable level and to help you maintain that weight.

NUTRITIONAL MANAGEMENT

In order to begin your own nutrition-management program, the Formula for Attaining Better Health (introduced in chapter 3) can be used as a systematic approach to behavior change.

FORMULA FOR ATTAINING BETTER HEALTH

Task 1. Assess your lifestyle and determine your goals.

Task 2. Choose one specific behavior in a lifestyle area where you desire some self-change.

Task 3. Observe yourself and gather information about your behavior patterns in this area.

Task 4. Identify and evaluate any thoughts, feelings, and attitudes that may either aid or hinder your efforts to change your lifestyle.

Task 5. Pinpoint the skills and tasks required to change your behavior and practice them.

Task 6. Constantly monitor the results of your self-change efforts and revise your behavior as needed.

◼ CASE STUDY

Ann P., aged fifty-five, lives alone. Her husband died a year ago, and in the same year her older sister moved to the Southwest to live closer to her son and his family. Last week, Ann's daughter, Marie, came from California for a visit and was appalled to find her mother looking pale and lacking energy. When her mother complained of back pain, Marie promptly arranged for her to see a doctor. A thorough physical examination of Ann revealed poor nutrition, weight loss, and anemia. Upon questioning, Ann indicated that she had lost interest in preparing and eating food. Her current diet consisted mainly of hot tea, toast, hot cereal, muffins, cookies, potato chips, and ginger ale. Occasionally she ate a hamburger.

Task 1. Assess Your Lifestyle and Determine Your Goals

Ann realized that it was important for her to do something about her condition—specifically about her diet. She agreed to spend the week of Marie's visit exploring ways to improve her food consumption. Working together, they wrote down each day what Ann would like to eat, what would need to be done if this food was to be available, and what choices Ann had to meet these needs. They tried to identify what had happened in the past few years that had changed Ann's interest in food.

In this review of Ann's daily eating, it was apparent that she was not eating sufficient meat, poultry, fish, fruits, vegetables, or dairy products. She used milk only on her cereal. She had always liked most foods and still did. However, when she broke her lower denture, she could no longer chew many foods. In addition, she had eliminated orange juice from her diet because the price had risen so drastically. As her energy level decreased, she had turned down invitations for lunch and dinner.

Task 2. Choose One Specific Behavior in a Lifestyle Area Where You Desire Some Self-Change

Ann decided she did not have the money now to go to the dentist and have a new set of dentures made, so she would have to stay with foods that were easy to eat and that could be delivered to her home. In looking over her choices of where to start, she elected to increase her intake of milk products by drinking two glasses of milk and eating one-half cup of cottage cheese or yogurt each day for the first week. These food items could be delivered from the deli two blocks away if she ordered them by phone. She could also get a pint of her favorite rice pudding there. This she could eat with fresh or canned fruit. Marie took Ann to visit the deli so she could think about the kinds of choices she could make over the next few weeks as she gradually built up her appetite and energy.

Task 3. Observe Yourself and Gather Information About Your Behavior Patterns in This Area

Ann took notes on her attempts to change her diet during the first week after Marie left. (See Appendix E for a full-sized, blank copy of the self-observation chart.) The entries for the first two days are shown on the next page.

Task 4. Identify and Evaluate Any Thoughts, Feelings, and Attitudes That May Either Aid or Hinder Your Efforts to Change Your Lifestyle

The old patterns of giving in to fatigue and doing things the "easy way" were still there for Ann. She was glad that Marie had gotten her to write out menus for what she would like to eat and had her order all the food in advance. This helped Ann eat more nutritiously. It cut down on decisions and made it harder for Ann to give in to her excuses.

Task 5. Pinpoint the Skills and Tasks Required to Change Your Behavior and Practice Them

Ann needed to decide what to put on her menu for next week from the foods the deli has available. She put a note on her calendar to remind her to place an order on Friday mornings.

Each week, Ann needed to decide where she could walk—starting in her own yard and gradually building up to the two blocks to the bank. She wants to be able to walk to the deli twice a week so she can look over her menu choices. She can also save the delivery charge. She wants to build up her endurance and strength, since she would like to feel up to a trip to California by Christmas.

Task 6. Constantly Monitor the Results of Your Self-Change Efforts and Revise Your Behavior As Needed

For the next few months, Ann will continue to be aware of the foods she

Self-Observation

Behavior: *Eat More and Healthier Food*

Date	Situation (Briefly describe where you were and whom you were with.)	Thoughts and Feelings in This Situation (Briefly describe how you were feeling and what you were thinking.)	Actions (Describe how you responded to the situation.)
Mon. 8/26	Home alone; fixed breakfast.	Not really hungry. Remembered Marie said to eat better food.	Cut up a banana on the cereal and added extra milk.
Tues. 8/27	10:30 A.M. – Home alone, read paper.	Felt hungry. Thought about cookies and tea.	Looked at the menu sheets and ate rice pudding and fruit.

eats, selecting a well-balanced diet of easy-to-chew foods from the four basic food groups. In the meanwhile, as soon as she can afford it, Ann will have new dentures made. Ann has recorded her plan as shown in the chart on pages 86–87. (See Appendix E for a blank self-change plan chart.)

Ann must note the results of her behavioral changes and review her specific behaviors from time to time so that her self-change goals can be achieved.

Self-Change Plan

Self-Change Goal	Specific Behavioral Change	Self-Observation	
To get stronger and have more energy.	Eat more dairy foods and vegetables — a healthier diet.	Keep a record of dairy foods and vegetables I eat for one week.	

Patterns that Aid or Hinder Self-Change Efforts	Skills and Tasks Required for Self-Change	Plan Summary
No interest in fixing meals only for myself. Lazy. Too tired to walk to the store for food. Not trying to eat meals with others. I want to get stronger to go to California and see Marie for Christmas.	Learn about nutrition. Make weekly menus and follow menu plan daily. Order deli food for the week each Friday morning, especially dairy foods and meats. Invite Joyce to lunch in 2 weeks.	Get library book on nutrition. Make weekly menus for next few months. Order good deli food for next few weeks. When stronger, go shopping more. Check with doctor in 3 months to see how anemic I am. Make appointment this week and mark calendar.

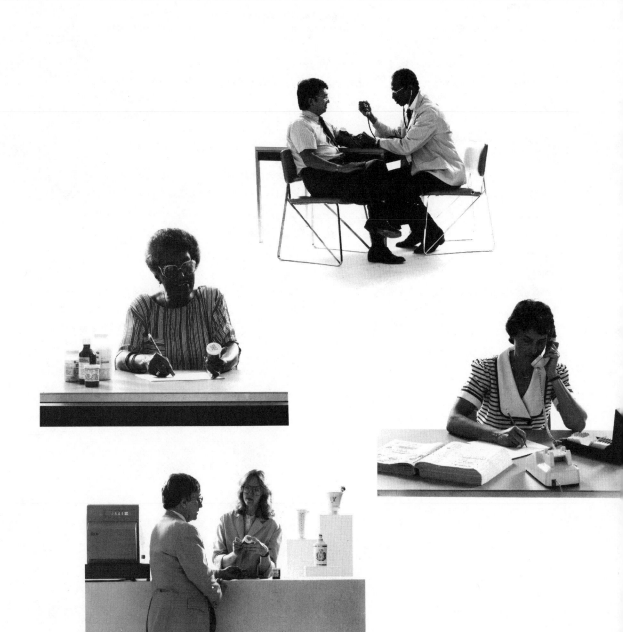

PART TWO

ORGANIZING SELF-CARE

Chapter 7

You and Your Physician

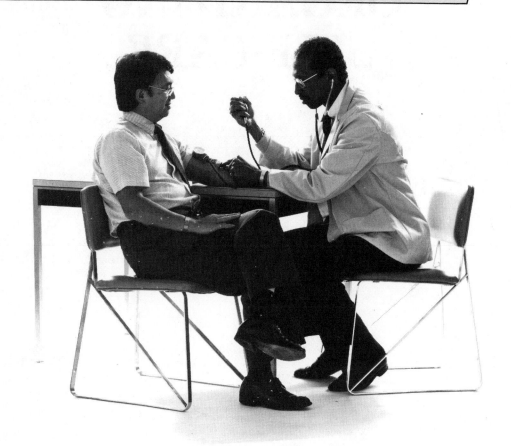

It is essential to establish an effective relationship with your primary physician—a relationship in which both you and the doctor can assume appropriate responsibilities for maintaining your health. Key elements in developing an effective relationship between you and your physician are (1) selecting a doctor who is right for you, (2) forming an active partnership, and (3) developing effective communication.

SELECTING A DOCTOR WHO IS RIGHT FOR YOU

The best time to find the right doctor for yourself is when you are well, not when you are sick or when you face a medical emergency. Most people have a doctor whom they like and trust. But there may come a time when you need to find a new doctor, for instance, if you move to a new location, if your current doctor moves or retires, or if you become dissatisfied with your present doctor. Everyone has his or her own "norms" for how his or her body functions and a unique history of illnesses, treatments, and responses. A doctor needs to have this information in advance to "read" effectively what is happening to you when you are ill. The following sources can aid you in selecting a new physician.

1. *Friends or Relatives*. If you have friends or relatives in the community, ask them about the doctors they know. This sort of personal recommendation can be a means of finding a good physician but also can be misleading if one friend or relative is your only source.

2. *Community Resources*. If you do not have a personal physician or are not satisfied with the one you have, you can call the secretary of the county medical society or the director of a local hospital and ask for a list of physicians who will accept new patients. Some emergency rooms maintain listings of practitioners who will assume primary care of patients.

3. *Your Current Physician*. If you are moving and are satisfied with your current physician, ask him or her to recommend a physician in your new area. Your present physician knows you, your personal style, and your health condition. He or she may know other physicians who would provide you with the same type of care you are currently receiving.

4. *Prepaid Medical Plans*. You may also want to consider joining a prepaid medical plan, where your yearly fee covers the costs of all your doctor visits as well as other medical services. These plans are called Health Maintenance Organizations (HMOs) or Independent Practice Associations (IPAs). Under these plans, you generally can choose, from among a panel of available physicians, an individual to be your personal physician. In some situations you may not be able to select a personal physician, but your health care should be well coordinated and efficient.

However, regardless of where you obtain your list of physicians, there are some important facts to consider: the location of the doctor's office, his or her credentials, and the way the practice operates.

Office Location

You will want answers to the following questions.

- Is the doctor's office close and/or convenient to where you live or to transportation?

- Is the office close to a good hospital and drug store?

- Is the office on the first floor? Is there an elevator, or do you have to walk up stairs?

Physician's Credentials

In the Yellow Pages of the telephone book, a physician is listed either as an M.D. (Doctor of Medicine) or a D.O. (Doctor of Osteopathy). If you are looking for a doctor who will consider all your health problems, you need to find a person trained as a generalist, a family practitioner, a general internist, or an osteopath. Other types of physicians are listed as specialists, meaning they have specialized skills related to some part of the body, such as a cardiologist for the heart and a dermatologist for the skin.

A specialist may be board-certified and is known as a diplomate of that board. If the physician has not taken the certification examination but has completed the specialty training, he or she will be considered board-eligible. Some primary-care practitioners have additional initials after their M.D., such as FACP (Fellow of the American College of Physicians) or ABFP (American Board of Family Practice).

To learn about a physician's credentials, you can call his or her office and ask the receptionist what medical school the physician graduated from, at what hospitals the general and specialty training was taken, and the dates of these educational experiences. Also, you can usually find the physician's diplomas and certificates on an office wall. Some people check the physician's credentials in the library in a reference book entitled *Directory of Medical Specialists*, which provides a current national listing of active medical practitioners. Your research will provide you with information you can use to compare the doctor's background with the backgrounds of other physicians you have had. You can ask other health professionals to help you evaluate this information. Credentials alone will not assure the right choice of a physician for you.

Operation of the Physician's Practice

When asking about the operation of a physician's practice, you will want to ask these questions.

- What are the office hours? On which days of the week is the office open?

- Does the physician make house calls? If so, under what conditions?

- Does the doctor have other physicians who will take phone calls and provide professional coverage for him or her when the doctor is not available (on vacation, on days off, and so on)?

- Which hospital(s) does the doctor use to admit patients? Is this convenient and appropriate for you?

- What are the standard fees for a

routine visit? a complete periodic examination? a house call? Does the charge for the initial physical examination of new patients include fees for laboratory tests? Does the practice accept Medicare assignment?

■ Does the doctor work with other clinical staff such as a nurse practitioner, nurse clinician, or physician's assistant?

■ Does the doctor or the doctor's office assistant submit insurance forms for you?

FORMING AN ACTIVE PARTNERSHIP

The advice your physician gives you depends a great deal on how you both understand each other's responsibilities. You both must be honest with each other, especially when you don't agree. The kinds of actions you both need to take to manage health problems and prevent illnesses require open discussion of problems and joint agreement on what to do. These decisions can involve physical and emotional discomfort, inconvenience, and expense You will want to minimize all of these.

A person consults a physician because of the doctor's special expertise. As a result, patients often believe that they should not question what the doctor recommends or seek more information from him or her. Although doctors do have knowledge and skill in diagnosing health problems and recommending solutions, they cannot be expected to know all your health-related problems, how you think about your health care, or whether you can or will follow their recommendations. Therefore, you must speak up and give this information. Tell the doctor if you have been given different advice in the past about your health problem(s)—both you and your doctor can benefit from this honest exchange.

Each person responds differently to medicines, medical procedures, and physical demands. Sometimes these differences are small, other times very great. However, when you have reactions to the medicine that are different from what the doctor told you to expect, you must let the doctor know. These unusual or adverse responses are often referred to as side effects. For example, itching and the appearance of a skin rash after taking penicillin for a sore throat suggests an allergic reaction to the drug. Unusual responses can also occur when the prescribed treatment fails to accomplish what it is supposed to; for example, bothersome diarrhea may not be controlled by a special diet and paregoric. In either case, the doctor cannot be effective in helping to manage your health problem if you don't report what is happening.

Like most people, you may forget to take your prescribed medication or may have been too busy to carry out a recommended treatment or simply couldn't find the suggested community resource. Any such omission may result in apparent treatment failure. If this occurs, the doctor needs to know the facts so his or her next decision is not to try still another treatment but rather to work with you in arranging ways for you to more readily follow the original treatment plan.

The list of what can go wrong when a doctor and a patient fail to communicate effectively is long—and the patient always pays a price. The problems cited so far represent patient failures. Equally important, the doctor must trust your judgment and understanding about what he or she tells you. Naive or passive patients often lead the physician to limit discussion and avoid explanations.

An active working partnership between you and your doctor implies that you will work together as a team and that both of you will assume appropriate responsibilities. Recent studies show clearly that sharing information and records leads to fewer illnesses, fewer hospital admissions, and significant savings of dollars. Your responsibilities as a patient might include the following:

■ Providing your physician with an accurate description of your symptoms and concerns; this may mean keeping records to improve your accuracy.

■ Reporting accurately and promptly all symptoms, even if you fear they indicate a serious disease.

■ Providing the physician with accurate information about your medical history, certain aspects of your personal life, and your family history.

■ Answering questions the doctor asks you about your daily activities, your family life, and your work and leisure.

■ Bringing a list of questions about your health concerns to your doctor, or arranging for a family member or friend to help in asking questions, and

getting those questions answered (see page 96).

■ Reading and asking questions to become more knowledgeable about your health in general.

■ Working with your physician to design a health maintenance plan that is consistent with your values and circumstances.

■ Carrying out the health maintenance and treatment plan you have developed together and reporting any problems you have encountered when doing this.

■ Notifying the physician's office when you are unable to keep an appointment.

■ Discussing your medical bills and any difficulties you experience in paying them.

In an active, working partnership with your doctor, the physician serves as the major source of expert advice. This advice is designed to educate you about your health care. *Together* you make informed decisions. To fulfill his or her role in the relationship, your physician's responsibilities as a partner might include these:

■ Obtaining a complete history.

■ Performing a physical examination when you first become a patient and repeating such an examination on a periodic basis.

■ Listening attentively to all your questions and personal concerns.

■ Involving you in decision making when the need for a consultation or special advice from a medical specialist arises.

- Involving you in deciding what treatment is safe, acceptable, and practical for you.
- Advising you on the potential hazards of treatment, including surgical procedures, and what your choices are—this is called *informed consent*.
- Helping you understand your health status and advising you how to enhance your independence, self-respect, and lifestyle as much as possible.
- Suggesting ways to lead an even healthier life.
- Discussing with you what family members should be told—or not told—about your health and illness.
- Maintaining complete confidentiality about the personal information he or she has until you agree (usually in writing) that the information may be released to others.
- Notifying you of new advances in medicine that can change your care.

An acceptance of these responsibilities can help each of you be more realistic about what to expect, be satisfied with your visits, feel calm when emergencies occur, and, over time, gain confidence and respect for each other. Like any partnership, this very personal relationship requires work, honesty, and mutual trust.

DEVELOPING EFFECTIVE COMMUNICATION

Developing an active partnership with your physician requires open and free-flowing communication. To achieve this kind of effective communication, several factors must be considered.

- Do you and your doctor come from similar cultural backgrounds? the same region of the country? If not, do you explore the differences in what words and ideas mean to each of you? In other words, do you really understand each other?
- Do you feel comfortable with the doctor's appearance, manners, and nonverbal communication?
- Do you get cues that the doctor does or does not feel comfortable with you?

Individuals respond to each other on the basis of what "image" each creates for the other. These images come from earlier experiences—associations made with personal appearance and mannerisms and with an undefined "body chemistry." Whatever it is that goes into your thoughts, it is well to recognize that unless you resolve uneasy feelings, you are unlikely to establish good rapport with each other.

Since you will need to be able to share very personal information and openly discuss potentially unpleasant topics with your primary physician, you need to select someone with whom you do feel comfortable. Go to your first visit with an open mind, and don't choose a physician on medical credentials only; decide if you can develop confidence, trust, respect, and openness with that person. If not, you are limiting your potential for an effective partnership.

Preparing for an Office Visit

A list of questions you might ask yourself follows.

Questions you will likely want to know the answer to by the time you leave the doctor's office are listed below.

TEN QUESTIONS TO ASK MYSELF BEFORE SEEING MY DOCTOR

1. What problem or symptom am I concerned about?

2. When did it begin? Did it begin suddenly or gradually?

3. How does it interfere with my life (for example, eating, sleeping, working, leisure, sexual activity)?

4. Is it related to time of day, time of week, time of month, time of year, time of life, meals, sleep, or anything else?

5. What helps?

6. What makes it worse or brings it on?

7. Could this be a side effect of any medication I'm taking, or is this a part of any known problem (for example, ulcer, migraine headaches, or depression)?

8. Since it started, is it the same, worse, or better?

9. What do I think or fear may be causing it?

10. What do I think needs to be done about it?

TEN QUESTIONS I MAY WANT ANSWERED BEFORE I LEAVE MY DOCTOR'S OFFICE

1. What is my problem called?

2. How does it affect my health?

3. What is likely to happen to me with or without treatment?

4. Are any further tests necessary? How long will they take? How much will they cost? Are side effects or pain likely?

5. Can something be done to treat the problem without medication?

6. What is the name of the medication? the dosage? How often do I take it?

7. What does it do? How long does it take to act? How long must I take it? What does it cost?

8. Are there any side effects, restrictions, or limitations of the medication's use?

9. How can I tell when I'm getting better? When am I likely to be well again?

10. How soon should I call or come in again for test reports, advice, or reexamination?

Getting a Second Opinion

When you do not have adequate information to make a decision about a recommended treatment, surgical operation, or special procedure, you should tell the physician this and ask for more information about the condition and the options. One option you should consider is seeking the opinion of another physician when elective surgery or some other special procedure is recommended. Studies report that in many cases of nonemergency surgery (for example, knee surgery, hysterectomies, prostatectomies), the costs and risks of surgery can be avoided without jeopardizing the health and well-being of the patient. It is wise to seek a second opinion (sometimes even a third), since there are legitimate differences in judgment among physicians.

The final decision of what you want to do is yours. You want to base this important decision on how you weigh the relative risks and benefits associated with the medical and surgical alternatives. Remember, there are many medical problems that cannot be totally cured even with the most aggressive and costly treatment. Sometimes receiving or asking for less medical treatment can give you just as good or better health results with lower risk of harmful complications.

Chapter 8

Keeping Your Own Medical Records

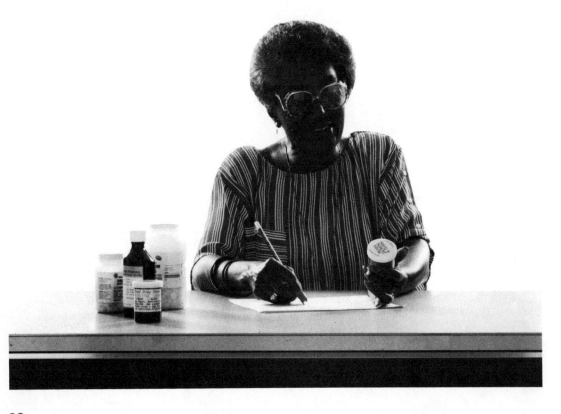

Doctors spend a great deal of time and care recording information in their patients' medical records. Physicians know that they cannot hope to give their patients top-notch health care without maintaining such records. Record keeping is essential for documenting important patient information such as past medical history and present treatment plans as well as future health maintenance considerations.

You can more intelligently manage your own health if you keep your own medical records. Keeping such records offers many pluses. You will be able, for example, to do the following:

- store critical information such as your blood type, any allergies, and emergency phone numbers you may have
- give yourself a picture of your past and present health
- help monitor your health status by keeping tabs on your prescribed medicines, laboratory test results, and any chronic problems
- improve communications between yourself and the health professionals whom you consult
- make your medical care more efficient and less costly

Starting your own medical records is not difficult. Just follow the steps given in this chapter and you will have a valuable tool that can help you for years to come.

You will need a notebook to store your medical records; a loose-leaf notebook works best. You should use something that is sturdy, since you will use it for many years. Use page dividers with tabs to separate each major section.

You will want to decide what you want in your medical records. In this chapter, you will find examples of forms that you can use "as is." Alternatively, you can use these forms as a guide to develop your own forms. Appendix C contains a complete set of blank medical record forms for your use.

Your medical records should be divided into four major sections:

1. Basic Facts
2. Current Information
3. Past Medical Care
4. Summary Information

A case example follows to illustrate how the forms in Appendix C can be completed. The subject is Jean Wilson, a sixty-eight-year-old retired office worker.

1. BASIC FACTS

Jean started her medical record using the basic facts sheet. (See figure 1.) It identifies Jean, shows where she lives, how she is insured, where she gets medical care, a few essential health facts such as allergies and blood type, and some emergency phone numbers.

Figure 1 shows Jean's basic facts sheet. She put her basic facts form at the front of her medical record notebook by taping it securely to the inside cover (see Appendix C, page 290, for a blank copy of the basic facts form). As you can see, Jean is married, has good medical supervision, has two allergies, and type O-positive blood.

Basic Facts

Name: Wilson   Jean   C.
    Last   First   Middle

Address: 125 Main Street   Anytown   IL   60600
    Street   City   State   Zip Code

Phone Number: 555-2131   **Social Security Number:** 000-00-000

Date of Birth: 3/15/18   **Place of Birth:** Placer, NH

Height: 5'2"   **Weight:** 118   **Marital Status:** married

Health Insurance: Medicare 000-00-000   3/1/83
       Identification Number   Effective Date

       Medicaid None
       Identification Number   Effective Date

       Other: GAP Insurance   Chicago, IL
       Company Name   Address

       000   00000   Jean Wilson
       Group Number   Certificate Number   Subscriber's Name

Main Doctor: Arthur Martin   General Practice
    Name   Specialty

    600 Spring Street   555-2345
    Address   Phone Number

Other Doctor: Francis O'Shea   Orthopedics
    Name   Specialty

    664 Spring Street   555-4321
    Address   Phone Number

Allergies: penicillin, shellfish

Drug Reactions: none except penicillin rash

Blood Type: O-Positive

Notify in Case of Emergency: James Wilson   husband
       Name   Relationship

       125 Main Street, Anytown   555-3131
       Address   Phone Number

Emergency Phone Numbers

Main Doctor:	555-1000	Police:	555-5000
Emergency Room:	555-2000	Fire:	555-6000
Hospital:	555-3000	Poison Control Center:	555-7000
Ambulance:	555-4000	Other:	

Figure 1

2. CURRENT INFORMATION

The second section of your medical records includes essential current health information: a chart for health problems, a chart for medications, and charts for chronic conditions and health maintenance.

Health Problems

Start off with a chart for health problems like the one shown in figure 2. (See Appendix C, page 291, for a blank copy of this chart.) This chart should include only significant health problems (1) that currently bother you, (2) for which you are under treatment, or (3) that have importance in health care (for example, allergic reactions in the past or surgical operations). Problems like high blood pressure, smoking, diabetes, arthritis, chronic anxiety, allergic reaction to penicillin, and appendix removal should be on the chart. Minor ailments or those that come and go quickly or that don't concern you or your doctor like colds, stomachaches, or periodic bouts of fatigue should not be included.

Figure 2 gives a sample of Jean's health problems. She has hypertension, had a cataract removed in 1981, and broke her right hip in 1984 when she tripped over her grandson's skateboard.

Health Problems *Jean Wilson*		
Problem	**Date Problem Started**	**Current Treatment**
High blood pressure	3/80	Inderal, 3 a day. Hydrodiuril, 1 a day
Allergic to penicillin	4/70	No more penicillin!
Cataract removed, right eye	11/10/81	Eye checkups
Right hip fractured	2/16/84	More calcium in diet
Arthritis in hands	1975	Ecotrin, 8 a day

Figure 2

Medications

The chart on medications is used to record the drugs that you currently take on a regular basis. (See Appendix C, pages 292–293, for a blank copy of the chart.) Include medicines prescribed by a doctor on the top half of the form and any medicines that you take on your own without a prescription (over-the-counter medications) on the bottom half. Figure 3 displays Jean's list of medications.

Medications (Medicines Prescribed by Doctor)   *Jean Wilson*

Name of Drug, Place Purchased, and Prescription Number	Reason for Taking Drug	Date Started Taking Drug	Date Stopped Taking Drug	
Inderal Jackson Drugs D 17-2880	*Blood pressure*	*3/80*	—	
Hydrodiuril Jackson Drugs D 17-2881	*Blood pressure*	*3/80*	—	

(Medicines Taken Without Prescription)   *Jean Wilson*

Name of Drug	Reason for Taking Drug	Date Started Taking Drug	Date Stopped Taking Drug	
Ecotrin	*Arthritis in hands*	*1975*	—	

Figure 3

It is very important to keep track of just what medications you take. This information should be kept on your medical chart. Use of medicines often changes quickly, *so your chart should be updated after each visit to a doctor.* It is also essential for any doctor you see to know what drugs, if any, you are taking that were prescribed by another physician. You can confirm name and dosage with your pharmacist if this information is not clear to you.

	Dosage and Schedule	Results or Side Effects	Cost of Drug
	1 tablet (40 mg) 3 times a day	Normal pressure	Don't know
	1 tablet (50 mg) each morning	Normal pressure	25¢ each tablet

	Dosage and Schedule	Results or Side Effects	Cost of Drug
	2 tablets 4 times a day	Ringing in ears	$5.60 for 60 tablets

At this point, you should throw away all drugs you are not using actively. There is neither economy nor safety in stockpiling old medicine.

Jean's medications are shown in figure 3. She is taking two prescribed medicines for her high blood pressure—Inderal and hydrochlorothiazide (Hydrodiuril)—plus coated aspirin for her minor arthritis.

Chronic Conditions

It is especially important to keep a medical record of any significant chronic condition that bothers you. Jean's hypertension is a chronic condition that requires frequent monitoring of her blood pressure to be sure her medications are appropriate. She bought a blood pressure kit at a drugstore so she can keep track of her blood pressure between visits to her doctor. When she goes for her annual physical exam, she takes her chart with her. The doctor is glad to have her provide this information. You can make up your own chart for any chronic problem. (See Appendix C, page 295, for a copy of a chart for this use.) Here's how to do it.

First, look at your chart of health problems and identify any ongoing chronic problems that are under treatment, for example, diabetes and hypertension. Second, set up charts—one for each problem.

Jean's blood pressure chart is shown in figure 4. (See Appendix C, page 294, for a blank copy of this chart.) The chart tracks her readings over a one-year period. It shows that her blood pressure was first measured on January 15, 1985,

when her level was 135/96 millimeters mercury (mm/Hg), and was last taken on December 10, 1985, when the level was down to 126/88.

You can use grid paper to make charts for other problems besides high blood pressure. For example, diabetes can be tracked with a chart that monitors the level of sugar in the blood (serum glucose level), and obesity can be followed by recording your weight on a chart.

Health Maintenance

Just as important as keeping tabs on your chronic problems is the use of charts to get an overview of how well you are doing at maintaining your overall health.

Doctors check many different aspects of your health when they take a complete history and perform a physical examination. In general, the doctor's health examination can be divided into four parts: (1) history, (2) physical examination, (3) laboratory tests, and (4) immunizations. Jean's health maintenance chart and the results of her last complete examination are shown in figure 5. (See Appendix C, pages 296–297, for a blank copy of the health maintenance chart.)

Figure 6 provides a set of recommendations for preventive health care. There is no one set of universally accepted guidelines for preventive care, but this gives you a reasonable framework to use.

The left-hand column lists the condition to be detected, the middle column indicates the recommended action, and the right-hand column tells you how frequently to repeat the procedure.

Blood Pressure and Weight	*Jean Wilson*			
Date	Systolic Blood Pressure	Diastolic Blood Pressure	Pulse	Weight
1/15/85	135	96	80	118
1/30	134	95	80	118
2/10	135	95	76	117
2/28	132	94	76	116
3/14	130	90	76	115
3/28	128	88	72	115
4/15	129	88	72	114
4/30	130	89	76	115
5/15	127	88	72	115
5/30	125	88	72	116
6/10	128	89	72	116
6/28	127	90	72	117
7/14	126	90	76	118
7/30	125	88	76	118
8/15	124	85	72	119
8/30	123	84	72	117
9/14	122	84	72	116
9/28	121	80	60	118
10/15	120	80	60	116
10/30	122	80	60	118
11/14	124	84	64	118
11/28	125	85	64	117
12/10	126	88	60	118

Figure 4

Health Maintenance   *Jean Wilson*

History Check (✓) appropriate column.	Yes	No	
Have you had major surgery in the last 5 years?	✓		
Have you had a weight problem in the last 5 years?		✓	
Do you take any prescription drugs?	✓		
Do you smoke?		✓	
Do you have any allergies?	✓		
Do you suffer from a chronic illness?	✓		
Does a member of your immediate family suffer from cancer, diabetes, chronic lung disease, or chronic heart disease?		✓	
Do you eat a balanced diet?	✓		
Do you exercise regularly?	✓		
Do you have regular dental checkups?	✓		
Do you give yourself a monthly breast self-examination (women)?	✓		
Have you had any serious health problems in the last 6 months? If so, list: _____ _____		✓	

Figure 5

Physical Examination Record Values in Shaded Box or Check (✓) If Normal	Date Checked 8/15	Date Checked 12/10			Laboratory Tests Record Values in Shaded Box or Check (✓) If Normal	Date Checked 12/10			
MEASURES					Cholesterol (circle if fasting)	210			
Height	62	62			Blood glucose (circle if fasting)	96			
Weight	119	118			Hemoglobin (Hgb) or Hematocrit (Hct)	40			
Blood pressure	124/85	126/88	/	/	Stool occult blood	✓			
Other _____					Mammography (women)	✓			
_____					Pap smear (women)	✓			
_____					EKG	✓			
_____					Other _____				
					_____				
					_____				
					_____				

SCREENING EXAMS					Immunizations Check (✓) If Done	Date 12/10			
Hearing		✓							
Breast (women)		✓			Tetanus				
Rectal		✓			Influenza	✓			
Vision		✓			Pneumococcal (high risk)				
Other _____					Other _____				
_____					_____				
_____					_____				
_____					_____				

Potential Health Condition	Action	Frequency of Action
Proneness to falls	Counseling based on review of total medical condition	Annually
Malnutrition or undernutrition	Counseling with nutritionist	Annually
	Height and weight measurement	Annually
Colonic cancer	Test of stool for occult blood	Annually
	Sigmoidoscopy	Every two years
Hearing defects	Screening	Every two years
Visual impairment	Screening	Every two years
Hypertension	Blood pressure determination	Every year, each visit
Breast cancer	Physician examination	Annually
	Counseling about self-examination	Annually and self-exam every month
	Mammography	Every two years
Cervical cancer	Pap smear	Every three years after two negatives
Anemia	Hematocrit/Hemoglobin test	Every two years
Syphilis	Blood test	Once in this age group
Tuberculosis	Skin test	Once in this age group
Diabetes	Blood test (glucose)	Every two years
Bacteriuria	Urinalysis	Every two years
Renal disease	Urinalysis and blood test (creatinine)	Every two years
Tetanus/Diphtheria	Immunization	Every ten years
Flu	Immunization	Annually
Pneumonia	Immunization	Once only
Dental caries and periodontal disease	Dental examination and cleaning	Annually
Poor-fitting dentures	Dental examination	Every two to three years or on complaint

Figure 6. Recommended Preventive Procedures for the Older Adult Years, Ages 60 to 74

3. PAST MEDICAL CARE

The three forms on the following pages—Hospital Stays, Medical Visits, and Health Providers—give you a way to keep track of your use of the health care system. (See Appendix C for blank copies of the forms.) On completing these forms, you will have a permanent record of whom you have seen, what you are supposed to be doing to maintain your health, and the cost of your care to date.

Hospital Stays

When you leave the hospital after an injury, operation, or illness, it is important for you to know your home care plan in order to speed your recovery. Filling out the information on the record of hospital stays will help ensure that you know clearly what needs to happen next. You will need to know the answers to questions like the following:

- *Medications.* What medicines do I take, and when?
- *Diet.* Are there any special instructions about what to eat or drink?
- *Services at Home.* After I go home, will I need any special services such as physical therapy, nursing, or housekeeping? Who will provide them?
- *Physician Follow-up.* When do I need to see my personal doctor again? Should I again see any of the doctors who helped care for me in the hospital?

Also, on occasion, you may need to recontact a hospital that you were in or get in touch with your main, or attending, physician. Keeping a record of hospital stays like the one Jean filled out after breaking her hip (see figure 7) will make it easy to do this. (See Appendix C, pages 298–299, for a blank copy of figure 7.)

Medical Visits

You may find it useful to keep track of your treatment by doctors, nurses, podiatrists, paramedics, or other health providers by using a medical visit form like the one shown in figure 8. (See Appendix C, pages 300–301, for a blank copy.) Before seeing the doctor or other medical person, you can fill in the first five columns. Then, after you leave, you can fill out the rest of the information, paying special attention to your treatment plan and follow-up. It is especially important to have a list of questions you want to ask your doctor or medical provider. Ten questions to ask yourself before seeing your doctor and ten questions you may want answered before you leave your

doctor's office are discussed in chapter 7, page 96. It is also a good idea to bring your own medical records to show the doctor what you are recording. For example, reviewing with your doctor any chronic problem chart that you have been keeping can be very useful.

A copy of Jean's most recent visit for her annual examination by Dr. Martin is shown in figure 8. Jean had been a little concerned about her frequency of urination and had questions about her heart getting more exercise, so she jotted these down in the fifth column, Questions to Ask Doctor or Other Health Professional, to help her remember to discuss these topics.

Health Providers

You may need to know what particular physician or health provider (dentist, optometrist, nurse, and so on) you saw at a certain time in the past or when traveling away from home. For example, your personal physician may wish to contact another doctor whom you saw while you were on a vacation or one who treated you in the past. A list of medical providers can come in handy. Following are the types of health providers whose visits you will want to record.

- audiologists
- counselors
- dentists
- dieticians
- learning specialists
- medical social workers
- mental health specialists
- nurses

Hospital Stays   *Jean Wilson*

Name, Address, and Phone Number of Hospital	Date Admitted	Date Discharged	Reason for Stay	
Mercy Hospital College Drive 555-6000	2/16/84	3/6/84	Hip fracture and operation	

Medications and Dosages Prescribed	Diet Instructions	Follow-up Services Needed at Home	
1. Aspirin, 2 tablets every 3 hours while awake	Regular with lots of fluids	Physical therapy, 2 times a week for 1 month	

- nurse practitioners
- optometrists
- paramedics

- physical therapists
- physicians
- physician assistants

	Name and Specialty of Main Doctor	Names and Specialties of Other Doctors	Major Tests and/or Treatment and/or Operation Performed
	F. J. O'Shea, orthopedics	*None*	*Pin placed in right hip*

	Physician Follow-up Appointments	Cost of Stay	Insurance Payment
	O'Shea — 3/20/85	*$7,820*	*$7,800*

- podiatrists
- psychiatrists
- psychologists

Jean's last visit to her physical therapist is detailed in figure 9. (See Appendix C, pages 302–303, for a blank copy of figure 9.)

Medical Visits	*Jean Wilson*			
Name, Address, and Phone Number of Doctor or Other Health Professional	Reason for Visit	Date and Time of Appointment	Specialty of Doctor or Other Health Professional	
Arthur Martin Mercy Hospital 555-1212	*1. Regular exam* *2. Frequent urination* *3. Heart problem?*	*12/10/85*	*General*	

Figure 8

Health Providers	*Jean Wilson*		
Type of Doctor or Other Health Professional	Name, Address, and Phone Number of Health Provider	Date of Visit	
Physical Therapist	*Marge Cannon, Physical Therapy Department Mercy Hospital 555-1212*	*12/7/85*	

Figure 9

4. SUMMARY INFORMATION

The final part of your own medical records can be used to keep background information on your health. It begins with a summary of your health "roots"— your family history—and goes on to register any illnesses, injuries, or surgeries you have already had as well as exposures to X rays or occupational hazards.

	Questions to Ask Doctor or Other Health Professional	Health Problem	Recommended Treatment Plan	Needed Follow-up	Cost of Visit	Insurance Payment
	Blood pressure level?	Yes	As before	Keep checking	$20	$18
	Infection?	No	Culture test	Call for results		
	Why skipping beats?	No	None	None		

	Reason for Visit		Health Provider's Recommendations	Cost of Visit	Insurance Payment
	Stiff fingers, some pain		More heat, more exercises	$13	$8

Family History

The value of your family history in assisting the doctor to make any specific diagnosis may decrease in importance as you age. It is still useful, however, to examine your family history to help spot diseases that can be prevented.

Figure 10 shows Jean's family history. (See Appendix C, pages 304–305, for a

Family History	*Jean Wilson*						
Blood Relatives	**If Deceased . . .**		**Selected Diseases and Conditions Linked to Family Background***				
	Year of Death	**Cause of Death**	**Alcoholism**	**Allergy**	**Cancer**	**Depression**	
Parents							
Mother	1970	*stroke*				✓	
Father	1962	?	✓				
Grandparents							
Dad Wilson	1910	?		DO NOT KNOW			
Mom Wilson	1921	?					
Uncles and Aunts							
Aunt Bea	1968	*stroke*		✓			
Uncle Bob	1975	*asthma*		✓			
Brothers and Sisters							
Frank				✓	✓	✓	
Anne				✓			
Children							
Bill				✓			
Susan							

*Check the box if any of your relatives had one of these medical problems.

Figure 10

blank copy of figure 10.) It shows that she may be at risk for stroke and that hypertension and allergies are common in her family. This knowledge has motivated Jean to do everything she can to control her blood pressure.

	Diabetes	Gout	Heart Disease	Hypertension	Mental Disorder	Stroke	Ulcers	Suicide	Other
	✓		✓	✓		✓			
			✓			✓			
			✓	✓	✓				
				✓					
				✓					

Major Illnesses, Injuries, and Surgeries

At times, you or your doctor may want to review quickly a list of the major illnesses, injuries, or surgeries you have had. This list should be recorded in chronological order. You need include only major health problems. Figure 11 illustrates Jean's history. (See Appendix C, pages 306–307, for a blank copy of figure 11.)

Major Illnesses, Injuries, and Surgeries	*Jean Wilson*		
Illness, Injury, or Surgery	Age at Occurrence	Place of Treatment	
High blood pressure	63	Home	
Right hip fracture	67	Mercy Hospital	
Cataract operation	63	Eye clinic	

Figure 11

Exposures to X Rays or Occupational Hazards	*Jean Wilson*		
X-Ray Exposure or Hazard	Place of Exposure	Age at Exposure	Treatment Received
Beryllium dust	Boston, MIT lab	27	None

Figure 12

Exposure to X Rays or Occupational Hazards

Your health can be threatened if you are exposed to certain human-made hazards. For example, exposure to X rays for medical diagnosis or treatment is generally not considered hazardous if the total amount of X-ray exposure is kept below certain levels. Likewise, exposure to certain chemicals or compounds used in the workplace or in pursuing hobbies may or may not represent a health risk depending on the substance, the amount of contact, and the frequency of contact. Other common hazards include exposure

	Major Complications	Long-Term Impact on Health	Comments
	None	Must always take medications	Monitor blood pressure regularly
	None	Some ache in hip	Take calcium supplements and exercise
	None	None	Need regular eye checkups

	Place of Treatment	Long-Term Impact on Health	Comments
	—	None known	Worked in research on new light bulbs — some friends had lung trouble

to dusts; exposure to high noise levels, such as noises produced from heavy machinery for extended periods of time; or repeated exposure to loud, short blasts of noise such as rifle fire.

You may not know whether you have been previously exposed to these hazards linked to your medical care, work, or hobbies. If you have been exposed, how-ever, and if you know this is the case, you can fill in an exposures form. Jean's completed exposures form is shown in figure 12. (See Appendix C, pages 308–309, for a blank copy of figure 12.)

The items in the chart that follows may be hazardous to your health if you are exposed to them above the levels thought to be safe.

Dusts	Gases	Metals	Physical Agents	Radiation	Other Agents
animal asbestos coal cotton fiber metal mica silica talc vegetable	alcohols/ ethers/esters aldehydes amines aniline benzene carbon monoxide chlorine cyanides fluorine halogenated hydrocarbons hydrogen sulfide organic solvents petroleum products sulfur dioxide	antimony arsenic beryllium cadmium chromium lead manganese phosphorus selenium	air pollution cold heat high humidity noise temperature change vibrating tools	infrared rays radioactive substances ultraviolet rays X rays	acids alkaline compounds cola tar dermatitis producers dyes hides inks lacquer/ varnish oils/fats/ waxes paints/ enamels salts sulfur

Figure 13. Common Environmental Health Hazards

If you keep your own medical records, you will be more informed and more able to be actively involved in your health care. You can use the ideas in this chapter—and the blank forms in Appendix C—to get started. If you want to keep a very close accounting of your health, use all the appropriate medical records forms in Appendix C. If you are not interested in so much detail, use selected parts of the medical records.

Most everyone will benefit by keeping at least these three critical forms up to date: Basic Facts, Health Problems, and Medications.

Chapter 9

Medications: What You Need to Know

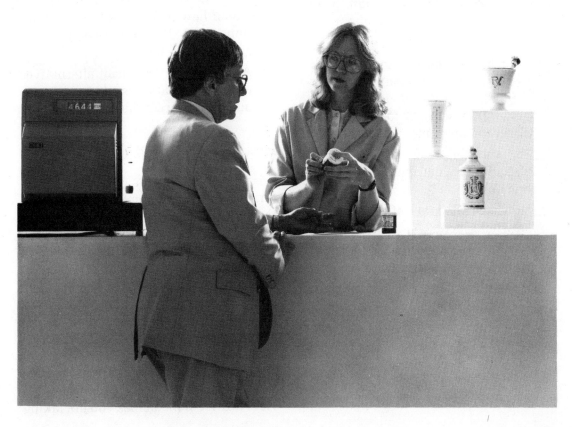

Your body is its own healer—it does take care of itself. In fact, a majority of the illnesses experienced in a lifetime either clear up spontaneously or persist in a chronic, nondisabling form. Therefore, drugs, which are foreign substances that affect the body, should always be given and taken with great conservatism and caution. You and your doctor must always weigh the cost-benefit balance of taking a drug. A prudent course to follow is to take as few drugs as possible, rely on diet and other modes of therapy as much as possible, and be alert to the possible effects of overdosage, underdosage, allergic reactions, and cross-reactions when taking drugs.

The following are important questions you should ask your physician, health professional, or pharmacist about each medication prescribed for you:

1. What is the name of the drug written on the prescription? Is the trade (brand) name listed or the generic name? (See page 123 for a discussion of generic medicines.)

2. For what condition is the medication prescribed? What should the medication do?

3. How much do I take of this drug, and on what schedule?

4. Should I get up in the middle of the night to take my medication?

5. How do I take it? On an empty stomach? With juice, food, or milk?

6. How much liquid should be taken with this medication?

7. What should I do if I miss a dose?

8. For how long do I take this medication? Should I take all of it, or should I stop taking it when the symptoms are gone?

9. Can I have alcoholic drinks while on this medication?

10. Will I be more susceptible to sunburn while on this medication?

11. Are there any precautions I should take?

12. What are the major side effects of this drug? What should I do if I notice any side effects?

13. Should I have any written information about this drug?

14. Can I take other necessary medicines with the new medication without complications? Can I continue to take the nonprescription drugs I use?

15. About how much does this prescription cost? Do you recommend a generic equivalent?

16. Are there any treatment alternatives to this medication, such as a change in diet or exercise habits?

GENERAL CAUTIONS

It is important that you receive, in legible writing from your doctor, the name of the prescribed drug and the directions as to how and when to take the medication. If you are obtaining medicines from more than one doctor, it is crucial that you tell each doctor exactly what medications you are currently taking. Whenever possible, bring *all* medications to the physician for his or her examination.

Discard any outdated drugs to avoid ineffective actions, adverse reactions, or excessive drug effects. In addition, review the list of medicines you are taking with your doctor at every visit. Be sure to tell your doctor about any past drug reactions.

Clinically it is very difficult to determine the amount of medicine needed by each patient to achieve a desired therapeutic effect. A doctor's prescription is based on the patient's weight, the patient's age, other medicines the patient is taking, the illness, and the overall physical condition of the person. Even with this careful determination of the correct medication and dosage, the doctor needs accurate reports from you on how the medicine is working for you. If you are not responding to the medicine as expected or if side effects develop, your doctor needs to know this so he or she can change the prescription. You need to report whether you were able to take the medicine as directed and the response you had to the medicine. You also need to tell the doctor whether the benefits from the medication were what the doctor told you to expect. Your physician needs this information to make a decision as to whether the medicine should be increased, decreased, or discontinued.

If you missed taking the medicine one or more times, it is very important that you tell your doctor. If necessary, he or she can help you establish procedures for taking your medicine that will reduce the likelihood that you will forget. Although it is essential that you take your medicine as prescribed, you should not try to make up for a missed dose by taking twice the amount the next time. The larger dose could be dangerous.

In addition, someone—a member of your family or a person with whom you share personal information—should know what medications you are taking and what potential reactions or side effects the doctor has described. These reactions may include changes in the level of your activity (more or less), physical functions (walking, eating, and so on), and/or mental behavior, including sleep. This person should know about the possible drug reactions so he or she can discuss his or her observations with you and, if necessary, report possible undesirable reactions to the doctor.

If you require assistance in using a particular medication, such as an injectable substance (for example, insulin) or eye drops (for example, timolol for glaucoma), the person who will help you should be instructed in the proper technique by the doctor or the office nurse. If this is not possible, the doctor can arrange for a visiting nurse to come to your home to help you take the medication or to instruct someone in your home in the proper technique.

Many drugs interact with other drugs, whether prescription or over-the-counter. They can also interact with foods and with alcohol. When you are taking prescription medicines, tell your doctor about any over-the-counter medicines you may be taking (for example, sleeping aids, cold remedies, diet pills, and/or laxatives) and about any alcoholic beverages (beer, wine, liquor) that you may be drinking.

If you fail to advise your physician about *all* your current medications, it is likely you will not receive the benefits from the therapy your doctor is prescribing. In some circumstances, the combination of medicines may be injurious to you. For example, the person taking anticoagulants (blood thinners) can experience serious bleeding if aspirin is also taken.

Finally, ask your doctor whether you should drive when you are taking a new medicine. Some medicines may make you drowsy, weak, and/or confused. These conditions interfere with safe driving.

INTERACTIONS OF DRUGS WITH FOOD

Older adults are at special risk from the effects of drugs on their nutritional status. First, older persons often receive several prescribed drugs concurrently and may add to this number several self-prescribed, nonprescription drugs. One study reported that at eighty years of age, the average number of drugs used was five. Second, older persons are often on special restricted diets, and their nutritional status may also be impaired by chronic disease. Drug effects may further alter nutritional status. Thus, it is especially important that older adults, in particular those with chronic conditions, discuss the problem of medications with their physicians.

Many different families of drugs are known to be capable of altering a person's nutritional status. In particular are the drugs commonly used in the treatment of chronic or long-term conditions. For example, the drug Digoxin (a heart stimulant) can suppress appetite; aspirin and other antirheumatic drugs can cause irritation of the stomach to produce nausea and vomiting; mineral oil laxatives can block absorption of vitamin D; and antidepressant medications can increase the appetite and lead to obesity.

Those drugs that have an effect on nutritional status require close monitoring by the physician. To maintain your nutritional health while you are taking such medicines, you should alter your food intake as instructed by the doctor. You also may be advised to take vitamin and/or mineral supplements.

INTERACTIONS OF DRUGS WITH OTHER DRUGS

The number of possibilities of drug interactions is great; however, three major types of drug interactions point up the importance of your doctor's being aware of all the medicines you take, both prescription and nonprescription.

First, the desired effect of one drug may be altered by another compound. For example, the use of alcohol when you are on an antidepressant, such as Elavil, can make you more heavily sedated. Or if you are asthmatic and you take propranolol for hypertension, you may have an attack of asthma because propranolol overrides the effect of a bronchodilator like aminophylline.

Second, one drug may change the way your body can use another drug. For example, antacids (Rolaids, Gelusil, and so on) alter your gastric (digestive) secretions, thus interfering with the absorption of aspirin and certain anticoagulants that are used to prevent blood clotting in cardiovascular patients. Antacids or milk products can bind the antibiotic tetracycline and prevent it from fighting infections effectively.

Third, drugs like cortisone may interfere with your body's ability to fight off infections, thus increasing the need for stronger antibiotics.

Any one of these three types of drug interactions is very serious. Once again, it is essential that you discuss the potential of your experiencing one of these problems with your doctor when you review all the medications you are taking. You should also ask your pharmacist to go over your list of medications and alert you to any potential problems.

ORGANIZING A SYSTEM FOR TAKING MEDICINES

A copy of the medications chart discussed in chapter 8 (pages 102–103) should be filled out and kept updated. Always show it to any physician who intends to prescribe a drug for you. This medication record can help your doctors prescribe drugs that are compatible, effective, and safe.

Using a medication chart can help assure that you take each medicine as directed by the physician. In addition, you may choose to make a daily calendar, where you can check off the medicine when you take it. You also can develop a code (a color or a symbol) you put on the medicine container and on your medication chart. This code can help you quickly match the correct medicine in the bottle and the instructions for taking it on the chart.

A final word of caution. *Never* mix pills in a bottle. This can add to confusion in taking and reordering medication.

GENERIC MEDICINES

Generic medicines are drugs of specific chemical structure that are equivalent in efficacy and safety to brand-name drugs. A brand name is a name given by a company for marketing purposes. A brand-name drug is usually higher priced than the generic drug. In many instances, a generic can be used in place of a brand-name medicine. By law, generic medicines contain the same chemical compounds used in the brand name (for example, acetaminophen is generic for Tylenol). The generic drug may be a different shape, size, or color than the brand-name drug. Ask your physician if he or she recommends the generic equivalent of the drug being prescribed for you and, if so, where you can purchase the generic drug. You can also discuss this drug choice with your pharmacist. Many states require pharmacies to provide generically equivalent drugs for Medicare or Medicaid recipients unless directed otherwise by the physician.

SAFETY PRECAUTIONS

Proper use of your medications is essential if you are to succeed in managing your particular health condition. In addition, intelligent use of medicines can help you control your health costs. To help you manage medication for safety and effectiveness, you need to be aware of shelf life for medications, proper storage, and safe disposal.

Shelf Life

The shelf life of a medication is the length of time the medicine retains its desired chemical properties in the form and amount it was originally prepared. The shelf life of medicines varies widely: antacids can be good for years, while antibiotics may lose their effectiveness in months. The Food and Drug Administration's requirement for effective shelf life for medications is generally two to three years. Do not keep or use old medications. When a medicine changes with age, it can become either dangerous or ineffective.

Storage

Refrigerate medications only if you are told to do so by your doctor or if the label on the container indicates that the medication should be refrigerated. Liquid medication, when not properly stored, can become thick, so the amount measured is inaccurate for the dose. Sometimes the cold air of the refrigerator causes moisture to condense on the inside of the container and thus affect your medication. The hot, humid air of the bathroom may make it a poor place to store medications. A dry, cool cupboard, perhaps near the kitchen sink, is a good location for the storage of medications.

Do not transfer medications from their original containers. These containers are specially designed to maintain the quality of medicine. Do not store medications in direct sunlight or near heat.

Disposal

You should throw away drugs when your doctor tells you to discontinue their use. When you dispose of the drugs, use the toilet, sink, or garbage disposal. *Never* put drugs in a place where children or animals can get to them and be poisoned. Also, destroy the labels so the prescriptions cannot be refilled.

The benefits of modern medicine in effecting cures and in reducing or eliminating uncomfortable and annoying disease-related symptoms can be lost by careless or ignorant behavior. Follow these ten safety precautions to avoid such problems and to obtain the desired drug benefits.

1. Keep an up-to-date list of all the medications you are presently taking. Show the list to all physicians you visit; this information is needed before another drug is prescribed for you.

2. Make certain you understand when each of your medications should be taken; timing can determine the success or failure of certain medicines.

3. If you skipped a dose of your medication, don't try to catch up by doubling the next dose on your own.

4. Don't stop taking your medicine when you start feeling better; this may cause a relapse or flare-up of the original problem (for example, not taking all the medicine for a urinary tract infection increases the likelihood of a recurrence).

5. Never exchange prescription medications with a spouse, relative, or friend, no matter how similar your illnesses.

6. Don't transfer a drug from its original bottle to another container.

7. A number of medications (for example, muscle relaxants) may cause dizziness or temporary drowsiness; be particularly careful when driving a car or operating any dangerous machinery if you are taking such medication.

8. Don't drink alcohol when on medication unless your doctor specifically says that it is safe to do so.

9. Keep the name and number of your druggist and closest poison control center near your phone.

10. Discard old, outdated, or unused medications.

TREATMENT ALTERNATIVES TO MEDICATIONS

Sometimes there are alternatives to taking medicines. Oftentimes a change in daily habits can improve the condition for which a person is taking medications. For example, if someone is a borderline diabetic or hypertensive, a change in his or her eating habits, weight, or exercise pattern may make the critical difference in the need for potent medications. Check with your doctor to see if there are any alternatives to medication, especially if you make lifestyle changes. These can include reducing your weight, decreasing your alcohol consumption, cutting down on your smoking, and increasing the amount of exercise you get.

Chapter 10

Community Resources

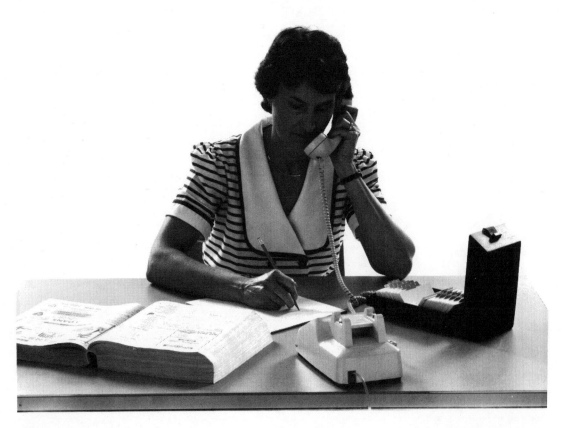

Communities will vary in the types, amount, and quality of services offered to the older adult. Available community resources can cover a wide range of services including telephone "hot" lines, friendly visitor programs, counseling, employment opportunities, equipment, escort service, transportation, respite care, hospice care, nutrition, home health care, mental health, housing, heating, homemaking, education, financial assistance, rehabilitation, foster grandparents, and legal assistance. Often these services are not utilized effectively because of lack of knowledge of their existence, misinterpretation of the eligibility requirements, pride or desire to resolve problems on one's own, or misconceptions that resources available to older persons are restricted to the indigent or underprivileged.

You can prepare for your future needs by exploring these resources before a problem arises. You may not have the time or energy to do this type of fact-finding when you are ill or in need of services. Intelligent use of the broad range of community resources can increase your ability to achieve and maintain functional health and contribute to containment of health care costs. When you identify gaps in services in your community, you can become an advocate for securing additional community resources and/or can become a volunteer to assist others in managing their health. You can help achieve the goal of independent living and an active and enjoyable life for older persons in your community.

GENERALLY AVAILABLE PROGRAMS AND SERVICES

Following is a description of the programs and services most widely available in all communities to the older adult with special needs. You might also review these resources for the possibility of your own contribution as a volunteer.

- *Area Agency on Aging* or *Council on Aging* is the local unit designated by the state Office on Aging. The unit is supported primarily by Older American Act federal funds and is used to redistribute these federal funds. Area agencies provide no direct service but subcontract for many services such as transportation and legal aid. They are required to maintain an information and referral service. They may be part of city or county government or a private nonprofit agency.

- *Senior centers* provide a variety of services (such as meals and educational programs), and their staffs will know what other services are available in the community.

- *City* or *County Public Health Departments* have information about health care services in the community.

- *Cooperative Extension Services* have county-level units with statewide staff supports located at state universities. The programs are developed in cooperation with the U.S. Department of Agriculture. The staffs provide a wide variety of informal educational programs on health, nutrition, economics, and so on, for urban and rural groups of all ages. The staffs also keep up to date on what community resources are available.

- **American Association of Retired Persons** local chapters maintain information about community programs. They have many publications about a full range of topics of concern to older persons. More than 26,000 volunteers take an active role in promoting a variety of services and educational programs, including Health Advocacy, Tax Aide, Widowed Persons Service, and Citizen Representation. Persons fifty and older may join AARP.

- **American Red Cross** local chapters, listed in your telephone directory, often provide a variety of services for older people such as friendly visiting and transportation. In addition, many chapters offer courses of interest to older people on such topics as nutrition, high blood pressure, family health, and home care and offer swimming programs for people with disabilities. First Aid and cardiopulmonary resuscitation (CPR) are also taught by their experts.

- **Voluntary health organizations** are listed in your telephone directory. The American Heart Association, the American Cancer Society, the American Lung Association, and the Arthritis Foundation have local chapters with educational materials and programs directed toward health problems of older persons.

- **Self-help groups.** There are nearly 150 major self-help organizations throughout the country. These organizations are formed by people who want to help themselves and one another share successful ways of coping with problems, provide support, and seek solutions to common problems and concerns. Among these self-help organizations are Alcoholics Anonymous, the American Diabetes Association, the Arthritis Foundation, Alzheimer's Disease and Related Disorders Association, the Epilepsy Foundation, the International Association of Laryngectomees, the Muscular Dystrophy Association, Stroke Clubs, and the United Ostomy Association.

To determine whether there is a self-help group in your community that you can join for support in managing a health problem, ask your Area Agency on Aging which ones are listed in their *Information and Referral Guide.* The social service department in your hospital will most likely know the self-help groups available in your community. If there is not one for your particular problem, the social service staff person may know of other persons interested in joining with you to start a self-help group.

RESOURCES TO MEET SPECIFIC NEEDS

Emergencies

- Emergency telephone numbers for the fire department, police department, poison control center, and, sometimes, ambulance services for medical emergencies are listed on the front inside cover of the telephone book. It is important that you post these numbers, as well as your physician's emergency number, by your telephone.

Transportation

- Transportation services have been developed in many communities to serve the needs of older and disabled persons who are unable to transport themselves. The arrangements include Red Cross volunteers serving as drivers, some special arrangements with bus and/or taxi companies, and specially equipped vans. The transportation service can provide rides to nutrition sites, health facilities, and shopping centers and can be used for outings. Information about the availability of transportation in your community can be obtained from the information and referral service of your Area Agency on Aging and your local American Red Cross chapter.

Meals

Several different types of meal programs have been designed for persons who have difficulty preparing meals.

- *Homemaker and home health care agencies* provide personal and homemaking services, which may include meal preparation and shopping.
- *Meals on Wheels* sponsors free delivery of hot meals (usually one per day, along with a cold meal) to those who are homebound. Red Cross volunteers, as well as volunteers from numerous other organizations, participate in the delivery of these meals. Some programs have age or income guidelines for eligibility; others do not.
- *Congregate dining programs* staff and operate nutritional centers that provide group meals.

- *Private catering services* are designed for those less restricted by financial considerations. Many private catering companies are listed in the Yellow Pages of the telephone directory. Special diets are available through some.

Health Care Equipment

Many commercial businesses rent or sell all types of health care equipment. These are listed in the telephone Yellow Pages under Hospital Equipment & Supplies. Local libraries may be able to provide more of this type of information.

Depending on the degree of disability and the outlook for recovery, equipment may be borrowed, rented, or purchased. Purchases of expensive devices should be delayed until there is a clear picture of what the need for equipment will be and perhaps until several types of borrowed or rented equipment have been tried.

Since your physician, a physical therapist, and/or an occupational therapist are the professionals best able to judge the type of equipment to be used, you should ask them for specific recommendations.

Home Health Services

Home health services typically include the professional skills of nurses (both registered nurses and licensed practical nurses), physical therapists, medical social workers, occupational therapists, and speech therapists. The nonprofessional home health services are usually provided by home health aides and homemakers.

A home health aide performs only the personal care activities included in a written assignment by a health professional. Tasks may include assisting the patient with personal hygiene, shaving, dressing, eating, and ambulation. A *homemaker* is responsible for duties such as preparation of meals, laundry, and shopping. These services are offered in several states by home health agencies, county social service agencies, and by some private nonprofit agencies.

The community organizations providing health-related care in a client's home are home health agencies and visiting nurse associations. Licensed home health agencies and visiting nurse associations are required to have a written plan of treatment established by the attending physician before a patient is accepted to receive health services. The agency must be capable of meeting the patient's specific needs in his or her home before the agency can accept the patient as a client.

A decision to terminate services should be made jointly by the client, the client's physician, and the agency. Before termination, a plan for referral or any necessary continuing care must be made.

Economic access to home health services must be a consideration. The vast majority of licensed agencies are almost totally dependent upon Medicare to pay for the services they provide.

Care from personnel of home health agencies and visiting nurse associations should be available at least eight hours a day, five days a week, and should be available on a need basis twenty-four hours a day, seven days a week.

Adult Day Programs

Adult day programs are often located at community centers, senior centers, churches and synagogues, and hospitals and clinics. Participation in an adult day program requires a support structure at home or the participants' ability to take care of themselves in the evening. Persons living alone, with family members, or in a congregate housing facility might take part in adult day programs.

These services are available to the frail elderly and, in some cases, the disabled adult. Trained supervision and rehabilitation programs are available for those who do not need the type or degree of care offered by nursing homes or home health agencies.

Many adult day programs provide transportation, social services, counseling, hot lunches, and recreation. A few offer medical screening services. Rehabilitation programs are also available in some centers. Persons with severe medical problems, those who are grossly incontinent, or those who wander cannot be cared for in most programs.

Major advantages of this type of program are the social and psychological benefits for people who would otherwise be isolated in the community or be placed in an institution for lack of necessary care. Structure, companionship, meals, and the availability of professional assistance allow people who need a protective environment to remain in the community.

Health Insurance

Some health care costs can be covered, at least in part, by health insurance. Most persons who are employed have coverage in a group plan with their employer. Others may carry private insurance. Those who are retired, however, generally have Medicare as their primary carrier. (See the white pages of your telephone book for the number to call for Medicare information, or call your local Social Security Administration office.)

Medicare

The Health Care Financing Administration (HCFA) administers the federally funded Medicare insurance program for persons who have reached age sixty-five and for some disabled persons under sixty-five. This insurance covers some, but not all, costs of hospitalization and physician care.

Medicare coverage of health care costs has many gaps that can add up to large out-of-pocket expenses. To overcome these gaps, you need to buy additional health insurance to assure more complete coverage of your potential health costs. Your local Social Security office has a publication, Your Medicare Handbook, which describes what portion of your health care bills Medicare will pay and what amount you must pay. Your payment covers deductibles, copayments (amount you pay as part of Medicare benefits), and the special restrictions and exclusions of services for which you must pay because they are not covered by Medicare.

Medicare consists of two parts: *Part A* is the Hospital Insurance (HI) that is financed through Social Security taxes; *Part B* is Supplementary Medical Insurance (SMI). It is financed through monthly premiums paid by Medicare recipients and federal government subsidies. These monthly premiums can be deducted from your Social Security checks. You pay a penalty for late enrollment in Part B. A 10 percent increase in premiums is added for each twelve-month period you delay enrolling after you are eligible for Medicare.

Eligibility. Anyone who has reached age sixty-five and is eligible for Social Security or railroad retirement benefits, has been entitled to Social Security disability checks for two years, or has end-stage renal disease is entitled to Hospital Insurance (Part A of Medicare). In addition, federal workers may now qualify for Medicare depending on the starting date of their employment and the length of that employment. Even if you continue to work, you are eligible, and you should file an application to enroll in Medicare at any Social Security office two to three months prior to your sixty-fifth birthday. You do not have to pay a monthly premium for Part A coverage, but you do pay Part B monthly premiums (in 1985 this was $15.50). Your spouse will be eligible for Medicare coverage at age sixty-five and must also file an application. A person who is not eligible for Social Security benefits can enroll in Medicare by paying the monthly premiums for both Part A and Part B.

Part A Coverage. The hospital and skilled nursing home care covered under Part A and the "deductible" (what you have to pay before Medicare begins to pay) have changed many times since the passage of the original Medicare legislation. It is very important that you keep yourself up to date on the changes that occur each year.

Part B Coverage. Your Supplementary Medical Insurance (SMI) has a deductible (it was the first seventy-five dollars in 1985). After the deductible is met, the SMI will pay only 80 percent of "reasonable" charges set by Medicare for physicians' services. The physician can agree to accept the amount defined as reasonable (that is, "accept assignment"), and you will pay the remaining 20 percent. If your doctor does not accept assignment, you must pay, in addition to the 20 percent coinsurance, the balance of the doctor's charges. Part B medical insurance also includes partial payment for emergency room and clinical outpatient services. Some of the services covered are doctors' fees; diagnostic tests; radiology and pathology; dental surgery; physical and speech therapies; prosthetic devices; medical supplies; and home health services. Laboratory services, medically necessary ambulance transportation, and such durable medical equipment as wheelchairs may also be covered, at least in part, by Medicare Part B.

Obtain Added Protection

In addition to paying your premium for Part B coverage of Medicare, you should obtain additional health insurance to cover Medicare gaps in coverage—the deductible and coinsurance charges. A good Medicare supplement insurance policy will pay the Part A hospital deductible; coinsurance charges for hospital and skilled nursing home stays; costs of one year of additional days in the hospital beyond those covered by Medicare for any one hospitalization, and the 20 percent coinsurance portion

of the Medicare-defined "reasonable" medical charges.

The health insurance policies that are sold include a variety of types of coverage: limited coverage (for example, fixed dollar amounts for hospitalization and/or skilled nursing home care), specified disease coverage (for example, cancer or heart disease), major medical coverage (for large expenditures, as much as $250,000 to $1,000,000 for a broad range of hospital and medical services), and comprehensive coverage. The latter combines features of both basic and major medical coverage; this is often not available after age sixty-five.

You are fortunate if your retirement insurance coverage is a continuation of your employer's group health insurance plan. In this instance, these rates are usually lower than individual rates, and the benefits in a group plan are likely to be more comprehensive than those provided by an individual program. If you need to buy individual health insurance, you should consider the following:

- Compare the costs, coverage, and benefits of several different policies. Your state insurance office may have information about individual health insurance policies available in your state.

- If you are not yet sixty-five, check the policy carefully for what changes occur when you reach sixty-five and how well the policy covers Medicare gaps. Avoid paying for duplicate coverage. When a health insurance plan has "coordination of benefits" clauses, this means the company will exclude payments for expenses that are paid by other health insurance coverage.

■ Check the length of time you must wait for the coverage to start for pre-existing health conditions (any sickness or injury for which you received medical advice or treatment). This should be six months or less from the time you purchase the insurance.

■ Select a policy that is "guaranteed" or "conditionally" renewable. The latter term means that the insurer agrees to continue to insure you as long as it continues to insure other persons in your state and you pay your premiums.

■ Ask what the insurance company's loss ratio is. This is the ratio between the income from premiums for the policy and the amount paid out in benefits. The federal government recommends that Medicare supplement policies sold to individuals have a minimum loss ratio of at least 60 percent.

■ You should always have at least ten days to review a policy. It should always have a clearly worded outline of the coverage provided.

■ Obtain the current list of services covered and the benefits provided by Medicare Hospital Insurance (Part A). Make a chart with a column that shows what Medicare pays for each benefit and, in a parallel column, list what the proposed insurance will pay. In this way, you can identify duplication and/or gaps in coverage.

■ Health Maintenance Organizations (HMOs) provide a wide range of health services for a flat fee paid in advance. Check to see if there is an HMO in your community that accepts Medicare payments. Does it provide the health services you need? The American Association of Retired Persons has a booklet, *More Health for Your Dollar: An Older Person's Guide to HMOs*, that offers information about how HMOs work in connection with Medicare and discusses the advantages and disadvantages of joining an HMO.

State and/or County Medicaid

You can obtain information about your state's participation in the Medicaid program by telephoning your city or county health and/or welfare department.

Medicaid is a federally, state-, and, in some states, county-funded program that helps low-income persons pay for their medical care. Each state has its own criteria for eligibility in Medicaid programs. Those who are disabled or already receiving welfare assistance may also qualify for Medicaid. Supplementary Security Income recipients, as well as persons who qualify under the low-income guidelines and are receiving Medicare, may also qualify for Medicaid. Services covered by Medicaid vary from state to state and may include inpatient and outpatient medical services, laboratory and X-ray services, physician services, transportation to obtain medical services, dental care, dentures, eyeglasses, hearing aids, care in a skilled or intermediate nursing home facility that is certified to accept participants in the Medicaid program, and medicines.

If medically necessary, home health care services are available to Medicaid recipients of any age in their own homes (this cannot be a hospital or nursing home). Nursing services by a registered nurse or a licensed practical nurse or personal care by a home health aide are covered. Services must be provided by a licensed agency participating in the Medicaid program. The Medicaid program, not the client, is billed for covered services and items provided.

All items and services provided to an eligible Medicaid recipient must be prescribed by the attending physician. Any supply, appliance, or equipment prescribed as a convenience item, as opposed to one that is "medically necessary," is not covered.

People who receive Medicare are eligible to have Medicaid pay the monthly premium of Part B of Medicare, part of the coinsurance and deductible for Medicare Part B, and the deductible for Part A of Medicare.

USING THE FORMAL NETWORK

Most persons have people to turn to in times of distress: a spouse, family, friends, neighbors, clergy. These people are called an "informal network" of helpers, and most people's needs are met through this informal network. However, when problems become too complicated for the informal network, it becomes necessary to approach professionals who have the knowledge and skills to help. Once a person goes to a professional—be it a doctor, lawyer, or social service worker—he or she is then using the "formal network" to help with his or her needs.

Oftentimes people are nervous about approaching agencies or the formal network because they don't know what to expect from them. The following steps need to be taken in working with the formal network.

Step One: Identify Your Need

First, you must identify your need and decide whether you wish to seek assistance. Such assistance can vary from seeking more information to arranging for a particular service.

Step Two: Locate the Appropriate Resources

Most people begin looking for support resources by asking for suggestions and names of contact persons from their informal network. A formal way to locate resources is to look in the telephone directory for a listing of the local community services and their telephone numbers.

In addition, many communities have a local resource directory distributed by the chamber of commerce, the United Way, the state or local Office of Elder Affairs, the Area Agency on Aging, the Council for Aging, or the community services or public relations department of an area hospital. Another good contact is your local librarian, who can assist you in locating appropriate resources.

Step Three: Contact the Resource

Visit or phone the resource to obtain information about its services and programs. Learn about the geographic areas served, the program eligibility, any waiting period to acquire service, the days and hours when services are provided, sponsorship (government or private, profit or nonprofit), the costs, the acceptance of third-party payments, and the availability of translators for non-English-speaking clients, if applicable to your situation. If this resource appears to be an appropriate one for you, you will need to discuss with a staff member the steps required to arrange for services.

A community resource may request these common documents in order to establish service eligibility.

- birth certificate, driver's license, or passport as proof of birth date
- Social Security card
- record of Social Security payments to establish income
- savings account passbooks and proof of ownership of other personal assets, including real estate
- health insurance cards such as those for Medicare, Medicaid, Blue Cross/ Blue Shield, and AARP Group Health Insurance

Step Four: Arrange for Services

Make an appointment with a staff member of the resource. Keep a record of date and time so you will be prepared for the visit, whether the arrangement is to meet at the agency or in your home. Call if you must cancel for any reason. In addition to having the necessary documents ready for the appointment, you may need to make arrangements for transportation and/or for a support person to be with you. Your goal is to make this person-to-person encounter productive and efficient. The initial meeting between you

and the staff member of the resource should lead to the development of a service plan. This plan should specify the services to be provided, the place they will be provided, cost of the services, and the conditions for service termination. Your active participation in developing this plan ensures that your real concerns and needs will be addressed. This input also helps the program personnel understand better you and your situation; together you then can explore alternatives for finding the service or program that best suits you. Since most agencies work closely with others in the community, one worker may suggest still other resources to explore. Your plan, for example, with a home health agency for an ill spouse may include arrangements for skilled nursing care, physical therapy, occupational therapy, and homemaker services.

Step Five: Monitor the Service

These supporting services and programs are meant to serve you, so be sure of your rights and responsibilities as a consumer. Once you are receiving services, you are entitled to see any part of the file being kept on you. If you wish to have a different agency person help you, or if you are dissatisfied with the service as delivered, you can appeal to a higher level person in the agency. Silence and frustration are not helpful to you, the agency, or other clients.

If you have difficulty following the recommended actions decided on in your original service plan, you should discuss this with the agency representative so other arrangements can be made.

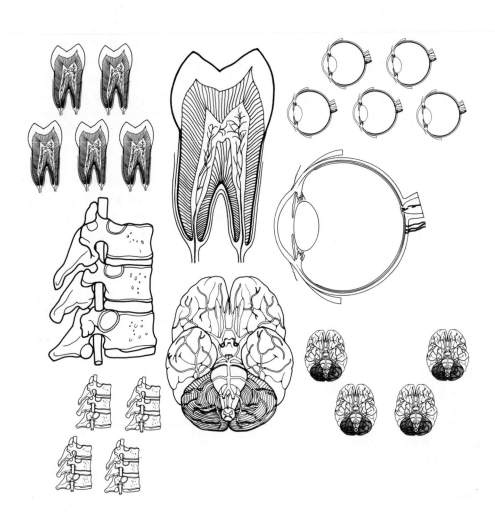

PART THREE

COMMON HEALTH PROBLEMS AND SELF-CARE TECHNIQUES

General Health Problems

■■ DEPRESSION

Everyone has felt depressed—that is, felt sad, mournful, or low as a result of a particular loss or disappointment, such as the death of a loved one or being passed up for a job promotion. This temporary feeling state or passing mood was appropriate to the situation. The reaction was neither wildly excessive nor prolonged enough to interrupt the other aspects of life.

Depression, in the medical sense, refers not to a mood or reaction but to a disease or condition that is distinctly abnormal. This medical disorder, the most common major emotional or psychological illness of adults, involves persistent abnormalities of mood or feeling, disturbances of bodily functions, and difficulties in thinking and other intellectual functions.

The basic, often overwhelming feeling experienced by depressed persons is that of sadness, gloominess, and "no joy." Although some of this despair may relate to a real loss or event, the reaction is exaggerated. Once this emotional state has developed, it tends to last with little daily variation for periods of weeks or months. (This is old-fashioned melancholia.)

Physical problems are numerous and dramatic. Typically, the depressed person complains of poor appetite, weight loss, constipation or diarrhea, and vague aches or pains. Sleep disturbances are common, that is, waking early in the morning and having trouble getting back to sleep. The early awakenings and sleep loss add to the basic emotional difficulty. Victims of severe depression complain of weakness and lack of energy and find little pleasure or satisfaction in activities they previously enjoyed. All too often, both the physician and the depressed person attribute these physical complaints to cancer or some other dreaded disease. Therefore, the individual often undergoes a series of unnecessary medical tests and procedures before the real culprit is recognized.

Mental functions are also affected by depression. Thinking is slow and inaccurate, memory is faulty, concentration is difficult, and the depressed person often considers himself or herself diseased, guilty, and beyond salvation. Predictably, suicide is a constant threat.

Many older people with depression have had one or more previous bouts of the condition in their early years, and some have a form of the disease that includes periods of excitability or overactivity—so-called manic-depressive disease.

WHAT CAUSES DEPRESSION?

Although the specific cause of this condition is still unknown, some experts believe that severe depressive illness results from chemical imbalance of the brain. In addition, emotional and psychological stresses, especially serious losses, seem to precipitate and prolong spells of true or abnormal depression. There is no evidence that normal moods or reactions of sadness and grief progress to lasting depression.

A few persons with specific medical conditions become depressed as a part of the disease process. Certain types of stroke, untreated disorders of the thyroid gland, and neurological conditions such as parkinsonism are likely to be accompanied by depression.

In recent years, literally dozens of drugs have been found to either contribute to or trigger spells of depression. This poses a special threat to older people who must use medications for control of other diseases or problems. Antihypertensives and sleeping pills, for example, are frequent offenders.

Equally important, many new and potent antidepressant drugs have been discovered, again suggesting that reversible chemical changes are important causes of this condition.

HOW CAN DEPRESSION AFFECT YOU?

The best descriptive word for depression is *pervasive*. Depression involves and affects almost every part of your life. Even so, depressed people vary widely in their responses, reactions, and behaviors.

Most often, depression is marked by vague but constant feelings of sadness, gloominess, and hopelessness. As a result, many persons seem overwhelmed, withdrawn, and disinterested in family, friends, and surroundings. Low energy levels make trivial tasks seem like major chores, and work performance often suffers.

Older people frequently develop nagging, rather nonspecific bodily complaints that mask and disguise the true nature of depression. Pain in the form of headaches, arthritic symptoms, and abdominal cramps may point toward depression. Unexplained weakness and weight loss may suggest the presence of depression. Depression may mimic dementia (see pages 241–242), producing memory loss, difficulty in concentrating, self-neglect, and loss of spontaneity. Treatment of the basic depressive condition typically reverses all these seemingly endless symptoms!

Unrecognized and untreated, depression may last from six months to more than two years, and most psychiatrists feel that the outlook for recovery worsens if the disease is neglected. Those people who receive an early diagnosis and have strong social supports have the best outlook. Although comprehensive medical treatment reverses depression in most cases, the tendency to develop depression should be considered a lifelong condition, one that can or should be recognized and the symptoms treated promptly and effectively.

■ Consult Your Doctor Now IF

■ You are experiencing prolonged (of more than three weeks' duration) unexplained sadness, weakness, or lack of interest in life that interferes with your normal activities.

■ You have feelings of hopelessness or guilt that cause you to think of dying or taking your own life.

■ Goal of Care

■ To recognize early signs and symptoms of depression and avoid a serious, prolonged bout of illness.

■ Self-Care Techniques

■ Take stock: (1) Have you had previous episodes of depression? (2) Is there a history of depression or suicide in your immediate family—parents, brothers, sisters, children? (3) Have you felt sad, helpless, or hopeless for the past three weeks or more? (4) Are you bothered by several aches and pains, poor appetite, weight loss, or severe fatigue? (5) Are you bothered by severe insomnia? (6) Have you experienced frequent personal difficulties at work during the past several months? (7) Do you think often about dying or ending your life?

While no quiz can always identify depression, people with positive answers to most or all of these seven questions can be considered prime candidates for this condition. If you answered yes to more than three questions, you might review the situation with your physician or other health professional.

■ Review your list of personal medications. Make note of antihypertensive drugs such as reserpine and Inderal. If you have questions about their possible side effects, consult your physician.

■ If you have had one or more periods of depressive illness in the past, be certain that family members and your physician are aware of this.

■ ALCOHOLISM

A majority of adults in the United States drink alcoholic beverages with some regularity, usually on social occasions. Most seem to enjoy the experiences—if not the beverages—and have no significant personal, medical, or social problems related to alcohol or its effects.

Unfortunately, a significant number of otherwise average people (six million or so) develop serious, sometimes life-threatening problems from addiction to alcohol. This addiction is known as alcoholism. Contrary to popular belief, an alcoholic is not just "anyone who drinks a lot." Alcoholism is a well-defined, chronic, progressive disease that has stages, complications, and treatments. Although the picture of alcoholism varies widely, the condition usually evolves over a period of ten or more years, with the gradual development of profound alcohol dependence, health problems, legal crises, and social stresses.

Unlike a social drinker, the true alcoholic is physically dependent on alcohol for performance and comfort. He or she cannot give up drinking to excess. The alcoholic must drink in the morning to "get started" and may even drink nonbeverage substances such as mouthwash or liniment for their alcohol content.

Health problems plague the alcoholic. Sudden withdrawal from drinking may cause convulsions and delirium tremens (DTs), a frightening neurological and psychiatric reaction that is occasionally fatal. Blackouts, total amnesia for events, may accompany bouts of heavy drinking. Other health problems especially common in long-term drinkers include stomach ulcers, inflammation of the pancreas, and progressive liver damage (cirrhosis).

The legal and social aspects of alcoholism are all too familiar. Arrests follow fights and other disturbances. Alcohol-related accidents account for more than 50 percent of all traffic deaths. Many alcoholics lose high-paying jobs. Families are often divided by anger, guilt, and extra expenses.

WHAT CAUSES ALCOHOLISM?

Inheritance is clearly important in the cause of alcoholism, especially in men. Children of alcoholic fathers are four times more likely to develop alcoholism than those of nonalcoholic fathers. The scientific basis for this family tendency is still unknown.

Many sociologists feel that family environments are very influential, but few facts support this notion. Although much has been said about the personality types of alcoholics, no studies yet have defined a "susceptible" personality—the personality that exists before the disease itself affects behavior.

Many potential alcoholics become active alcoholics when drinking is used to relieve the tension of family crises, illnesses, or other stresses. A few studies have shown that *older alcoholics* are of two general types: One type begins drinking heavily in youth when family tendencies, social pressures, and personal failures combine to cause addiction to alcohol. The second type drinks little or no alcohol until late-life personal or social stresses such as retirement, loss of spouse, poverty, or illness trigger alcohol abuse.

HOW CAN ALCOHOLISM AFFECT YOU?

Early in the course of the disease, most individuals consider themselves social drinkers, paying the price of hangovers for occasional bouts of heavy drinking.

As the drinker consumes increasing amounts of alcoholic beverages, he or she alternates more and more between binges of drunkenness and periods of uncomfortable withdrawal. Sooner or later, alcohol, a strong brain depressant, produces blackouts, or loss of memory for hours or days of drinking—clear indications that early brain damage has occurred.

If heavy drinking continues for five to ten years, serious nervous and medical complications begin to appear. Trouble going to sleep or other sleep disorders (see "Insomnia," pages 144–147) develop, leading to late-night drinking. Early-morning anxiety and withdrawal symptoms (so-called morning shakes) soon follow, requiring more alcohol. Stomach dysfunction interferes with nutritional food intake, and vitamin deficiencies may occur. Liver damage is often progressive, with resulting intestinal bleeding, coma, and death. Alcohol-induced brain disorders usually involve intellectual loss and a form of dementia.

At all stages of this disease, interpersonal conflicts, social difficulties, and economic tensions are commonplace. The end results of long-standing alcoholism are grim. Death occurs on the average ten years prematurely. In addition, the death rate is two to three times greater among alcoholics than among nonalcoholics of the same age.

▩ *Consult Your Doctor Now* <u>IF</u>

▪ You feel that you have a problem with alcohol, especially if there is a family history of alcoholism.

▪ Your family feels that you drink excessively.

▪ You have experienced significant personal, family, legal, or employment difficulties because of your drinking.

▩ *Goal of Care*

▪ To recognize the early features of alcoholism and prevent its progression.

▩ *Self-Care Technique*

▪ The Brief Michigan Alcoholism Screening Test (MAST) is a widely used device for recognizing heavy drinkers who show signs of becoming true alcoholics. If you are concerned about your drinking and its effects, answer these questions honestly and add up your total score.

THE BRIEF MICHIGAN ALCOHOLISM SCREENING TEST

Read each question at the left. Decide whether the answer is yes or no. Then draw a circle around the number next to the correct answer.

1. Do you feel you are a normal drinker? Yes 0 No 2

2. Do friends or relatives think you are a normal drinker? Yes 0 No 2

3. Have you ever attended a meeting of Alcoholics Anonymous (AA)? Yes 5 No 0

4. Have you ever lost either male or female friends because of drinking? Yes 2 No 0

5. Have you ever gotten into trouble at work because of drinking? Yes 2 No 0

6. Have you ever neglected your obligations, your family, or your work for two or more days in a row because you were drinking? Yes 2 No 0

7. Have you ever had delirium tremens (DTs), experienced severe shaking, heard voices, or seen things that weren't there after heavy drinking?   Yes 2   No 0

8. Have you ever gone to anyone for help about your drinking?   Yes 5   No 0

9. Have you ever been in a hospital because of drinking?   Yes 5   No 0

10. Have you ever been arrested for drunk driving or driving after drinking?   Yes 2   No 0

Add all the numbers circled to determine your score.

If your score is greater than 5, you have a significant problem with alcohol and are at risk for developing alcoholism. You should discuss this problem with your physician or other health professional. Most experts suggest that you participate in a program such as Alcoholics Anonymous (AA).

■ INSOMNIA

Most healthy young adults sleep between seven and eight hours a night. As people reach middle age, many find that they need less sleep. After age forty-five or fifty, depth, or soundness, of sleep also decreases. (Deep sleep that accounts for 20 percent of sleep time in teenagers may disappear completely in normal elderly persons.)

Insomnia, reported by about 30 percent of all adults, refers to any bothersome or distressing decrease in the duration or depth of sleep. Three major types, or patterns, of insomnia may afflict healthy people: (1) a frustrating delay in falling asleep; (2) repeated brief awakenings that may occur throughout the night; and (3) awakening very early in the morning and not being able to fall back to sleep.

Sleep experts point out that most people overestimate their sleep problems, greatly exaggerating the amount of time it takes them to fall asleep and the amount of time they lie awake.

WHAT CAUSES INSOMNIA?

Environmental changes obviously influence sleep patterns. An overheated room, a change in work schedule, or unfamiliar noises may give rise to two or three restless nights.

Many bouts of transient insomnia result from everyday emotional stresses that are upsetting and lead to unpleasant internal reactions. Anxiety over approaching retirement, anger provoked by a family argument, or sadness following a major loss often leads to restless nights and drowsy days.

Almost any form of physical distress may contribute to loss of sleep. A nagging headache, a throbbing toothache, or the deep ache of arthritic joints may prevent effective sleep. Itching or the frequent urge to urinate can affect both depth and duration of sleep.

Few older persons realize that many drugs alter sleep patterns. Prolonged use or sudden withdrawal of most sleeping medications leads to a period of poor sleep. Although alcohol may seem relaxing and induces sleep, it often fragments and disrupts critical rest later in the night. Some drugs used for the treatment of hypertension, lung disease, or arthritis cause altered sleep.

Many diseases also produce insomnia. Psychiatric conditions like depression may have early awakening, inability to fall asleep, frequent awakenings, or combinations of any of the three as major features. Persons with chronic bronchitis may have more difficulty breathing at night than during the day. A few older persons with disrupted sleep and daytime sleepiness suffer from some form of sleep apnea (literally, not breathing). Most often these persons experience restless behavior and loud snoring at night, morning headache, and severe daytime drowsiness. Some have partial blockage of their upper airway passages, often complicated by mild brain dysfunction, which leads to the nighttime breathing difficulty and loss of sleep.

HOW CAN INSOMNIA AFFECT YOU?

Lack of sleep at night can make an individual feel sleepy, or certainly not well rested, during the day. The body, however, quickly compensates for a night or two of poor sleep with daytime naps and added hours of "good" nighttime sleep. More serious bouts of insomnia may have more serious effects. First, fear of not falling asleep may itself produce so much bedtime anxiety that sound sleep is not possible, creating a vicious cycle of insomnia. Second, a series of sleepless nights is often followed by days of drowsiness, unwanted (and even dangerous, as when falling asleep at the wheel) catnaps, irritability, and mental dullness. Third, prolonged sleep loss may result in confusion and faulty judgment. Finally, persistent insomnia and its ill effects lead, all too often, to trials of alcoholic nightcaps and sleeping pills, followed by the very real hazards of drug dependence.

Consult Your Doctor Now IF

- New or unexplained insomnia has lasted more than seven days.
- Daytime symptoms of drowsiness, falling asleep, or mental difficulties have become frightening or have interfered with work or other activities.
- Nighttime restlessness and snoring have caused concern in a bed partner or family members.

Goals of Care

- To discover the factors—environmental, personal, or medical—that led to sleep disruption.
- To design a program of sleep management that promotes regular refreshing sleep of proper duration and depth.
- To avoid dependence on sleeping medications of any sort.

Self-Care Techniques

- Keep a careful log, or chart, of your sleep behavior for seven to ten days. Include the date, the amount of time taken to fall asleep, the number of awakenings during the night, the number of hours slept, the quality of the rest, the time slept during the day, and all medications you are currently taking. (See Appendix C, page 310, for a sleep chart to use for your medical records.)

- Review the documentation of your sleep chart carefully, preferably with your doctor, noting the actual time spent asleep and napping in each twenty-four-hour period.

- Schedule your wake-up times. Establish a regular awakening time, waking yourself up with an alarm if necessary. This consistent point in your schedule helps create a regular sleep cycle in most cases. Spending too much time in bed may make your sleep shallow. Getting up at regular times, even if you still feel a bit drowsy, may help you fall asleep more easily at night and sleep more soundly as the week goes on. Getting up earlier than your scheduled time won't hurt you.

- Don't try to force sleep when you cannot; you will just become angry and more wakeful. If you are still awake after twenty minutes have passed, read, watch television, or do something else relaxing until your body calms down and you feel sleepy.

- Establish a regular pattern of exercise. Try to exercise regularly every day,

even if you are tired. If you keep yourself on a daily exercise program, you will sleep more soundly. Your sleep will improve as your exercise program continues over weeks and months (see chapter 5).

- Hunger can keep you awake or disturb your sleep. On the other hand, if you eat too much or snack on heavy foods, your body will be too busy digesting the food to relax. Experimenting with bedtime snacks of warm milk, cheese, and other dairy products may help you relax. A little sugar helps some people relax. If this is true for you, try milk and cookies or a glass of fruit juice or a bowl of lightly sugared cereal and milk before bed.

- Omit caffeine at least eight hours before you plan to sleep. Caffeine in coffee, tea, chocolate, and many soft drinks can keep you awake or interfere with your sleep.

- Omit beer and alcohol at bedtime. Alcohol may help you fall asleep fast, but it won't help you sleep well. Your sleep will be light and disturbed, not deep and heavy. Beer wakes you up faster because it increases your need to urinate.

- Quit smoking. Heavy smoking, above two packs a day, disturbs sleep because your body begins to react to withdrawal after three hours without a cigarette. If you give up smoking, you will sleep poorly until your body adjusts; then your sleep will improve.

- If your self-help program is unsuccessful after two weeks or so, contact your doctor. If sleeping medication is prescribed by your doctor, be sure not to take it with alcohol. Alcohol and sleeping medications should never be taken together. Avoid mixing any prescribed sleeping medication with over-the-counter sleeping drugs.

◼ FORGETFULNESS

Many psychologists now recognize three levels of memory: immediate memory, recent memory, and remote memory. *Immediate memory* refers to the recollection of names or events within seconds of hearing or seeing them, such as repeating a telephone number just given to you by the operator. *Recent memory* involves the ability to learn and retrieve information for minutes, hours, or days, such as remembering the names and faces of the two new Rotarians you met last week. *Remote memory* is the ability to recall accurately happenings of years ago, such as still remembering details of your high-school prom.

Most complaints of forgetfulness by otherwise healthy adults involve recent memory. In fact, more than one-half of older people questioned in a large community survey reported some problems with recall of recent events. Immediate and remote memory functions seem to change very little with age.

This "benign forgetfulness" that happens to approximately 20 percent of the population may become noticeable as early as age thirty-five. It is an aging process that typically worsens very slowly in the decades to follow. Four features set this recent memory loss apart from the more serious problem of dementia (see pages 241–242). The features are as follows:

1. Minor events and trivial details (for example, names of people met at a party) are most often forgotten while critical items are well preserved.

2. The memory gap is not absolute, as the missing names or items are often recalled later on.

3. The forgetful person recognizes and worries about his or her memory problem, whereas the individual with significant brain damage or dementia is usually unaware of his or her mistakes.

4. Forgetfulness is the only sign of mental difficulty; reasoning, judgment, use of language, and orientation are all normal.

WHAT CAUSES FORGETFULNESS?

Most people have some problem in remembering details of recent events, and many studies suggest that such difficulties are part of normal aging. Other bodily actions and reactions may become less brisk and efficient as people reach the later decades, so delays in complex mental processes should be expected.

Special psychological tests show that much of the recently learned but "forgotten" information is still stored, so it may be that only the retrieval process is slow. Training and practice usually lead to improved recall, while anxiety, depression, and stress increase the difficulty. In fact some severely depressed persons have loss of memory as their major problem.

There is no evidence that simple forgetfulness is caused by hardening of brain arteries, vitamin deficiencies, or serious mental illness.

HOW CAN FORGETFULNESS AFFECT YOU?

The immediate effect of forgetting names, facts, or faces is embarrassment—and more stress. Some people, uncomfortably aware of their poor memory at parties and other gatherings, begin to avoid social events. A few withdraw completely from normal activities and become victims of their own anxiety.

One common belief is that people with simple forgetfulness are doomed to develop progressive loss of other intellectual functions, eventually reaching a vegetative, demented state, or "senility." This is not so! Several careful studies have shown that adults with simple recent memory loss do not become demented more frequently or die sooner than other persons of the same age.

■ *Consult Your Doctor Now* <u>IF</u>

- You have one or more episodes of *total* loss of memory for any recent event or situation.

- You experience frightening or dangerous mishaps, such as driving on the wrong side of the road, as a result of memory lapses.
- Trouble with recent memory has caused significant difficulties with your work or other duties.

■ *Goal of Care*

- To develop habits and practices that keep forgetfulness and its effects to a minimum.

■ *Self-Care Techniques*

- Make your home an orderly, everything-in-its-place environment. Place essential objects such as keys, wallet, purse, and/or notebook in a convenient location—by the telephone or near the front door, for example. Place a label at each location stating which object is to be kept there.
- Write down in a notebook with a calendar the full schedule for each day, noting names and other relevant information beside each event. Consult your notebook just before and during the event. Add any new information that will help remind you of important names, places, or dates (for example, Ed Smith, doctor; Ann Watson, receptionist).
- Use your notebook as a sort of memory diary, noting situations and circumstances in which significant lapses of memory occurred. You will probably find that stress, fatigue, and distraction are the common elements that helped defeat you.

- Organize a pocket notebook to serve as a memory book.

- Use a small tape recorder as your personal secretary. Dictate each day's schedule, complete with important names, addresses, and topics (for example, "11:00 A.M., meet Helen Hobbs and Dorothy Baker at main library checkout desk—discuss fund raising, work schedule, and Saturday picnic"). Add summaries of these events, reminding yourself of decisions, future appointments, and unanswered questions.

◼ DIZZINESS

An individual is constantly aware of the position of his or her body in relation to the environment or immediate surroundings. The brain instantly detects and corrects for changes in either body position or surroundings; for example, if a person stumbles or if a door swings in his or her face, the person automatically adjusts to protect himself or herself.

Dizziness, or vertigo, in the most general sense, is a feeling of poor balance or an actual loss of coordination between the body and its surroundings. Whether momentary or continuous, the feeling of dizziness may be that of a spinning or turning movement ("I thought the room was spinning around"), the sensation of faintness or weakness ("I was giddy and nearly blacked out"), or a sense of loss of balance ("I was unsteady and stumbled"). Many people have real difficulty in describing the experience, using such words as "light-headed," "fuzzy," or "woozy."

If the spell of dizziness lasts more than a few seconds, the individual may feel anxious, nauseated, and sweaty.

WHAT CAUSES DIZZINESS?

Almost any condition that affects certain brain centers, vision, the internal ear, various bodily senses of position, or the general circulatory system may produce dizziness. Most cases of dizziness, however, fall into one of the following categories: (1) true vertigo; (2) poor vision; (3) overbreathing, or hyperventilation; (4) emotional distress; or (5) specific medical and drug-related conditions. *True vertigo* is a brief spinning sensation, with or without nausea, that occurs after rapid changes in body position or as a result of mild damage to the balance center of the inner ear. (When this spinning sensation is complicated by hearing loss and ringing in the ears, the condition is called Ménière's disease.) Many people with *poor vision* of any sort feel dizzy or unsteady while walking or turning, especially if they also have deafness, arthritis, or nerve weakness that makes walking slow and awkward. Almost one-quarter of the people bothered by dizziness, faintness, or light-headedness suffer from spells of *overbreathing.* Hyperventilation is usually triggered by anxiety, pain, or other stresses. These spells of overbreathing accompanied by dizziness and faintness may last for as long as thirty minutes and are often accompanied by feelings of numbness and tingling in the fingers and lips. Constant dizziness or fuzziness that lasts for weeks or months most often results from *emotional stress,* such as from prolonged depression (with difficulty in concentrating and weakness), anxiety (feelings of fright and tension), or concern about one's own health. In addition, a large number of *medical and drug-related conditions* may cause occasional bouts of dizziness. These conditions include strokes, viral infections, heartbeat irregularities, and drug reactions (especially to alcohol).

HOW CAN DIZZINESS AFFECT YOU?

Whatever its cause, a dizzy spell is startling and frightening and leaves the victim shaky and weak. Severe spells, especially those associated with feelings of spinning about (self or surroundings), may be accompanied by nausea, vomiting, and heavy sweating.

On occasion, the dizzy or light-headed person stumbles, misjudges the position of objects around him or her, and falls to the ground. Injuries such as a broken wrist may occur as a result.

Many individuals affected by frequent or severe dizzy spells understandably become leery of situations that are potentially hazardous to themselves and others, for example, driving an automobile, climbing steep steps, swimming alone, and working near flames or machines.

▰ Consult Your Doctor Now IF

- You have two unexplained dizzy spells in a week.
- You experience dizziness or faintness that could produce significant injury to yourself or others.
- You have dizziness accompanied by true blackouts, loss of hearing, ringing in the ears, or significant headaches.

▰ Goals of Care

- To understand the major cause of bothersome dizziness.
- To control dizzy spells and prevent their complications.

▰ Self-Care Techniques

- Maintain a dizziness chart or record for one month. Include the following information: the date of the episode; the time it began and ended; the situation you were in when the spell occurred—moving? standing up? bending over? walking?; any accompanying symptoms such as ringing in the ears, headache, nausea, vomiting, sweating, or falling; whether or not there was a spinning or turning sensation; and all medications presently being taken. (See Appendix C, pages 312–313, for a dizziness chart to use for your medical records.)
- Try to avoid overstimulation of your visual and balance systems. Avoid

looking out of rapidly moving vehicles and the stop-and-go motions of buses and other vehicles.

- Practice arising from chairs very slowly and turn carefully and deliberately while walking.

- Arrange to hold on to safe supports in dangerous areas like stairs.

- Use a light cane or walker for balance and reassurance while walking.

- Correct any visual problems that make walking difficult or uncomfortable.

■ WEAKNESS

The English language provides dozens of words to describe that tired, used-up feeling—*exhaustion, fatigue, weakness, weariness, listlessness,* to name a few. In most instances, a person can relate the feeling or effect to an obvious cause—a sleepless night, an overwhelming grief reaction, or a taxing cross-country trek. In other instances, however, this feeling develops without apparent cause. In these cases, it must be regarded as a feature of some underlying condition, as a manifestation of illness, and not as a disease in itself.

Although many cases of general weakness cannot be analyzed and classified precisely, some cases can be described as being in the category of (1) tiredness, (2) fatigue, or (3) listlessness. The term *tiredness* refers to the feeling that appropriate rest and relaxation would cure. *Fatigue* usually suggests general muscular exhaustion and a sensation of being "all in." The term *listlessness* implies somehow that motivation is lacking or that the basic difficulty is more mental than physical.

Whatever the term applied, many people experience periods of weakness and exhaustion that are disabling and often frightening to all concerned.

WHAT CAUSES WEAKNESS?

About half of all adults who complain of weakness and feelings of exhaustion have a largely psychiatric or emotional condition. Of these, a majority suffer from some form of depression (see pages 139–141). Other adults seem to experience episodes of weakness as poorly resolved parts of grief reactions or interpersonal conflicts—a sort of "neither fight nor flight" response to stress (see pages 40–43).

There are, of course, numerous physical causes of weakness, but most of these are accompanied by some other signs of disease. For example, metabolic difficulties, especially those involving the thyroid or adrenal glands, may lead to profound weakness in addition to weight changes and mental symptoms. Untreated diabetes mellitus may, on occasion, present as unexplained weakness and easy fatigue. Advanced or poorly controlled kidney or liver failure is often associated with profound weakness. Disorders of nerve or muscle function such as parkinsonism may begin as general weakness.

Many infections, especially viral conditions such as influenza, have profound fatigue as a prominent feature. Congestive heart failure, especially in the very old, may be accompanied by crippling weakness and tiredness.

Finally, the most common cause of bothersome weakness in older adults may well be simple lack of muscle use—idled muscles lose strength and tone in a matter of days. All too often, a minor hip or knee injury leads to immobility, which leads in turn to muscle wasting and still more inactivity in a depressing downward spiral.

HOW CAN WEAKNESS AFFECT YOU?

Weakness and feelings of exhaustion, whatever the cause, are demoralizing. Depression (if not already present), frustration, loss of appetite, and disordered sleep often appear if the problem persists. Attempts to override the weakness by sheer willpower and physical effort rarely succeed. As a rule, only specific management of the underlying condition, whether emotional or physical, relieves the weakness.

Muscle weakness itself is rarely permanent, even when it is extensive and severe. Thus, the person with disabling thyroid gland deficiency typically regains muscle strength and energy as the disorder is treated. When heart disorders are corrected, muscle tone and general vigor return promptly.

Some of the weakness of disuse atrophy can be prevented. Control of joint pain, careful isometric exercises of muscles surrounding an injured joint, and local heat treatments can often keep muscle wasting to a minimum.

■ *Consult Your Doctor Now IF*

■ You have unexplained weakness that is limiting your activities or causing personal concern.

■ *Goals of Care*

■ To understand and correct the cause, or causes, of weakness.

■ To prevent the complications of weakness.

■ *Self-Care Techniques*

■ If you have any symptoms associated with diabetes (see pages 245–246), a sudden weight change, or problems with kidney function, make an appointment with your doctor for a physical examination.

■ If you have experienced a personal loss and have not been able to resolve your grief, seek counseling from a health professional and/or member of the clergy. Also review chapter 4, pages 35–49.

■ If you have been physically inactive because of injury, review the flexibility exercises in Appendix A and start using the idle muscles again.

■ UNEXPLAINED WEIGHT LOSS

Once healthy adults reach full body maturity, occurring at ages twenty-five to thirty, they tend to maintain a fairly stable body weight. Barring major changes in the level of physical activity or in dietary practices, appetite should regulate food intake so exactly that body weight should vary less than 5 percent from year to year.

While many people fight the battle of being overweight or even obese, others find themselves unable to maintain their "ideal" or desired body weight. An unexplained weight loss of more than 5 percent of one's usual weight that occurs in less than six months can be considered as involuntary weight loss.

WHAT CAUSES WEIGHT LOSS?

Body weight drops when caloric supply fails to meet body energy demands. Mental or emotional states can affect appetite and food intake. Anxiety or depression often causes the appetite to fail; mealtimes lose their appeal, the individual eats less, and thus body weight drops.

Many medical and surgical conditions are complicated by loss of appetite, failing energy, and weight loss. Cancer, especially when it involves the organs of the chest or abdomen, may cause rapid loss of weight. Uncontrolled metabolic disorders such as diabetes mellitus and thyroid gland dysfunction may result in unexplained weight loss. Most individuals recovering from serious injury or major surgical operations temporarily lose considerable weight from failure to eat full diets. Persons recovering from the effects of fever and from side effects of medication may also temporarily lose considerable weight.

Critical sources of energy are lost when vomiting and diarrhea are present, so conditions like diarrhea (see pages 214–216) regularly lead to weight loss and wasting. Finally, simple "mechanical" and economic difficulties may prevent an older person from consuming a well-balanced, energy-rich diet. Dental problems can prevent complete chewing of nutritious food; the disability of arthritis can make food preparation slow and painful; low income may mean skimpy or skipped meals.

HOW CAN WEIGHT LOSS AFFECT YOU?

Weakness is the major complaint of people who experience undesired weight loss. Lack of energy produces the feeling of muscular weakness and easy tiring. Many persons also report drowsiness and the lack of ability to concentrate. Understandably, frustration and feelings of depression often accompany both unexplained weight loss and its associated diseases.

Although weight loss itself can produce symptoms, most of the problems experienced are related to underlying conditions. Emotional illnesses such as depression (see pages 139–141), tumors of various sorts, and gastrointestinal diseases affect general health in many ways—weight loss being one. This situation improves when the basic condition is corrected.

▰ Consult Your Doctor Now IF

▪ You experience unexplained loss of 5 percent or more of your usual body weight in less than six months.

▪ Your appetite becomes noticeably poor, and weight loss develops.

▰ Goals of Care

▪ To determine the cause of unexplained weight loss.

▪ To correct the underlying condition and restore normal or "ideal" body weight.

▰ Self-Care Techniques

▪ Use a weight-loss chart that includes dates; weights, in the morning before breakfast, twice a week only; complaints, such as loss of appetite, nausea, vomiting, diarrhea, pain, or weakness; and all medications being taken, including both prescription and nonprescription drugs. (See Appendix C, page 311, for a weight-loss chart to use for your medical records.)

▪ Review your eating habits and be certain you (1) eat well-balanced, attractive, and unhurried meals three times a day and (2) do not interfere with your appetite by snacking or by having more than two to three alcoholic drinks a day.

▰ FEVER

The internal temperature of the healthy body is maintained within a narrow range, "normal" temperature being regarded as 98.6° F, give or take one degree Fahrenheit. The centigrade equivalent is 37.0° C, give or take 0.5 degree centigrade. Controlled by a special nerve center deep in the brain, the body processes that produce heat (metabolic processes, burning of foods, and muscle action) are closely balanced by processes that release heat (sweating, radiation of heat from skin surfaces, and loss of warm air through the lungs). Body temperature may vary as much as two degrees Fahrenheit during a day; it is usually higher in the evening and lower in the early morning hours. In adults, temperature measured with a rectal thermometer tends to be one degree Fahrenheit higher than the oral temperature. Some older people have body temperatures that consistently run one or two degrees Fahrenheit lower than normal. It also has been noted by doctors that in some older persons, the absence of a higher temperature does not necessarily mean the person has no illness usually associated with fever, such as pneumonia.

Elevation of body temperature by disease is called fever. Although warm environments (such as hospital rooms) may cause body temperature to rise a degree or so, and vigorous exercise increases body heat for twenty to thirty minutes after exercising, continued elevation of temperature always suggests the presence of disease. Like pain, fever is a symptom of some medical condition, not a disease in and of itself.

Very mild fever—an increase in temperature of less than one degree Fahrenheit—may be part of many common illnesses and simply cause a bit of sweating at night. Most often in adults, fever of two degrees Fahrenheit occurs at the beginning of an infection or skin rash, fading in two or three days as the inflammation subsides. Fevers that persist beyond one week or climb by more than three degrees Fahrenheit often indicate more serious infections or generalized conditions that require prompt study and treatment.

WHAT CAUSES FEVER?

Many conditions change the balance between heat production and heat loss to cause a higher body "thermostat" setting. The common feature in most instances is body tissue damage. Chemicals from the injured area, from blood cells, and from hormones used in body defense stimulate the brain's temperature-control center to set a new balance level.

Infections of all sorts account for most fevers in adults. Viral infections like the common cold may be accompanied by a day or so of low-grade fever, whereas severe attacks of influenza are often accompanied by fevers to 103° or 104° F. Tuberculosis may cause low-grade fevers—accompanied by nightly drenching sweats—that last for weeks before other symptoms appear. Small localized infections like conjunctivitis (see pages 172–174) usually do not cause fever.

Many patients with cancer complain of feverishness, often before the growth itself has been discovered. Tumors of the lung often cause moderate fever, in some cases because pneumonia has developed around the site. New growths in the blood (leukemia) and lymph nodes (lymphoma) may cause persistent and uncomfortable fever.

Drug reactions now account for many cases of fever. In most instances the fever is part of an allergic reaction that sometimes also causes skin rash, arthritis, or other symptoms. In other instances drugs like sulfonamides, antihypertensives, and antidepressants may produce fever without other signs or reactions.

Medical conditions are often accompanied by fever. Most types of arthritis, some gallbladder diseases, kidney inflammation, and postoperative states may produce fever.

HOW CAN FEVER AFFECT YOU?

Some experts believe that fever itself improves the body's defense responses, thereby helping the body overcome invading viral and bacterial organisms. Others argue that these possible benefits are outweighed by the discomfort and the stress on the heart and circulatory system produced by increased body temperature.

Most people are made uncomfortable by an increase of one to two degrees in body temperature: the face is flushed, the head feels congested, muscles and joints ache, and perspiration makes them feel both hot and cold. In addition, fever often causes restlessness and leads to a sense of weakness and fatigue as the body temperature rises and falls.

Some fevers, especially those related to serious bacterial infections, are associated with chills or tremors. Here, the body's muscles contract for minutes at a time in an uncontrolled fashion, causing shivering, shaking, and chattering of teeth. As a result, body heat production increases rapidly, and temperature climbs.

In most cases, fever subsides or is controlled by drugs, so the major problem is that of the underlying condition. When fever continues for more than a week, weakness, weight loss, and a feeling of depression may occur. Very high fever (much greater than 104° F) may lead to temporary confusion (delirium), seizures, or even circulatory shock.

Consult Your Doctor Now IF

- You have fever greater than 100° F, when taken orally, that lasts more than three days without an obvious cause.
- You have shaking and chills.
- You have a fever greater than 103° F.

Goals of Care

- To document the presence of fever and determine its cause.
- To minimize the discomfort and hazards of fever.

Self-Care Techniques

- Keep a fever chart as long as your fever continues plus two more days—in case it recurs. Include the following: (1) The date and the times of four temperature readings each day. (See pages 340–342 for instructions. Temperatures may be taken by mouth or by rectum, which provides more sensitive values, and should be taken at the same times each day. At least one reading should be made in the evening, 6:00 P.M. to 12 midnight, and one in the early morning, 6:00 A.M.–8:00 A.M.). (2) Pulse rate (see pages 56–57 for instructions on how to take your pulse). (3) A list of accompanying symptoms, such as chills, sweating, pain, or nausea. (4) Dosage and timing of all medications taken, such as antibiotics, aspirin, Tylenol, and sleeping pills. (See Appendix C, pages 314–315, for a fever chart to use for your medical records.)

- Unless your doctor tells you otherwise, drink at least ten glasses of fluid each day to replace the water and salts lost by sweating. Cool water, fruit juices, and colas are excellent.

- If approved by your doctor, especially if the cause of fever is known, take aspirin or Tylenol in some form (usually two tablets, or 650 mg) every four hours while awake to keep the body's temperature lower and to relieve the aches and pains associated with fever. Several important points must be remembered: (1) take these medications with generous volumes of liquid; (2) take buffered aspirin (for example, Ascriptin, or Ecotrin), or Tylenol if you have an upset stomach or a history of stomach ulcers; and (3) take these drugs at regular intervals of four hours while you are awake to avoid distressing upward and downward swings in temperature.

◼ ACCIDENTAL HYPOTHERMIA

All vital functions of the brain, heart, and other organs depend on very specific levels of body temperature. The delicate balance between body heat production (by metabolic processes, burning of foods, and muscle action) and heat loss (by sweating, radiation of heat from skin surfaces, and loss of warm air through the lungs) maintains an internal temperature of about 98.6° F (or 37° C). Normally, this critical temperature is maintained in spite of dramatic extremes of climate, physical activity, or body weight.

When body temperature falls below 95° F (or 35° C), the life-threatening condition of hypothermia is said to exist. Accidental hypothermia is a condition seen most often in elderly persons, and it generally occurs as a result of their being in their own home settings.

WHAT CAUSES ACCIDENTAL HYPOTHERMIA?

Most adults who experience an episode of accidental hypothermia have slow and often inadequate body heat production systems. In rooms as warm as 65° F, they feel chilly but shiver little or not at all, and their body temperatures drift down from 98.6° F to 95° F and lower.

Most persons who experience accidental hypothermia have more than one existing medical problem or risk factor, and the addition of a small insult—an extra sleeping pill, an alcohol binge— may precipitate a serious crisis.

Any disease that restricts physical activity also cuts down on body heat production. Therefore, crippling arthritis, strokes, parkinsonism, and muscle weakness may prevent normal body movements, thus contributing to the development of accidental hypothermia.

Inadequate body heat production can develop as a result of poor brain function, which can occur from conditions like strokes and dementia or from drug effects (from antidepressants, sleeping medications, and alcohol). This poor brain function may alter the critical balance between heat production and heat loss, thus contributing to the development of accidental hypothermia.

HOW CAN ACCIDENTAL HYPOTHERMIA AFFECT YOU?

As body temperature reaches 95° F, most victims experience chilliness without shaking chills. Arms and legs seem heavy, weak, and stiff, and thinking processes become slow and fuzzy. Since cold skin, stiff muscles, and drowsiness may be the only findings on medical examination, the diagnosis may be missed at first.

If the metabolic rate continues to decline and body temperature falls still farther, the person often becomes confused and even unconscious. Blood pressure soon falls to dangerously low levels, the heartbeat is slow and irregular, and breathing grows progressively slower. At body temperatures much below 80° F, serious damage to vital organs usually occurs, and some individuals do not survive despite vigorous treatment. In fact, the mortality from this condition among elderly persons ranges from 40 to 80 percent.

Success of treatment of accidental hypothermia depends on early diagnosis, and diagnosis depends on the use of a thermometer that registers these abnormally low body temperatures. Most instruments in common use are not marked below 94° F (about 34° C), so the condition is often not recognized.

Consult Your Doctor Now IF

- You are exposed for more than eight hours to temperatures of less than 60° F, especially if you (1) have a history of accidental hypothermia; (2) have mobility problems, for example, arthritis; (3) have thyroid deficiency; or (4) take tranquilizers or are receiving antidepressant therapy.

- Your oral temperature is recorded at less than 95° F (35° C).

Goal of Care

- To modify personal and environmental factors to prevent accidental hypothermia.

Self-Care Techniques

- Avoid prolonged exposure to damp or windy cold.

- When it is cold outside, always wear a hat or cap to cover your head. Forty to 50 percent of body heat loss may occur through the face and scalp.

- Keep your living quarters at or above 65° F, especially if you have mobility problems.

- Be certain the telephone numbers of a close friend, family member, doctor, and ambulance service are conveniently displayed in several parts of your home.

- Arrange, if possible, daily call-ins if you are ill or disabled.

- Inspect the safety and support aspects of your home. Remove objects that might contribute to falls and install railings or supports where needed.

- Take immediate action if your home's heating system breaks down.

- Take immediate action if anyone threatens to turn off your gas or electricity.

The Skin

■ DRY SKIN AND ITCHINESS

Normal aging of the skin causes (1) thinning of its outer layer of cells, (2) a decrease in the skin's elasticity, (3) a reduction in the secretion of protective oils, and (4) a delay or slowness in the healing process when the skin is cut, injured, or bruised. As a result of this aging process, the skin of older persons tends to be shiny, wrinkled, rough, and dry and prone to irritation, especially in areas exposed to sunlight.

Itchiness is that bothersome tingling sensation that demands a scratch. Itchiness may occur in any area of the skin, including the scalp, that is either injured or irritated. With advancing age, the skin becomes more sensitive to numerous substances. This hypersensitivity results in part from the condition of the outermost layer of cells. If looked at microscopically, the skin cells are jumbled or piled rather than flat, causing the skin to be rough or scaly. This roughness, which gives the impression of dryness, leads readily to irritation and itching.

Over half of older adults experience dryness and itchiness of the skin, usually over the lower legs, the forearms, and the hands. Prolonged dryness and scratchiness of these areas often lead to more irritation, with redness and cracking of the affected skin.

WHAT CAUSES DRY SKIN AND ITCHINESS?

Anything that irritates the skin can cause dryness and itchiness. The irritation may be very localized, as with a mosquito bite, or widespread, as seen in allergic reactions to penicillin. Almost any type of contact or mild injury—such as the chemicals in poison ivy, the heat produced by wearing heavy clothing, the scratchy surfaces of woolen clothing, and roughened skin itself—can stimulate tiny nerve endings in the skin to produce itchiness.

In addition, a few general medical conditions can cause generalized or total body itchiness. Some of these conditions include prolonged kidney failure, certain liver diseases, thyroid trouble, and drug reactions. If itchiness is caused by a medical condition, the itchiness generally occurs without an obvious rash or other change in the skin.

Itchiness, more than almost any other sensation, is affected by your emotional state. When you are alert and busy, an itching spot on your back is all but forgotten; when you are tired and fretful, you cannot sit still because of the itch.

Many other factors increase the irritation and itchiness of dry skin. Hot water, detergents, and cold dry air, for example, often trigger so-called winter itch.

HOW CAN DRY SKIN AND ITCHINESS AFFECT YOU?

The intensely annoying local sensation of itchiness produces an almost uncontrollable desire to scratch, with the subsequent scratching often increasing the irritation process. Relatively thin, rough skin is injured by repeated scratching. The injured skin may develop cracks, ulcers, and/or scarring. The open surface wounds can become infected with bacteria, which can then lead to serious illnesses.

Consult Your Doctor Now IF

- Itchiness and scratching have led to loss of sleep for more than two or three nights or if scratching has produced breaks in the skin.
- Itchiness involves most of the body without obvious cause or obvious rash.

■ You have an unexplained itchy rash that is spreading.

Goals of Care

■ To prevent itchiness.
■ To control dry skin and/or itchiness, should either occur.

Self-Care Techniques

■ If the following applies to your condition, most likely there is no need to seek immediate medical advice:

1. The itchiness or dry skin involves the lower legs, the forearms, and/or the hands.
2. The skin appears dry and rough and has fine scales, patchy redness, and/or welts.
3. The itchiness increases after a warm bath, at night, or during stressful experiences.
4. The itchiness is made worse by rough clothes, perspiration, and/or overheating.

■ Avoid sun exposure, which increases dryness, roughness, and itching.
■ If the dry skin and itchiness are localized, soak the involved areas with cold, wet compresses for fifteen minutes three times a day. Pat the area partially dry and then apply a mild, nonalcoholic lotion or cream containing lanolin or glycerin.
■ Bathe every other day in cool water, using only very mild or no soap if the skin is generally dry or itchy. After bathing, pat the skin partly dry and apply a mild body lotion. (Body lotions placed in the water are less effective and create hazardous slippery surfaces.)
■ During the day, lotions (Vaseline Intensive Care or Keri, for example), ointments (Aquaphor, for example), or creams (Nivea and Keri, for example) may be applied to dry and itchy skin.

SKIN RASHES

A rash (sometimes referred to as dermatitis or an eruption) is simply any sort of irritation or inflammation of the skin accompanied by visible breaking out and often accompanied by itchiness (see pages 158–160). Three types of rash are of special importance to older adults—seborrheic dermatitis, acne rosacea, and intertrigo.

About one-third of people sixty-five and older have some form of *seborrheic dermatitis*. Small reddish yellow scaling and slightly raised patches occur generally in skin areas that are oily: the scalp (as dandruff), around the ears, the eyebrows and eyelids, the face, and the chest. Although seborrheic dermatitis may begin in childhood, the rash comes and goes without significant scarring and often increases during winter months. It may appear in persons with parkinsonism and first may be noticed following certain types of drug therapy.

Acne rosacea usually begins spreading subtly in middle age as red, slightly raised spots or patches over the nose and cheeks, often resembling the acne eruption of adolescence. As the condition progresses over periods of months to years, the reddened areas merge, the inflamed skin becomes thickened and pebbled, spots of infection develop, and the rash expands to involve the entire nose, the cheek area, and the eyelids. In extreme cases, the unfortunate person becomes a W.C. Fields look-alike, with a large knobby nose. Insult is added to injury when observers attribute the condition to an excess of alcohol.

Intertrigo (literally, "a rubbing together") is a rash that occurs in and around the body's skin folds, most often appearing in the groin, armpits, and lower abdomen and under the breasts. This bothersome type of local dermatitis may appear anytime the skin folds are subject to prolonged heat, moisture, and friction. The irritated skin surfaces become reddened, weepy, and itchy, and secondary infection may follow. Obese individuals, especially those with complicating medical illnesses like diabetes or incontinence, are commonly affected.

WHAT CAUSES SKIN RASHES?

Seborrheic dermatitis, often a lifelong problem, may result from overactivity or some other abnormality of the skin's oil-producing glands. Some studies suggest that this form of dermatitis runs in families, and it frequently appears in individuals with parkinsonism. What-

ever its causes, seborrheic dermatitis tends to flare up during emotional or physical stress.

The actual cause of *acne rosacea* is not known. However, the rash regularly increases if the victim's face flushes repeatedly, as with drinking hot coffee or eating hot, spicy foods. Although folklore links alcoholism with the red nose of rosacea, the main effect of alcohol is simply to stimulate flushing. Untreated secondary bacterial infection of the inflamed skin nodules may lead to scarring or pitting.

Intertrigo seems to begin as local inflammation caused by prolonged friction of skin that is softened by excessive heat and moisture. Skin wastes and bacterial products collect in these inflamed areas, leading to more irritating reactions that often extend deeper into the skin.

HOW CAN SKIN RASHES AFFECT YOU?

Beauty may be only skin-deep, but extensive or unsightly rashes tend to make both victim and onlooker anxious and uneasy. In addition, most forms of dermatitis cause itching, which adds to the existing discomfort and tension.

With prompt and effective treatment, seborrheic dermatitis and intertrigo may heal with no traces. Persistent or severe acne rosacea may, if not treated vigorously, leave the skin of the face thickened, scarred, and discolored.

Any rash that breaks the protecting surface of the skin may permit bacteria, yeast, and fungi to attack deeper areas. In such cases, boils may form, and bloodstream infection may occur. Infection in the skin near the eyes or nose is especially serious, since it can permanently damage surrounding tissues.

None of these common rashes or pigment changes is known to lead to skin cancers.

Consult Your Doctor Now IF

- A new or unexplained skin rash spreads, especially if it affects the skin near the eyes or nose.

- A skin rash becomes secondarily infected—with local areas of warmth, tenderness, swelling, and increased redness—or if fever and chills develop.

- Your usual medication is no longer effective in controlling the skin rash or if the skin irritation seems to increase.

Goals of Care

- To recognize and understand the nature of common skin rashes and discolorations.

- To design and use treatment programs for specific skin rashes to promote healing, prevent complications, and avoid recurrences.

Self-Care Techniques

- Carry out a skin survey (see page 164) and become familiar with your skin and its problem areas.

- Learn to recognize the *earliest* signs of flare-ups—for example, a small red spot of acne rosacea on your cheek or the first patch of intertrigo in your groin. Delays in recognition may make the difference between a few days of simple treatment and weeks of frustrating effort.

- Make the prescribed treatments an important but routine part of your daily activities. For example, apply cold-water compresses to areas of itching intertrigo while watching the morning and evening TV news, and always allow time for your coffee and tea to cool to avoid the flush-and-flare effects of acne rosacea.

- If a prescribed treatment program seems ineffective, carry out a simple experiment: (1) Select a small, inconspicuous area of the skin rash; (2) if possible, circle it with a fine felt marking pen; (3) avoid treating it for several days; and then (4) compare its appearance to that of treated areas. If the untreated area appears the same as the treated areas, the prescribed treatment is obviously not working. If the untreated area looks better than the treated areas, the treatment may be having an adverse effect. In either case, consult your doctor or other health professional.

■ SKIN TUMORS

The Latin word *tumor* means "a swelling or lump." Most skin tumors of adults are essentially harmless—"benign" in medical terms. A significant number, however, have the capacity to spread and grow into normal skin and into the muscle and bone below it. These tumors are malignant, or cancerous.

All adults have one or more skin tumors, and many have dozens, so the basic challenge is to distinguish harmless from malignant tumors.

Four types of harmless tumors are especially common in persons over fifty years of age. These types are seborrheic keratoses, skin tabs, cherry angiomas, and sebaceous hyperplasias.

Seborrheic keratoses are circular, buttonlike, brownish black, waxy-looking, pebbled tumors found most often on the face, neck, and trunk. Approximately 90 percent of people past middle age have seborrheic keratoses tumors. *Skin tabs*, or tags, are fleshy, sacklike, painless little lumps of normal-appearing skin that tend to develop on the face, neck, chest, and arms. *Cherry angiomas* are pinhead-sized, flat, reddish purple spots that appear most often on the trunk. *Sebaceous hyperplasias* appear as small, soft, yellowish bumps over the face, especially the forehead. These tumors are benign growths of the oil-producing glands of the skin.

Skin cancers, which make up more than 50 percent of all cancers in the United States, develop most often in sun-exposed areas of the skin such as the face, ears, neck, or hands. A majority of these cancers begin as small, reddish, painless nodules that may bleed or become ulcerated as they enlarge. Unlike benign tumors, most cancers feel firm or hard to the touch, and they tend to enlarge and grow into surrounding structures. A few skin cancers arise from the brownish-colored pigment cells that make up common moles. These tumors, melanomas, are especially dangerous, for they may grow rapidly and tend to spread to lymph glands and other areas of the body.

WHAT CAUSES SKIN TUMORS?

No single or specific cause is known for either harmless or malignant tumors of the skin, but several interesting facts have now been established. First of all, the incidence and prevalence of skin tumors (and of most skin cancers) increases steadily after age forty and probably decreases somewhat after age eighty. Thus, aging itself is a factor.

Second, people who are fair (blond or red hair, light skin, and blue eyes) are especially susceptible to skin tumors, whereas dark-skinned people are relatively resistant. Third, the common malignant tumors occur most often in areas of skin that have been exposed to sunlight (to ultraviolet rays) for many years—areas such as the face, the ears, the neck, and the hands. Finally, some skin tumors tend to arise from skin that has been irritated for years—for example, on the nose under the frame of glasses or in skin near some chronic infection.

Although most skin cancers do not develop from the four previously mentioned benign tumors, melanomas often arise from pigmented moles that have seemed "innocent" for years.

HOW CAN SKIN TUMORS AFFECT YOU?

Benign tumors present no health hazard, but rather a cosmetic problem. Since these tumors tend to appear on the face, neck, and arms, many people attempt to remove them or cover them with various powders, creams, or lotions. True cancers of the skin, small and inconspicuous at first, must be treated with respect. The abnormal cells may invade surrounding skin, burrow into underlying muscle and bone, and escape to nearby lymph glands (the term *rodent ulcer* captures their behavior quite well). Even after apparently successful surgical removal of skin cancer, the cancer-bearing areas should be examined regularly, for tumor cells may remain behind in the scar. Equally important, the discovery of one cancer in sun-damaged skin increases the chance of a second malignant tumor.

Consult Your Doctor Now <u>IF</u>

- You have a new or unexplained skin lump, ulcer, or sore that has been present two weeks or more.
- You have an unusual or changing skin spot in an area of irritation or sun-damaged skin (see page 163).
- You feel that a mole is changing—that is, enlarging, bleeding or oozing, changing color or shape, or itching.

Goals of Care

- To prevent the development (or further development) of unattractive benign tumors and malignant cancers.
- To recognize and treat promptly all cancers of the skin.

Self-Care Techniques

- Begin a sun-protection program by following commonsense rules for exposure, wearing a hat, and using an effective sunscreen (see pages 166–167).
- Carry out a skin survey: (1) In a brightly lit room, with skin surfaces well exposed, examine all sun-exposed skin, paying particular attention to areas such as the forehead, a bald head, the ears, the nose, the eyelids, the lips, and the backs of the hands and forearms. (2) Make a note, perhaps by drawing a sketch of each area, of each skin abnormality, recording its size, color, and feel, and the presence of itching, scaling, or bleeding. (3) Continue the skin survey to include *all* areas of your body if you find lumps or tumors of the sorts described earlier. (4) If any of the lumps you have mapped is anything but "classical," or typical, make an appointment for an examination by a primary physician or dermatologist. (5) Repeat appropriate parts of this survey in eight to ten weeks. If you detect any significant change in any of the original tumors, consult your physician. The physician will examine all skin changes carefully and may urge you to have a tiny piece of the changed skin, or lesion, removed for microscopic examination (a biopsy). If this simple test shows definite or possible cancerous changes, the entire lump should be removed by freezing (liquid nitrogen) or by a surgical procedure under local anesthesia. Unlike many cancers, cancers of the skin can be seen, diagnosed, and cured.
- Follow medical advice in treating any benign skin tumors.

SUN-DAMAGED SKIN

Many undesirable, even disfiguring changes in the skin after middle age result from the action of the sun's rays on the skin. Most of what is termed premature aging in the skin of the face and hands is, in fact, damage produced by years of exposure to the effects of ultraviolet (UV) rays of sunlight.

The most familiar and obvious form of sun damage is sunburn. Within hours after overexposure to the sun's rays, the skin becomes red, painful, and sensitive to the touch. Suntan, a darkening and thickening of the outer skin layers, begins several days after exposure and deepens through the next two to three weeks.

Injury to deeper layers of the skin results in a loss of the skin's elasticity and in the formation of fine and coarse wrinkles. Color changes are especially prominent in people with fair complexions. Freckles and the larger tan "liver spots" may appear and alternate with spotty areas of white skin over the face, hands, and forearms. Sun damage to tiny blood vessels in the skin leads to dilation of tiny facial veins and thus to easy bruising.

Then, years and sometimes decades later, the more dramatic and even dangerous sun-related problems appear. The damaged skin becomes rough or dry to the touch, often with thick, scaly, red patches known as actinic (sun-caused) keratoses. More important, the sun-damaged areas of the skin are the most common sites of both benign and cancerous tumors (see pages 162–164).

WHAT CAUSES SUN-DAMAGED SKIN?

The type and severity of exposure-related damage depend on both the nature of the exposure and the person involved. Most experts now agree that the most damaging rays from the sun are the ultraviolet rays (so-called UV-A and UV-B bands). Ultraviolet rays are the energy-containing beams that are not visible to us as light. Individual skin cells and fibers are injured by exposures to ultraviolet light, and repair is often incomplete. Therefore, repeated heavy doses of sunlight lead to an accumulation of skin damage. Ultraviolet rays are only partly blocked by clouds and window glass. They may be reflected back to the skin by white sand, water, and snow.

Individuals vary tremendously in their ability to tolerate such irradiation. The dark pigment cells of normal skin either block or absorb much of the radiation from ultraviolet rays. Therefore, blacks and dark-skinned Asians rarely burn and subsequently develop far fewer later complications from sun-damaged skin. Blonds and redheads are notoriously sensitive to the ill effects of sun exposure. In addition, long hair helps protect the scalp from sun damage. Finally, certain drugs (for example tetracycline, thiazide diuretics, and some tranquilizers) tend to sensitize skin to the action of ultraviolet rays (so-called photosensitivity). Therefore, even very brief exposure to the sun may result in violent skin reactions.

HOW CAN SUN-DAMAGED SKIN AFFECT YOU?

Most adults are all too well acquainted with the effects of severe sunburn. The involved areas of skin are painful, tender, and swollen for twelve to twenty-four hours. The skin may blister; in a few days, peeling, or shedding, of dead skin takes place. Extensive sunburn, especially in fair people, may cause serious illness with fever, weakness, and fainting.

Years after the last summer tan has faded, the thinning, drying, and wrinkling of sun-damaged skin begin to appear. These changes, along with benign tumors (see pages 162–164), often have a serious effect on appearance and morale, prompting costly searches for magic creams or other potions that will somehow restore youthful complexions.

The most serious late effects of prolonged sun exposure are growths, or skin cancers. Ninety percent of skin cancers are directly related to earlier sun damage. These malignant tumors, which are often multiple, tend to be slow-growing. However, if not treated properly, they may cause serious disease and even death.

■ Consult Your Doctor Now __IF__

- You have a one- or two-day-old sunburn that affects more than one-quarter of your skin surface or is accompanied by fever and other general symptoms.
- An unexplained spot or lump on a sun-exposed area of your skin has persisted for more than two weeks.

- A skin tumor or patch is changing—that is, the patch is enlarging, bleeding, or oozing, changing color or shape, or itching.

■ Goals of Care

- To prevent additional sun-related damage to exposed skin.
- To detect possible skin cancers early.

■ Self-Care Techniques

- Protect yourself from (more) sun exposure, for evidence now suggests that some damage can be reversed: (1) Keep exposure to direct or indirect sun rays to a minimum. Avoid outdoor activities during the brightest part of the day (10:00 A.M. to 2:00 P.M.), especially in the summer. Beware of reflected ultraviolet rays from sand, water, or snow. (2) Cover exposed areas when in the sunlight; bald heads, the tips of ears, the face, and the arms are most at risk. (3) Be especially careful about exposure to direct sunlight if you are taking drugs such as tetracycline, thiazide diuretics, and certain tranquilizers.
- Use a special sunscreen cream or lotion that is effective for your skin type.
  1. Determine your skin type. Type I is the most sensitive, sure-to-burn skin of redheads. Type VI is the resistant, never-burn skin of blacks and some Asians. Most people fall in the middle range of II to V.
  2. Find the proper sunscreen for your skin type. Effective screens are

graded by the Sun Protection Factor (SPF) ratings, which range from 2 to 15. Redheads (Type I) and blonds (Type II) should rely on screens rated as 15 (for example, PreSun 15 and Total Eclipse). Dark-skinned people who always tan (Types IV and V) may use preparations with lower ratings such as 6 (for example, Pabafilm and Block Out).

3. Apply the cream or liquid generously to high-risk areas of skin before going outdoors. Reapply the screen after swimming or perspiring heavily.

4. If the screen produces burning or a rash (see pages 160–162), consult your doctor or ask your druggist for another type of screening agent.

■ Carry out a skin survey (see page 164).

The Eyes and Vision

■ VISUAL LOSS

Normal vision depends on the proper functioning of a set of very complex and delicate structures in the eye (see figure 1). First, light rays from objects reach the outer transparent surface (cornea) of the eyeball. These light rays are then funneled through the rounded opening (pupil) to the lens. The lens is a crystal-clear disc that further bends light rays and focuses them on the retinal layer. The retinal layer—a very thin, delicate membrane made up of light-sensitive cells—transforms the light rays into electric, or nerve, impulses. These impulses then travel along the optic nerve to the brain, allowing a person to "see" a visual image.

Improper functioning of any of these elements may cause some form of visual loss. The loss can vary. It may be a temporary one, caused by mild injury, or a permanent one. Visual loss is not always obvious to the affected person; for example, glaucoma may cause loss of sizable areas of vision before the person realizes it. Fortunately, people can compensate or make up for most early forms of eye difficulty with eyeglasses. Thus vision may be quite good despite visual changes.

WHAT CAUSES VISUAL LOSS?

By age fifty most people, as a result of the aging process, have the following minor changes or losses in vision: a decrease in the sharpness (or acuity) of vision, a decline in the ability to see small objects clearly, and an increasing difficulty in distinguishing objects of similar shades of lightness or darkness. A motorist, for example, may have

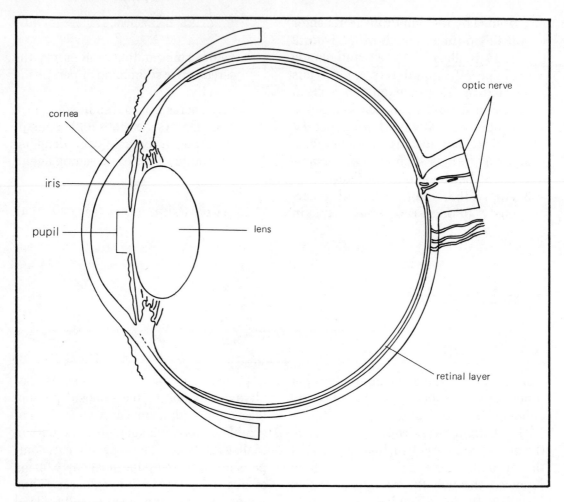

Figure 1.   The healthy eye

trouble distinguishing the figure of a pedestrian standing in front of a background hedge. However, there is no need for alarm, since these features of normal aging are not causes of blindness. Also, blindness and/or eye damage are *not* caused by eyestrain from reading, improper glasses, or poor lighting.

Three diseases of the eye—cataracts, glaucoma, and senile macular degeneration—are, however, of great importance,

for they are the most common causes of partial or total blindness in adults. All three can be treated if recognized early. Cataracts, or clouding of the lenses, may affect up to three-quarters of the population after age seventy-five (see pages 170–172). Glaucoma, a condition that damages the retinal layers and nerves of the eye by increased fluid pressure within the eyeball, can lead to blindness if not detected early (see pages 174–176).

Senile macular degeneration is scarring of the most sensitive area of the retinal layers (see pages 177–178). Almost 10 percent of people aged sixty-five and older have evidence of this condition.

Many other diseases can damage some part of one or both eyes and affect vision. In addition, the eye lens can be impaired from direct injuries such as from a blow, from strong chemicals, from intense sunlight, or from electrical shock. Certain general medical conditions such as diabetes, high blood pressure, temporal arteritis, and drug reactions can cause a decrease in visual acuity.

HOW CAN VISUAL LOSS AFFECT YOU?

Most conditions that cause visual loss in adults tend to progress slowly and to affect both eyes. As a result, most people adapt or adjust to visual loss. Tasks requiring sharp vision are avoided, brighter lights are used for reading, and corrective over-the-counter glasses are changed. In some cases, unfortunately, this adjustment leads to serious delays in diagnosis and treatment.

Partial visual loss affects people in very different ways. Many young persons who rely heavily on full vision may have to make major changes in their personal and professional lives. Numerous older persons, retired and less competitive, may accept some loss of sight gracefully by modifying their work and recreational habits; sharing more responsibility with family and friends; and learning to make use of special glasses, large-print publications, and other aids.

A few persons, especially the socially isolated and very old, find visual loss a terrible burden and become seriously depressed.

▰ Consult Your Doctor Now IF

- You experience any sudden changes in vision, especially blurring or double vision.
- One or both eyes are red or in pain.
- You see halos around lights at night.
- You receive a direct injury to the eye, such as from a blow or from a strong chemical.

▰ Goals of Care

- To prevent or control conditions that may cause visual loss.
- To restore maximum vision.

▰ Self-Care Techniques

- Arrange for periodic eye examinations. If you have no family or personal history of major eye disease, seek a three-part eye checkup every two years. This should include testing for visual acuity (the usual chart with letters and numbers), direct examination of the inside of the eye (with an ophthalmoscope), and measurement of eye pressure or tension (a painless procedure with a small instrument called a tonometer). If you have a personal or family history of significant eye disease, consult an ophthalmologist and arrange for an annual eye examination.

- Prevent direct damage to your eyes by wearing protective glasses or goggles when exposed to flying objects.

- Take proper care of general medical conditions, such as diabetes and high blood pressure, that may affect your vision.

- Avoid prolonged exposure to direct sunlight or wear protective sunglasses that filter out ultraviolet rays.

- Report any visual difficulties to your doctor or ophthalmologist.

- Once specific eye treatments have been prescribed (eyeglasses, drops, or salves), continue them without interruption unless your doctor or ophthalmologist recommends a change.

■ CATARACTS

Sharp, precise vision depends greatly on the shape and structure of the eye lens. This crystalline lens is a disclike, transparent body that bends and focuses light rays from an object onto the retina, thus allowing vision (see figure 2). The lens, especially during the first four decades of life, is slightly elastic. This elasticity allows the lens to change shape in order to focus clearly on both near and far objects. The lens is said to develop a cataract when it grows progressively denser, has less ability to change shape (focus), and becomes faintly cloudy. Cataracts usually affect both eyes. They develop at widely varying rates, most taking several years to reach a stage of complete cloudiness, or "ripeness." Careful studies indicate that about 90 percent of people over the age of seventy-five have some type of cataract.

WHAT CAUSES CATARACTS?

With advancing age, especially after age fifty, most of the changes seen in the lens—the thickening, hardening, and loss of transparency—seem to be part of the normal aging process. This age-related cataract, known as a "senescent" cataract, is the most common variety of cataract seen in the United States. As a matter of fact, by the age of sixty-five, more than 50 percent of all adults have some signs of cataract development.

For reasons that are not clear, certain groups of adults tend to acquire cataracts at earlier ages. American Indians, persons with diabetes mellitus, and some persons with a history of steroid (for example, cortisone) drug treatment for other medical conditions are known to be at high risk for early lens changes.

Direct injury to the eyeball may lead to the development of a cataract over a period of months or years. A blow to the eye, many types of chemical burns, electrical shocks, and exposure to strong sunlight may damage the lens. In addition, some types of cataracts are present at birth.

HOW CAN CATARACTS AFFECT YOU?

Fortunately, a majority of people with early cataracts experience no significant

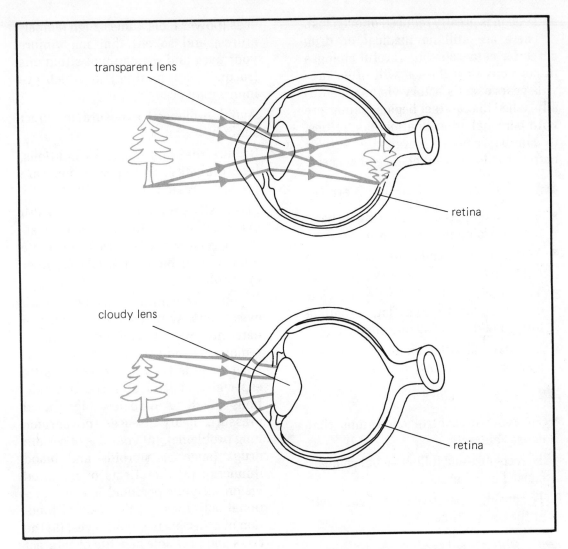

Figure 2. Cataracts affect the ability of the eye to focus. As the lens grows denser, it becomes cloudy or opaque and blocks the passage of light rays.

change in their vision. The cataract is simply discovered during a periodic eye examination. In these cases, the eye doctor, or ophthalmologist, recommends regular follow-up evaluations to monitor visual function.

As the cataract develops and the lens becomes more dense and cloudy, the individual may begin to notice problems with vision. Distant vision is typically more affected, and individuals often describe the problem as blurring, haziness, or "looking through a screen." Some individuals, usually those with cloudiness of the back of the lens, experience a harsh glaring reflection in their eyes that makes reading especially difficult and interferes with outdoor activities. If the cataract is allowed to progress, or "ripen," the entire lens eventually becomes milky, and vision is greatly reduced or even lost.

There are still no medical or drug cures for cataracts, but careful changes in corrective eyeglasses will often provide years of satisfactory vision. Eventually, when the cataract begins to interfere with personal or occupational activities, it can be removed surgically with a better than 95 percent chance of success.

▬ *Consult Your Doctor Now* <u>IF</u>

- You are bothered by blurring or haziness of vision in one or both eyes.

- You note increasing difficulty with night vision.

- You receive a direct injury to your eye, such as from a fist, a ball, a foreign body, or a strong chemical.

- You have diabetes mellitus or hypertension that is poorly controlled.

▬ *Goals of Care*

- To avoid or control conditions that cause cataracts.

- To recognize and follow visual changes caused by cataracts.

- To consider operative cure of cataracts at the proper time.

▬ *Self-Care Techniques*

- Use protective eyeglasses or a mask when exposed to occupational hazards (power tools, fumes, high temperatures, and so on) that may injure your eyes and recreational situations (racquet ball, hunting) in which eye injury may occur.

- Avoid prolonged exposure to direct sunlight.

- Be sure that any medical conditions, like diabetes or hypertension, are properly treated and controlled.

- Establish a program of periodic health examinations that includes vision testing at least every two years (or more often if you have cataracts or other eye problems).

- If you have cataracts in one or both eyes, work with your eye doctor to determine whether and when surgical removal is indicated. Factors to consider include (1) your general health, especially control of medical conditions (such as diabetes, high blood pressure, heart disease, and chronic lung problems); (2) your use of certain drugs (such as steroids and blood thinners); (3) the effects of impaired vision on your personal and occupational activities; (4) the state of function of other parts of your eyes; (5) the risks and probable benefits of cataract removal; and (6) the types of eyeglasses, contact lenses, or implanted lenses that can be used after surgery.

▬ CONJUNCTIVITIS

The conjunctiva is the thin, pinkish, slightly moist layer that covers the white part of the eyeball and lines the inside surfaces of the eyelids (see figure 3). Normally bathed in tears, this remarkable structure protects the eye (and

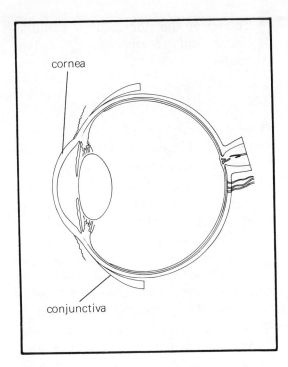

cornea

conjunctiva

Figure 3. Conjunctivitis occurs when the conjunctival surface of the eye becomes irritated and inflamed.

vision) in several ways. First, it traps and washes away irritating particles that might scratch the surface of the cornea. Second, its secretions keep the corneal surface moist and clear. Third, it produces special secretions as needed to kill bacteria and/or to help neutralize toxic chemicals. Conjunctivitis occurs when the conjunctival surface becomes irritated and inflamed.

WHAT CAUSES CONJUNCTIVITIS?

Conjunctivitis is the most common eye disease in the United States. This is understandable, as the conjunctiva is constantly exposed to the environment. Therefore, bacteria and viruses of all sorts lodge in the folds of the conjunctiva, where they may multiply and thus produce inflammation. Direct injury to the surface of the eye (for example, by a foreign body or from scratching) may start irritation; the irritated surface then becomes infected by bacteria. In addition, most chemicals (in solid, liquid, or gas forms) are readily dissolved in eye secretions and can become powerful irritants. Many internal conditions such as allergies or general infections may inflame the conjunctival lining, causing conjunctivitis. Injuries or diseases that interfere with the normal flow of tears predispose to various types of conjunctivitis, and age-related changes in the formation of tears may lead to dryness of the eyes and a conjunctivitis-like condition. Some skin conditions such as acne rosacea (see page 161) cause inflammation of the eyelids and the conjunctival lining. Damage to the surface of the cornea leads to an especially painful form of conjunctivitis.

HOW CAN CONJUNCTIVITIS AFFECT YOU?

Mild conjunctivitis of the sort caused by common viral infections or allergies is simply bothersome. With mild conjunctivitis, the eyelids become red and slightly swollen, and the affected eye feels itchy or scratchy and is plagued by episodes of watery tears, which, if excessive, may interfere with vision. When more serious bacterial infection causes the conjunctivitis, the eyelids are typically bloodshot and fiery red (so-called pinkeye), the tears tend to be cloudy and thicker, and the eye stings or feels raw. At night, the discharge from the eyelids often dries around the lid margins, causing the sticking together of eyelids on awakening. If direct injury or inflammation involves both the conjunctiva and the deeper parts of the eyeball, the symptoms are more striking. The eye is deep red in color, painful to the touch and painful on movement. Direct light often causes pain and blinking, and vision may be slightly blurred or weak.

Most cases of mild or even moderately severe conjunctivitis heal completely, with or without medical treatment. However, the prompt use of antibiotic medications, soaks, and comforting eyewashes does hasten relief. Medical help should be sought when the inflammation is more severe and persists for more than a few days, especially if it produces eye pain and blurring of vision. Severe conjunctivitis can damage the cornea, resulting in patchy loss of vision.

Consult Your Doctor Now IF

- You develop acute conjunctivitis following known or possible direct eye injury from particles, fumes, or heat.
- You have conjunctivitis with pain and light sensitivity in one or both eyes.
- You have conjunctivitis with blurred vision in one or both eyes.

Goals of Care

- To prevent injury or infection that produces conjunctivitis.

- To relieve the symptoms of conjunctivitis and prevent damage to the cornea.

Self-Care Techniques

- Protect your eyes from chemical, particle, and fume irritation by using proper goggles or safety glasses.
- If an irritant enters your eyes, act immediately to irrigate the eye(s) with large volumes of cool water until the irritation subsides. Do *not* use chemical antidotes. Then cover the inflamed or irritated eye with cold, moist compresses for twenty minutes of each hour. Consult your doctor promptly.
- Avoid the use of handkerchiefs, towels, or gloves that have been used by other individuals with acute conjunctivitis.
- Avoid rubbing your eyes with your hands or any objects that have been in contact with sores or infected areas of the skin.
- If acute conjunctivitis is mild and not caused by direct injury, follow these procedures: (1) Apply cold compresses every three hours and as required for itching. (2) Gently rinse your eye(s) each morning and evening with a mild sterile solution (such as Murine, Visine, Liquifilm Tears, or Tears Plus). (3) Cover the affected eye(s) with a soft cloth patch if it is sensitive to light or air.

■ GLAUCOMA

A small amount of clear, colorless fluid normally fills the space between the corneal surface and the front part of the lens of the eye (see figure 4). Formed

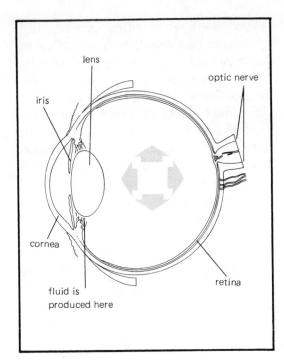

lens

optic nerve

iris

cornea

retina

fluid is
produced here

Figure 4. Glaucoma is a combination of high fluid pressure in the eye, nerve damage, and visual loss.

before one has even noticed any visual loss. Glaucoma ranks as a major cause of blindness. It occurs mainly in the population of persons fifty years of age and older, and in many cases much eye damage is preventable with routine eye checkups.

WHAT CAUSES GLAUCOMA?

Any condition that damages the filtering canal, which lies along the angle between the back of the cornea and the front of the iris, may lead to glaucoma. A few glaucomas are "secondary" to direct injury to the eye or to local infections. However, the majority of glaucoma cases are "primary"; that is, they develop without obvious, previous injury. The most common form of primary glaucoma is called open-angle glaucoma because the filtering canal appears open even though it is scarred or narrowed deeper in the eye. The filtration blockage and elevated eye pressure may exist and increase very slowly for many years before the abnormal pressure begins to destroy the vital retinal and nerve tissues. Even then, the destruction and resulting patchy loss of vision may go unnoticed, and the diagnosis is often not made until the person is permanently and almost totally blind in the eye. Many people with open-angle glaucoma have a strong family history of this condition. It is now known that use of corticosteroids may precipitate damage in susceptible people.

behind the iris, or colored part of the eye, this fluid flows out through a narrow filtering canal behind the margins of the cornea.

Any blockage of the delicate filtering canal prevents normal drainage. If blockage occurs, pressure, or tension, within the front of the eye builds up as the fluid continues to be formed but is unable to drain properly. This high pressure soon damages the sensitive retinal layers of the optic nerve, thus causing progressive loss of sight. The combination of high fluid pressure, nerve damage, and loss of sight is called glaucoma. Glaucoma is a particularly bad disease, for the eye damage is irreparable, and there are no forewarning early symptoms. Therefore, much of the eye impairment occurs

Some primary glaucomas are called acute angle-closure glaucomas because the filtration angle is blocked by a swelling, or pushing forward, of the iris.

The pushing forward is probably a life-long defect, one that predisposes to closing of the angle. Sudden change, by actions of drugs like antidepressants, narrows the angle even more. Patients with this condition apparently have small or shallow eye spaces behind the cornea, an abnormality that causes no difficulty until the iris is suddenly pushed forward against the edge of the cornea. Then, as eye pressure rises rapidly to very high levels, the affected eye becomes inflamed, its tissues undergo rapid and serious injury, and vision is threatened. Without prompt treatment, acute glaucoma produces permanent blindness. Some attacks of acute angle-closure glaucoma are brought on by drugs that dilate the pupils of the eyes—drugs such as those used in treating nasal congestion (for example, Neo-Synephrine and Sudafed) or diarrhea (for example, Lomotil).

HOW CAN GLAUCOMA AFFECT YOU?

The slightly increased eye pressure of open-angle glaucoma produces no symptoms and may persist for years before retinal layer and nerve cells are destroyed. Then, although tiny blind spots develop around the field of vision, the glaucoma may progress unnoticed until only a small island of vision remains. *Early detection is essential!*

The picture of acute angle-closure glaucoma is quite different. Here, the sudden rise in eye pressure causes blurring of vision, the appearance of rings around lights, and severe pain in and around the eyeball, often accompanied by nausea and vomiting. The surface of the involved eye appears foggy or cloudy, and the eyeball becomes red and inflamed. Without prompt treatment, acute glaucoma causes complete blindness in a matter of hours or days. It is important to realize that 50 percent of the persons stricken with acute glaucoma will experience an attack in the "normal," or second eye, within weeks of the original illness.

▆▆ *Consult Your Doctor Now **IF***

- You have sudden pain or blurring of vision in either eye.
- You are aware of any blind spots in your vision or have difficulty seeing objects located at the edge of your vision.

▆▆ *Goals of Care*

- To detect abnormally high eye pressure before loss of vision occurs.
- To prevent eye damage and visual loss by proper treatment of glaucoma.

▆▆ *Self-Care Techniques*

- Continue treatment exactly as directed, since omission of medication may lead to a sudden rise in eye pressure.
- Do not take new medications without first consulting your doctor, druggist, or other health professional.
- Be certain that members of your immediate family (brothers, sisters, and children) have their eye pressures checked regularly.

■ SENILE MACULAR DEGENERATION

Senile macular degeneration (SMD) is the scarring of the most sensitive area of the eye, the central retinal zone. SMD is the combination of loss of retinal cells and impaired vision. The retinal layer is a very thin, delicate membrane that lines the inside of the back of the eyeball (see figure 1). The retinal layer is made up of specialized nerve cells that are remarkably sensitive to light. The lens focuses rays of light from outside objects onto the retinal cell layers, causing some cells to register black or white and others to register various colors. Nourished by tiny blood vessels entering the back of the eyeball, the cells of the retinal layer are easily damaged by almost any change in nourishment.

Normal aging of the eye involves weakness and gradual loss of some of these retinal cells. Research studies have shown that more than one-third of biologically normal persons age sixty-five to seventy-four had significant changes in retinal cells. Some of these individuals had measurable loss of visual acuity as well.

Most adults with SMD experience slow, almost unnoticeable loss of sight as retinal cells weaken and die. After years of progression, the damage of SMD may destroy central vision in one or both eyes, leaving the person greatly disabled for reading. Other people have more rapid retinal cell loss and scarring, and legal blindness may develop in both eyes in a matter of weeks.

SMD is now the leading cause of blindness in the over-sixty-five population. Approximately 10 percent of persons sixty-five and older have evidence of some senile macular degeneration. Early recognition and vigorous treatment of certain forms of SMD will stop or slow its progression, but no therapy now available will restore sight. *Therefore, prevention is essential!*

WHAT CAUSES SENILE MACULAR DEGENERATION?

The actual cause of SMD is unknown. While it is clear that some retinal cell loss occurs during normal aging, the extensive damage and scarring in the center of retinal layers are distinctly abnormal. Changes in small blood vessels that nourish the light-sensitive cells have been seen. However, the changes in these small blood vessels are not known to be a result of such diseases as high blood pressure, stroke, hardening of the arteries, or diabetes.

With rare exceptions, SMD does not run in families, or, rather, it is not hereditary.

HOW CAN SENILE MACULAR DEGENERATION AFFECT YOU?

Since this condition destroys nerve cells in the central, most sensitive part of the retinal layers, distortion and loss of central vision are the most prominent features. Early in the course of SMD, the individual may complain only of slight blurring of vision while reading, especially when reading under bright lights. Because the outline of objects cannot be focused sharply on the scarred retina, many persons note ᵗ at straight objects like doors or fences appear wavy or curved.

As SMD progresses, central vision in one or both eyes fails, eventually leaving large blind spots in the areas where vision should be sharpest. Even with advanced disease and legal blindness, persons with SMD can see well enough to the side (side vision) to walk and do unskilled work.

Recent advances in laser treatment techniques permit expert ophthalmologists to seal or coagulate the areas of retinal damage in selected cases of SMD. Early detection of progressive SMD and careful laser treatment will stop or slow visual loss in more than half the persons treated. Other medical and surgical therapies have not been effective, but many devices are now available to help compensate for the visual loss (for example, special glasses, hand lenses, and large-print publications).

Consult Your Doctor Now IF

- You have begun to experience trouble-some blurring of vision while reading or doing fine work.
- Straight objects like fence posts and doors seem wavy or curved.
- You have a history of significant visual loss in one eye.

Goals of Care

- To detect senile macular degeneration before significant visual loss has occurred.
- To prevent senile macular degeneration from progressing to the point of blindness.

Self-Care Techniques

- Arrange for periodic eye examinations (see page 169).
- Be alert for problems such as blurring of vision while reading or looking at faces, or curving and unevenness of straight objects.
- If you have had laser treatment for senile macular degeneration, maintain a regular examination schedule with your ophthalmologist and check your visual acuity at home with a lined card or grid, following instructions from the doctor.

The Ears and Hearing

■ DEAFNESS

Normal hearing depends on proper functioning of a complicated apparatus—the human ear. Physical structures in the middle ear (the eardrum and a chain of small bones) capture sound waves for a wide variety of sounds, amplify them, and change these sound waves into fluid waves. Inner nerve elements respond to these waves and convert them into electrical signals, which travel to the brain, where they then become recognized and understood (see figure 5).

Deafness or hearing loss refers to (1) the loss of sensitivity of one or both ears to some or all sounds ("Speak up. I can't hear you!") and (2) the loss of selectivity or understanding of sounds ("Talk slower. I can't make out your meaning!").

Deafness can involve either one or both types of the aforementioned hearing losses. Most deaf or hearing-impaired persons are not totally deaf; they can still hear certain types of sounds. Therefore, the majority of individuals may

benefit from the use of hearing aids. In addition, hearing tests (audiograms) show that most normal older persons have a slight loss of hearing for high-pitched sounds.

However, any hearing loss that interferes with personal or social activities is definitely abnormal and should be evaluated carefully. Also, hearing problems that are accompanied by ringing in the ears (tinnitus) or dizziness (vertigo) always require medical care.

WHAT CAUSES DEAFNESS?

Most hearing loss in older persons results from very slow damage to nerve cells in

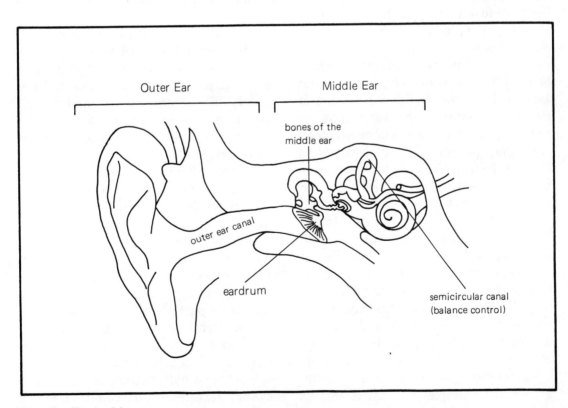

Figure 5. The healthy ear

the inner ear. This normal hearing loss, known as presbycusis, usually affects both ears equally and tends to run in families. Typically, this hearing impairment is not recognized for months or years by the affected person. Individuals with this condition complain that some sounds, especially high-pitched ones (for example, soprano voices), seem faint or dim. However, their main problem lies in distinguishing spoken words. Noisy surroundings increase their difficulty in hearing accurately.

Hearing loss may result, in some instances, from the damage of prolonged exposure to loud noises. Many studies have shown that miners, construction workers, and truck drivers have more late-life deafness, especially if no precautions were taken to protect their ears from the sound damage associated with their work.

An important, and often curable, cause or poor hearing is blockage of the outer ear canal. Earwax buildup, infection of the skin lining of the ear canal, or plugging by cotton swabs or small blood clots may produce partial deafness in one ear. Here, all sounds are decreased, and the affected ear may feel stuffy or full (pages 183–184).

Some adults are partially deaf in one or both ears as a result of repeated or prolonged infections of the middle ear during childhood. A history of earaches, draining ears, and perforated eardrums may be clues to this problem. Fortunately, unlike infants and children, older adults rarely develop acute or severe middle ear infections that affect hearing.

Certain drugs—neomycin and gentamycin, for example—can cause serious and lasting deafness, while others, like aspirin, can produce a temporary decrease in hearing and ringing in the ears if taken in too large a dose.

Many other less common conditions, from nerve tumors to changes in skull bones, can damage hearing.

HOW CAN DEAFNESS AFFECT YOU?

Most people fail to appreciate the magic of hearing until they begin to lose their hearing. Their daily lives are engulfed by a sea of sounds that keep them alert, delight them, educate them, and generally keep them aware of their world. They can compensate for mild hearing losses by careful listening or watching for visual cues, but loss of hearing acuity soon becomes a burden and a frustration.

As the hearing disability increases, the individual often becomes suspicious, socially isolated, and even depressed. In some cases, job performance suffers, family life becomes tense, and friends begin to question the person's mental health. On occasion, failure to hear leads to serious traffic accidents.

Many conditions that damage the physical structures—conditions such as middle-ear infections and ruptured eardrums—can be treated and remedied by medical or surgical means. Permanent damage to the sensitive nerve cells and fibers, however, such as occurs following prolonged exposures to loud noises and/or as part of the normal process of aging, often requires the use of an artificial booster—the hearing aid, one of the miracles of modern medical technology. While this small, battery-driven device cannot restore the nerve's function, it does provide a substitute channel for the sound passage and helps strengthen the impulse that reaches the brain.

More than three-quarters of older people with permanent hearing loss can benefit from the use of a hearing aid. One study showed that careful personal instruction in the use of aids reduced the nonuser rate from 20 percent to 3 percent. Yet only about one in five hearing-impaired adults actually wears one! Vanity, anxiety, and a lack of understanding seem to account for this reluctance to wear the device. In general, once significant deafness is recognized as a problem or disability, expert advice from the individual's personal physician or from an ear specialist (audiologist or otolaryngologist) should be sought before the disability becomes oppressive and limits the person's ability to relate to others.

Basic elements of the hearing aid include a microphone, an amplifier, a receiver or earphone, an ear mold, and a power battery (see figure 6). The microphone, the outermost part, serves to pick up or receive sound waves (like the cuplike part of the ear) and convert them into electrical impulses. Powered by the tiny battery, the amplifier increases the intensity of these sound waves as needed. Then these electrical impulses, or signals, are converted once again to sound waves by the receiver unit, which directs them into the outer ear canal through the ear mold. From there, the sounds move along normal pathways to reach the eardrum.

Hearing aids are adjusted to the special needs of each user by controls that affect loudness and sensitivity. Modern aids may fit directly into the outer ear, behind the ear, or into the frames of special eyeglasses.

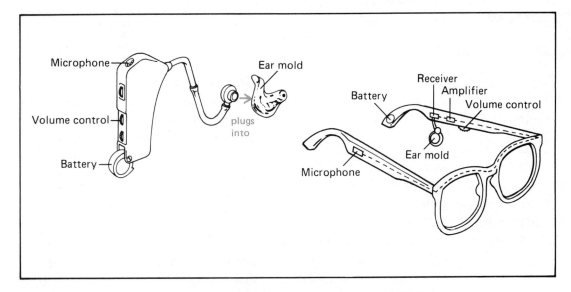

Figure 6. The hearing aid on the left shows a popular model that fits behind the ear; the one on the right is built into the frame of special eyeglasses.

Most people with a moderate degree of deafness, especially those who are eager to improve their hearing for personal or professional reasons, experience improvement. Faint sounds are now easily heard, and "fuzzy" conversations become sharp and clear. Others find that uncomfortably loud or harsh sounds are filtered out by the hearing aid. Many previously skeptical hearing aid users report that "life is real again," even though normal hearing has not been restored.

Other helpful devices are being developed every day. Fire alarms and other warning devices for the deaf may be installed in homes. Special amplifiers and teletypewriters are now available for improving telephone use. (Additional helpful information can be obtained from organizations like the American Speech-Language-Hearing Association, Rockville, Maryland, and Self-Help for Hard of Hearing People, Inc., Washington, D.C.)

Consult Your Doctor Now IF

- You think you are becoming deaf. There are simple tests that could be a part of your regular checkup. If there is evidence of impaired hearing, you should have an examination by a specialist (otolaryngologist) in addition to full audiometer testing.

- You develop *sudden* hearing loss in one or both ears, that is, a decrease in hearing that intensifies within a matter of days to weeks.

- You experience hearing loss associated with ringing in the ear, dizziness, pain in the ear, headache, or escape of fluid from the ear.

- You have a head injury, and it leads to hearing loss.

- You cannot hear a wristwatch ticking two to three inches from each ear.

Goals of Care

- To maintain optimum natural hearing.

- To determine whether a hearing aid will improve hearing loss significantly.

- To restore maximum hearing by effective use of modern hearing aid devices.

Self-Care Techniques

- Avoid exposure to loud or painful sounds, such as from explosions, large machines, jets, and drills. If this exposure is unavoidable, always wear approved earplugs or ear guards.

- Never attempt to remove earwax with mechanical objects, such as cotton swabs or paper clips. For earwax extraction, follow the warnings and steps on how to irrigate the ear given on page 184.

- If your family or friends have commented on your lack of hearing, poor attention, or failure to respond, or if you, yourself, are aware of difficulties in hearing or in understanding common sounds (for example, conversations and television programs), seek medical advice.

- If you have been diagnosed by a doctor as having a hearing deficit, discuss the pros and cons of hearing aids with him or her. If indicated, a carefully selected hearing aid should be obtained, and you should be given training in its use. The final decision about using one of the several types available to you is yours, so educate yourself fully and be prepared to work for better hearing.

■ If you choose to use a professionally fitted hearing aid, be aware that your personal physician must evaluate your general medical status to rule out contraindications to the use of a hearing aid. In addition, each hearing aid must meet very strict federal performance standards. You may want or need a hearing aid orientation and čounseling program, a series of personalized discussions and demonstrations that can help you obtain maximum benefit from the hearing aid.

■ EARWAX BLOCKAGE

The specialized skin cells that cover the bony outer ear canal manufacture wax, or cerumen—a yellowish, dense, sticky material that tends to accumulate inside the ear canal. Normally as wax builds up, its outer surfaces exposed to air turn brownish black, become hard in consistency, and tend to stick to the lining of the canal. In time this exposed wax dries, forming flakes or particles that are then discharged through the outer ear opening. If the hardened wax accumulates, the narrow ear canal may become obstructed or blocked, with interruption of the passage of sound waves to the drum.

Earwax's stickiness and waterproof properties make it an excellent protective barrier for the sensitive ear canal and eardrum. Dirt, insects, and other foreign bodies are trapped in the wax and are eventually pushed out from the canal. Water droplets are kept out by air bubbles that form between the wax and the ear canal wall.

WHAT CAUSES EARWAX BLOCKAGE?

The bony structure of the ear canal, as well as the rate of wax formation, varies greatly among individuals. As a result, some people with very narrow ear canals tend to build up wax plugs rapidly. As the wax accumulates, the air-filled tunnel that connects the eardrum with the outside world progressively closes until complete blockage occurs.

Wax buildup and blockage are especially likely to occur in people who are sick, weak, and not aware of their increasing problem.

HOW CAN EARWAX BLOCKAGE AFFECT YOU?

Since conduction of sound waves from the environment to the eardrum depends on an open ear canal, complete obstruction by wax (or any other material) decreases hearing acuity. Typically, the blocked ear feels stuffy or full, and all sounds seem distant or muffled.

Occasionally the wax becomes extremely dry and hard, and it may actually injure the lining skin, with resulting inflammation, infection, and pain.

All too often, attempts are made to remove harmless wax with objects such as cotton swabs or paper clips with injurious results. These attempts can often scratch the lining of the ear canal, producing bleeding and sharp pain, or wedge hardened wax against the eardrum, leading to hearing difficulties and/or the pain of an earache.

■ Consult Your Doctor Now IF

- Hearing loss or stuffiness of your ear has lasted more than three or four days.
- Pain and soreness or bleeding from your ear occurs.
- Probing with an instrument has produced decreased hearing.
- You think a foreign body has blocked your ear canal.

■ Goal of Care

- To prevent or correct blockage of ear canals.

■ Self-Care Technique

- Irrigate the ear. Follow these warnings and steps.

Caution: Never irrigate your ear or put drops in your ear canal if you have any history of middle-ear infections or drum perforation unless directly approved by your doctor or nurse. If in doubt, have your ears examined before irrigation.

Step 1: Hardened wax blocking the ear canal may be softened by gently dropping four or five drops of an ear solution containing peroxide and glycerin into the ear canal. (Do not put the tip of the dropper inside the ear canal.) Insert a small plug of soft cotton into the ear to prevent leakage of the solution. This should be repeated two to three times each day for about four days. The softened wax should then escape. Use of the ear drops once each week should prevent another blockage.

Step 2: If the obstruction is not relieved after four days of treatment, you may float the loosened material out by *gently* irrigating the ear canal with one tablespoonful of slightly warm (95°–105° F) water. Draw the warm water into the ear syringe; then gently squirt it in a slightly circular motion into the canal. Allow the ear to drain. (Caution: The use of colder or warmer water may produce dizziness.)

Step 3: If gentle irrigation does not remove the wax, consult your doctor, for wax and other material may have become wedged against the canal wall.

Teeth and Gums

■ *PERIODONTAL DISEASE*

The normal adult tooth—often considered a dull, lifeless rock—is, in fact, a living jewel! The enamel, its whitish outer cap, is the hardest material in the human body. Both the tooth and its enamel are beautifully suited for the function of chewing (see figure 7). The roots of the tooth are firmly embedded in the gum and are surrounded and supported by the cementing substance, the periodontal ("around the tooth") ligament, and the jawbone. With proper care and preventive measures, most persons should enjoy good dental health well into advanced age.

Unfortunately, even though dental science has gone far toward conquering caries (cavities) in the young, periodontal disease continues to be the leading cause of tooth loss, especially in persons over thirty-five. Bacterial organisms, mouth secretions, and food particles stick to the tooth surfaces as dental plaque. In time, toxic materials from the plaque work their way downward through the gum, where they inflame and destroy the critical supporting tissues that nourish and protect the tooth. The gums become swollen and red, bleeding occurs, teeth are loosened, cavities form in the roots nerves are inflamed, and unpleasant tastes are experienced. This is the description of periodontal disease (pyorrhea).

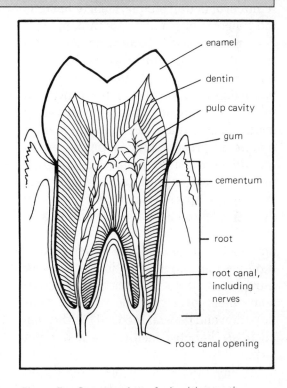

Figure 7.   Cross section of a healthy tooth

WHAT CAUSES PERIODONTAL DISEASE?

Some age-related changes in the mouth seem to set the stage for gum disease. The saliva itself may become less effective in cleaning the tooth surfaces and in controlling bacterial growth. Some older persons note a bothersome dryness of the mouth, a condition that may predispose individuals to gum infection and

185

damage to the periodontal areas. Medications, such as those used to treat hypertension and depression, may cause dryness of the mouth and lower local resistance. Finally, poor oral hygiene, especially lack of attention to *daily* removal of dental plaque, clearly hastens the progress of gum and tooth damage.

Certain specific factors seem to accentuate periodontal difficulties. The buildup of dental plaque is the most important one, for this material permits bacterial organisms and their irritating products to attack the gums. If dental plaque is present and is permitted to remain, periodontal damage follows in a matter of weeks to months. Teeth that are poorly spaced fail to meet evenly during chewing. The resultant misdirected chewing places excessive pressure on weakened teeth. Some experts attribute certain gum infections to weak immune, or protective, reactions seen in some older persons. The roles of malnutrition and general medical conditions, such as diabetes mellitus, are not yet clear.

At any rate, most of the general and specific factors that act together to cause periodontal damage can be identified and managed by close cooperation between an individual and his or her dentist.

HOW CAN PERIODONTAL DISEASE AFFECT YOU?

With periodontal disease, the gums pull back from the roots of the teeth. Inflammation begins inside the gum margin that has receded, often producing reddened, swollen, and sore gums that bleed easily on brushing. In addition, partial plates or tooth caps or crowns that fit poorly may add to the gum irritation and tooth root damage. When periodontal disease occurs, the dentist will often clean the teeth carefully, correct periodontal defects, such as areas of infection, and develop a full program of tooth maintenance.

Neglected periodontal disease leads eventually to discomfort and loosening of the affected teeth. Now the question is difficult—fight to save remaining teeth, or admit defeat, extract the teeth, and aim for artificial dentures, with variable levels of success? Dental restorations are successful, but the length of time the teeth may be retained and the expense involved must be considered when making the decision to extract teeth or restore them to function. However, neither patient nor dentist should delay full extractions when hopeless teeth begin to interfere with nutrition, social exchange, and general health (see chapter 6).

Consult Your Doctor Now IF

- You have a bad taste in your mouth or you have bad breath.
- You have painful, reddened, swollen, or bleeding gums.
- You have drifting or loosening of any teeth.

Goals of Care

- To prevent periodontal disease and loss of teeth.
- To establish a healthy mouth for a lifetime.

Self-Care Techniques

- Maintain a dental chart that includes the date of each dental visit; examination and treatments performed—x rays, cleaning, fillings, and so on; all symptoms of periodontal and other dental problems that you may be having (bleeding gums, toothache, dry mouth, loose teeth, poorly fitted dentures, sores in mouth, and so on); and home treatments such as flossing and rinsing the mouth. (See Appendix C, pages 316–317, for a dental chart to use for your medical records.)

- With the help of your dentist and/or dental hygienist, establish and follow a careful home program that includes (1) effective brushing using a soft toothbrush and a toothpaste that is not too abrasive and that contains fluoride, preferably in the morning and evening; (2) dental flossing, with floss or tape, at least once daily; (3) use of a recommended mouthwash, preferably one containing fluoride or an antiplaque agent; and (4) use of a disclosing solution—which stains, and thus reveals the presence of, plaque.

- Have routine professional examinations by a dentist.

TOOTHACHE

Few symptoms are as distressing as pain in or around the teeth. The ache itself is uniquely distressing—constant, throbbing pain that seems to be made worse by anything the sufferer does!

Toothache may complicate any number of conditions that affect the teeth and mouth. Classically, dental caries, or cavities, cause pain by eroding the tooth enamel and exposing the dentin layer, a sensitive zone surrounding the central pulp of the tooth (see figure 8). In a similar fashion, loss of a permanent filling or crown or direct injury to a tooth often leaves a sensitive tooth surface. On occasion, a sound, well-placed filling may begin to cause a toothache if the filling presses on sensitive areas near the pulp.

Inflammation of the sinuses of the face, such as may occur with the common cold, may irritate the roots of teeth in the

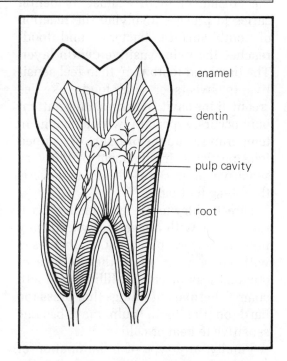

Figure 8. An inflammation of the dentin layer or of the pulp can cause toothache.

upper jaw to produce pain that is perceived as toothache.

WHAT CAUSES TOOTHACHE?

Basically, any process that irritates or injures the pain-sensitive parts of the tooth will trigger a toothache. The protective enamel coat is not especially sensitive, but the dentin, pulp cavity and canal, and the supporting bone and gum are well supplied with nerves. Once a pain-sensitive part of the tooth is irritated, almost any additional stimulation will increase the pain. Heat, cold, direct pressure of chewing, and the congestion produced by lying down tend to make the ache worse.

Most often, toothache occurs when the erosion of tooth enamel by dental caries (a process involving the reaction of tooth surface, bacteria, and food) reaches the pain-sensitive dentin layer. The damaged tooth may then feel sensitive to sweets or cold foods like ice cream. If the cavity enlarges, intermittent pain occurs, especially with a change in temperature and the pressure of trapped food particles. Involvement of the very sensitive pulp cavity leads to severe, throbbing toothache.

Direct injury to the teeth (as by forceful contact with a steering wheel) may produce severe pain that is increased with chewing, even in the absence of obvious loss of crown, filling, or tooth enamel. Permanent fillings that press too hard on the tooth pulp may become sensitive to heat or cold.

Finally, any type of inflammation of the gums or bone tissue surrounding the teeth may give rise to tooth pain. For example, sinus infections that complicate colds and X-ray damage to the jaws of persons with tumors may give rise to local pain resembling toothache.

HOW CAN TOOTHACHE AFFECT YOU?

With rare exception, a toothache tells you, in no uncertain terms, that a tooth has been damaged and demands care! The aching pain and increased sensitivity to temperature changes may come and go at first, but an untreated cavity, a small crack in the tooth, or a missing filling will soon cause constant pain. Unlike many types of local ache or discomfort, simple toothaches tend to be *worse* when treated with hot or cold applications, so aspirin or Tylenol and a trip to the dentist are always in order.

Severe, continuous, and throbbing tooth pain, increased by lowering the head, usually means that the inflammatory or infectious condition has involved the root pulp and nerve root. This sort of distress is often intolerable, and only strong medication, ice packs, and immediate expert dental care will provide relief.

The acute distress caused by recent loss of a tooth crown or filling may be partly controlled by covering the exposed surface and surrounding teeth with a wad of sealing wax.

■■■ *Consult Your Doctor Now* <u>IF</u>

■ You have significant acute tooth pain of any sort.

■ You experience any mouth or facial injury that may have damaged the teeth.

Goals of Care

■ To maintain the health and integrity of your teeth.

■ To control or remove conditions that cause toothache.

Self-Care Techniques

■ Maintain a self-care dental chart. (See Appendix C, pages 316–317, for a chart to use for your medical records.

■ With the help of your dentist and/or dental hygienist, establish and follow a careful home program that includes (1) regular brushing, preferably in the morning, evening, and after each meal, using a fairly soft toothbrush and a toothpaste that is not too abrasive and that contains fluoride; (2) use of recommended mouthwash, preferably containing fluoride; and (3) dental flossing, with floss or tape, at least once daily.

The Respiratory System

■ COUGH

The body carefully protects the airways and lungs from blockage or contamination that would interfere with the vital flow of oxygen. No protective device or mechanism is more sensitive and effective in this defense than the cough. For practical purposes, a cough is a sudden, forceful expiration, or breathing out— a rapid release of pent-up air under pressure in the lungs through the air passages, windpipe, and mouth.

The main functions of a cough are to remove secretions (as in bronchitis), solid materials (as a peanut), or irritating gases (such as cigarette smoke) from the respiratory tract.

Sputum, the material brought up by coughing, usually consists of mixed secretions from the lungs, upper airways, and mouth. Normally, sputum consists of small amounts of water along with clear and colorless secretions that are swallowed unnoticed. With infections like bronchitis and pneumonia, the sputum increases in amount, becomes thicker, and appears yellowish or greenish. Bloody sputum may appear with many conditions; cancer of the lung, pneumonia, tuberculosis, and chronic bronchitis are the most common causes of red or brownish sputum.

A cough may be voluntary or involuntary. In either case, the stimulating factor is usually irritation of either the lungs themselves, the highly branched bronchial tree (the bronchial tubes), or the upper air passages (larynx or windpipe). (See figure 9.)

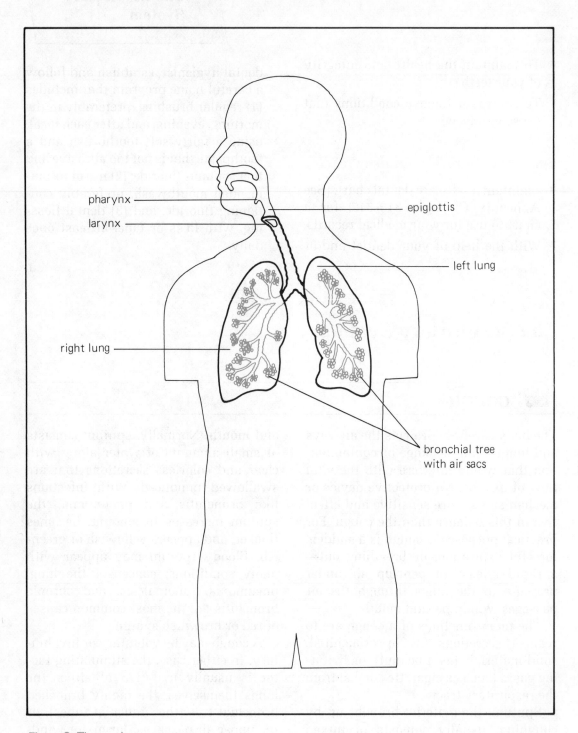

pharynx

larynx

epiglottis

left lung

right lung

bronchial tree
with air sacs

Figure 9. The respiratory system

WHAT CAUSES COUGH?

Almost any mechanical (physical) or chemical stimulation that irritates the airways, from the back of the throat to the lowest part of the lungs, will stimulate the cough response. Thus, inflammation of the larynx (by the common cold), bronchitis (such as influenza), and pneumonia (infection of the lungs themselves) are typically accompanied by severe cough. Lung congestion caused by heart failure is an important cause of persistent cough.

Many irritating particles that are inhaled into the air passages or respiratory tree trigger a protective cough. Cigarette smoke, smog, chemical fumes, and dust account for many chronic coughs in our society. Blockage of or abnormal pressure on any bronchial passages leads to cough. Cancer of the lung has replaced tuberculosis as the most common cause of this blockage. Some tense and anxious individuals cough repeatedly as a sort of nervous tic or spasm. Finally, cough itself may cause more cough; the airway irritation caused by frequent and violent coughing may trigger even more reflex coughing.

HOW CAN COUGH AFFECT YOU?

Strong, brisk coughing serves to force irritating or potentially dangerous material upward toward the mouth for disposal. Such a cough is lifesaving when a bite of steak lodges in the windpipe. The sticky bronchial secretions of asthma attacks are cleared effectively by coughing, and more effective air passage into the lungs follows. This sort of acute cough should not be suppressed or stopped until the basic condition improves.

Prolonged bouts of vigorous coughing such as may occur with influenza (see pages 196–197) are physically and emotionally exhausting. Sleep is interrupted, chest and abdominal muscles become sore, and nutrition suffers. Treatment of the underlying condition and careful use of cough-suppressing drugs lead to relief.

Very forceful coughing, which may characterize the morning cough of smoker's bronchitis, can, on occasion, produce a painful fracture of a rib. Violent coughing spells have also been known to slow the circulation and cause fainting.

Cough that lasts more than three weeks always requires careful evaluation. In addition, a change in a chronic cough—more coughing, sharp chest pain, more sputum, or blood in the sputum—should receive prompt medical study. Cancer of the lung is now the most common malignant tumor among men in the United States and is rapidly overtaking breast cancer as the most common cancer in women. Very early diagnosis and treatment offer the best chance for cure.

Consult Your Doctor Now IF

- You have an unexplained cough that has lasted more than three weeks.
- Your chronic cough changes—that is, it becomes more forceful or frequent, chest pain appears, or your sputum appears reddish or bloody. (See page 189.)

■ Goals of Care

- To understand the cause of a bothersome cough.
- To control an acute cough safely.

■ Self-Care Technique

- If you have a distressing or tiring cough due to an acute condition like viral bronchitis or the common cold, (1) drink a lot of fluid (ten or more glasses each day) to keep bronchial secretions liquid; (2) use a room humidifier or a steam kettle to decrease bronchial irritation; (3) avoid rapid or vigorous work or exercise; and (4) use a commercial cough preparation as directed. Cough syrups that loosen bronchial secretions while dulling the cough reflex are more satisfactory (for example, Robitussin-DM and Vicks Formula 44). Remember that some preparations contain drugs that cause drowsiness and other ingredients that can interact with other prescription items.

■ SHORTNESS OF BREATH

Shortness of breath is the personal, or subjective, feeling of difficult or uncomfortable breathing. The medical term for shortness of breath is *dyspnea*. It is a sensation that is described by the following complaints: "I can't catch my breath"; "I'm suffocating"; "I'm breathless." Next to severe pain, breathlessness is said to be the most uncomfortable and anxiety-producing symptom a person can experience.

The sensation is, of course, not always a sign of disease. Whenever individuals exert themselves beyond their customary exercise tolerance, they experience shortness of breath. Also, many intense emotional experiences may be accompanied by overbreathing. Thus, shortness of breath must be considered in the proper context. Is the breathlessness excessive for the activity or situation involved? Does shortness of breath appear with less exertion than before—after one flight of stairs instead of three? Is it present even at rest? Does it wake the individual from sleep?

WHAT CAUSES SHORTNESS OF BREATH?

Four general types of medical conditions give rise to the symptom of breathlessness:

1. *Physical changes in the lungs and airways.* Scarring of the lungs, as often occurs in emphysema and chronic bronchitis (see pages 197–199), increases their stiffness and the work of breathing. Congestion produced by heart failure makes the lung tissue heavy. The extra work required to expand the tissue is recognized as breathlessness. Any form of pneumonia may involve acute shortness of breath. The severe weakness of chest muscles that may occur after a stroke

often produces breathlessness even when the work of breathing is basically normal.

2. *Chemical abnormalities of the blood.* The brain center that controls breathing is exquisitely sensitive to certain chemical conditions. It normally responds to low blood oxygen concentrations by increasing the breathing drive. As a result, conditions that lead to falling oxygen levels (for example, pneumonia, asthma, or airway blockage by a foreign body) are associated with the symptom of breathlessness.

3. *Excessive demands on the entire respiratory system.* On occasion, even though the lungs provide normal amounts of oxygen, bodily demands for the gas become excessive, and overbreathing results. Diseases of the thyroid gland and prolonged fevers may produce this type of shortness of breath.

4. *Chronic states of anxiety.* Finally, individuals with chronic anxiety states often complain of breathlessness and have a dramatic, sighing style of breathing that does not reflect disease of the heart or lungs.

HOW CAN SHORTNESS OF BREATH AFFECT YOU?

Abnormal breathlessness, that not associated with simple overexertion, produces a profound sense of anxiety and distress that only the affected person can appreciate and describe. Typically, the individual sits up, often near an open window, with shoulders hunched forward, obviously working to "get enough air." Exertion, especially when it involves use of the arms, is undertaken reluctantly and slowly. Food intake is decreased, and needed sleep is interrupted. In short, the entire body focuses on the driving need for air.

Fortunately, shortness of breath is only a symptom of disease, so it subsides as the underlying condition is controlled. People with known chronic lung diseases, heart trouble, or muscular diseases are usually keenly aware of the meaning of increasing breathlessness and decreasing exercise tolerance, so prompt attention to details of management relieves them of this distress. Other problems such as cough, ankle swelling, and weakness usually represent secondary effects of the underlying condition.

Consult Your Doctor Now IF

- You develop significant unexplained shortness of breath.
- Shortness of breath causes progressive difficulty in carrying out your usual tasks.

Goal of Care

- To prevent or control the symptom of breathlessness.

Self-Care Techniques

- The most direct approach in controlling or decreasing shortness of breath involves the redistribution of work and necessary tasks. Program your day so that activities can be carried out most efficiently. For example, do all upstairs cleaning and housekeeping in one trip and make only one trip to town for shopping, banking, and other errands. Delegate tasks to family members or friends. Heroic efforts on your part are counterproductive.

■ If you have a chronic medical condition that predisposes you to shortness of breath, monitor that condition. Maintain a chart that warns you of potential problems. For example, gradual weight gain may be an early

clue to heart failure that will progress to produce breathlessness. Review and work with your doctor to improve your medical management.

■ If your doctor agrees, design an exercise program that will improve your muscle strength and cardiovascular fitness. Inactivity and weakness make you less able to function efficiently and more likely to experience breathlessness.

■ ASTHMA

During normal breathing, air flows in and out of the bronchial tubes (bronchial tree) that lead from the windpipe to the lungs (see figure 9). Quite predictably, even temporary narrowing or partial blockage of large numbers of the smallest bronchial tubes creates a dangerous situation. The work of forcing air along the bronchial tubes increases; the volume of air, and oxygen, reaching the lungs and other parts of the body decreases; and the lungs themselves may be damaged. Reversible narrowing of these small airways along with attacks of difficult breathing, coughing, and wheezing (noisy, prolonged exhalation, or breathing out) is termed *asthma*.

Asthma is not a single or specific disease; rather, it is the situation produced by one or several conditions that trigger narrowing of the critical bronchial passages and block air flow. In most instances, the narrowing results from a combination of factors: spasm of the muscles that surround the bronchial walls, swelling of the lining membranes

of the bronchial passages, and abnormal secretions into the central bronchial passages. The typical attack begins gradually, often with a slight cough and sense of anxiety. As wheezing and shortness of breath follow, the asthma victim becomes fearful and exhausted. With prompt treatment, the wheezing tapers off and breathing becomes normal. On occasion, however, the overworked lungs become infected, and pneumonia results.

WHAT CAUSES ASTHMA?

Although many different diseases and body reactions can lead to asthma attacks, two general types of asthma can be recognized—allergic asthma and idiosyncratic, or nonallergic, asthma. *Allergic asthma* tends to occur in families, usually develops during childhood, and is often accompanied by allergic skin conditions like eczema and hives. More than half of these allergic persons outgrow this condition, which tends to be seasonal and related to the release of pollens like ragweed pollen. These asthma sufferers have a wide variety of underlying conditions such as aspirin sensitivity, in which compounds containing aspirin trigger attacks, and environmental sensitivities, where metal fumes, plastic vapors, tobacco smoke, and other substances cause bronchial spasms and asthma attacks. In some individuals, brisk physical exertion is followed by wheezing and coughing.

Nonallergic asthma may begin in adult life, often during or following a mild respiratory infection. These patients tend to have more severe attacks of asthmatic difficulty that occur throughout the year. Many develop new sensitivities to chemicals and environmental irritants, and eventually resemble patients with allergic asthma.

It should be emphasized that the coughing, wheezing, and shortness of breath produced by temporary narrowing of the bronchial passages—that is, acute asthma attacks—are only rarely produced by a single insult. Most often, the individual and his or her family can identify three to four conditions that interact to start and sustain a spell. For example, the pollen season is in full swing, exposure to cigarette smoke starts a spell of coughing, and the anxiety produced by severe shortness of breath adds fuel to the flame. In almost all forms of bronchial asthma, emotional upset is a common stress that may precipitate or worsen asthma attacks.

When asthma attacks first appear in adult life, about 20 percent of the persons affected recover completely within a few years, and another 40 percent improve significantly with or without treatment.

HOW CAN ASTHMA AFFECT YOU?

Many individuals with mild allergic asthma in childhood learn to avoid the pollens and dusts that trigger attacks, and they have no real difficulty in later life. Still others suffer repeatedly with acute asthma, becoming dependent on various medications for year-round comfort and productivity.

Acute attacks may consist of only a few minutes of hacking cough and labored breathing, or they may progress rapidly to frightening, day-long spells of labored wheezing, profound shortness of breath, constant cough, and overall exhaustion. Some asthmatics seem destined for difficulty, but the underlying problem usually determines the nature of individual attacks. Vigorous treatment of the acute episode with medications that decrease bronchial spasm and swelling (for example, theophylline tablets and Isuprel spray), drugs that block allergic reactions (for example, corticosteroids), and general supportive measures usually produce impressive results. There are now many practical lifestyle and medical programs that can prevent recurrences of otherwise crippling asthma.

Consult Your Doctor Now IF

- You develop acute asthmatic symptoms for the first time.
- You have recurrent symptoms of asthma that fail to respond to usual treatments.

Goals of Care

- To control the symptoms of an acute asthma attack.

- To prevent the major complications of recurrent bronchial asthma.

Self-Care Techniques

- Use an asthma chart, which should include this information: the date and time of day the attack occurred; how long the attack lasted; how the attack developed—rapidly or slowly, with or without exposure to known irritants, with or without specific treatment; the treatments used and whether they were effective or ineffective; and any complications. (See Appendix C, pages 318–319, for an asthma chart to use for your medical records.)

- Stop smoking.

- Working with your doctor, design a careful plan to anticipate and prevent acute asthma attacks. You should know in advance the conditions to avoid, the danger signals to note, and the medications to use.

- Always have an annual influenza vaccination.

- If your doctor advises it, have a single Pneumovax immunization to decrease the chances of developing certain types of lung infection or pneumonia.

INFLUENZA

Influenza, also known as the grippe or the flu, is an acute infectious disease caused by a virus. After the virus enters the body, usually in inhaled water droplets, fever (to 103° F), headache, and overwhelming body ache occur. If pneumonia (lung inflammation) develops, cough, chest pain, and shortness of breath soon add to the general discomfort. A secondary, or additional, lung infection by bacteria is a special threat to older persons and to those with chronic lung problems. In uncomplicated influenza infection, patients recover from their major symptoms in six to eight days, but many are left with marked general weakness and low resistance for several weeks.

WHAT CAUSES INFLUENZA?

Influenza is caused by influenza viruses. The viruses are labeled types A, B, and C. Type A agents are the viruses that tend to produce widespread epidemics and severe disease. For example, in 1968, more than one-quarter of the entire United States population was infected within three months. Since these viruses usually enter the body in inhaled water droplets, the viruses are easily transmitted from person to person by coughing. There is even some evidence that certain animals (for example, birds and swine) may help spread the infection. In addition, the Type A strain of virus changes its makeup almost yearly, thus setting the stage practically each year for a new wave of influenza.

Older people and individuals with underlying medical problems (for example, heart disease, diabetes, emphysema, and other chronic diseases) are clearly at high risk for contracting influenza infection and for developing serious complications like pneumonia. In some nursing homes, for example, 60 percent of the older residents developed influenza in one outbreak, and 30 percent of those infected later died! History tells us that outbreaks tend to occur in the United States generally between the months of October and April.

HOW CAN INFLUENZA AFFECT YOU?

Young and healthy adults may develop no symptoms of influenza infection but may serve as virus carriers. Some experts feel that unvaccinated medical workers may actually help spread the disease among patients.

Most adults who are otherwise well experience a six- to seven-day illness with fever, headache, generalized aches and pains, and weakness, followed by a short period of recovery. If the initial phase is complicated by pneumonia, the fever climbs higher, and the individual becomes seriously ill. Advanced age and most medical conditions add greatly to the risk of lung complications.

During the last twenty years, medical scientists have developed effective influenza vaccines. These vaccines are concentrated solutions of inactive (killed) viruses that provide excellent protection against the disease and its most serious complications. People who are at high risk should receive this safe and painless inoculation *each* fall because the exact nature of the current infecting viruses changes almost yearly.

Consult Your Doctor Now IF

■ You have not received an annual flu vaccination and are at high risk for influenza and its complications. High-risk persons are those sixty-five years of age or older or those who have heart or lung disease.

Goals of Care

■ To prevent the development of influenza infection.

■ To reduce the chances of developing pneumonia and other complications of influenza.

Self-Care Technique

■ Keep a vaccination chart that includes the date and type of each annual influenza vaccination you receive (See Appendix C, page 320, for a chart to use for your medical records.)

CHRONIC OBSTRUCTIVE LUNG DISEASE

Like so many other medical disorders, chronic obstructive lung disease is not a simple condition with a single cause. Rather, it typically results from two major diseases that work together to damage the lungs and airways, obstructive emphysema and chronic bronchitis. *Obstructive emphysema* causes progressive weakening and ballooning and the eventual destruction of the millions of tiny air sacs that make up the lungs (see figure 9). Once established, emphysema produces progressive shortness of breath as its main symptom. The second disease, *chronic bronchitis*, is a persistent inflammation or irritation of the bronchial passages (see figure 9). These air-conduction channels become scarred, narrowed, and clogged with secretions, producing the symptoms of cough, increased sputum production, and shortness of breath. The end result of these two conditions is chronic obstructive lung disease—a persistent, usually progressive, often crippling lung disease that is difficult to treat. The prominent features of chronic obstructive lung disease are cough, unusual amounts of sputum, shortness of breath, and repeated bouts of pneumonia.

Next to coronary heart disease, chronic obstructive lung disease accounts for more severe disability and untimely deaths than any other health-related problem in the United States. By conservative estimates, between 10 and 25 percent of adults in the U.S. suffer from this frustrating condition.

WHAT CAUSES CHRONIC OBSTRUCTIVE LUNG DISEASE?

One fact is certain: cigarette smoking is a major cause of both emphysema and chronic bronchitis. It seems likely that the irritants in tobacco smoke inflame and eventually weaken the bronchial and lung tissues, making them more susceptible to damage by bacterial infection. Thus, individuals with chronic obstructive lung disease are predisposed to attacks of pneumonia that leave them with even more lung damage and disability. Although many of the lung changes of chronic obstructive lung disease are permanent, improvement in symptoms and signs of disease often follows discontinuation of smoking.

Industrial pollutants seem to be associated with some cases of emphysema. Prolonged exposure to cadmium or certain airborne fibers favors the later development of chronic obstructive lung disease.

Perhaps 1 to 2 percent of the population with chronic obstructive lung disease has a family history of similar lung trouble.

HOW CAN CHRONIC OBSTRUCTIVE LUNG DISEASE AFFECT YOU?

Most "healthy" adults who are heavy smokers can be shown to have significant abnormalities of their breathing function upon special testing. Of great importance, from both the personal and public health viewpoints, is the fact that breathing function will often return to normal if cigarette smoking is discontinued.

It is known that smokers have more respiratory infections than do nonsmokers. These infections contribute to the progressive lung damage of chronic bronchitis and emphysema. As the bronchial passages become more irritated and narrowed, cough becomes a problem. At first the cough occurs primarily on arising in the morning, producing small amounts of clear sputum. Later the chronic obstructive lung disease victim coughs throughout the day, and the sputum production increases in volume. When an acute respiratory infection occurs, the cough becomes even more severe, and the sputum produced appears greenish or grayish. Significant permanent lung damage is present when shortness of breath occurs during usual, light exercise. Vigorous treatment at this stage usually controls the major symptoms. The treatment consists of nonprescription syrups for controlling the cough; antibiotics given for acute lung infections; and theophylline-derivative drugs, which are helpful in controlling shortness of breath.

In most cases, the lung and airway destruction progresses slowly but surely over a period of several years. Eventually the hacking cough is present to the point of exhaustion, shortness of breath is bothersome even at rest, and signs of heart failure and brain dysfunction appear. At this stage of chronic obstructive lung disease, therapy is designed primarily for comfort and for temporary control of secondary complications.

Consult Your Doctor Now IF

■ You experience a sudden or dramatic increase in the symptoms of chronic obstructive lung disease—cough, shortness of breath, and production of discolored sputum.

Goal of Care

■ To prevent the development and progression of emphysema, chronic bronchitis, and chronic obstructive lung disease.

Self-Care Techniques

■ Stop smoking!

■ Get an annual influenza vaccination (see page 197). Obtain a pneumococcal (Pneumovax) inoculation against the complication of certain types of pneumonia, if your doctor agrees.

■ Drink ten or more glasses of fluid each day, especially during an acute respiratory infection, since proper fluid balance increases sputum flow.

■ Treat acute respiratory infections promptly and vigorously. Discuss with your doctor the advisability of taking a brief course of antibiotics, such as Bactrim or Ampicillin, in order to prevent secondary bacterial infections.

■ If your cough disrupts sleep, work out a careful program that controls the cough but does not block the effective removal of infected sputum. Steps in this program might include (1) drinking two glasses of water or other fluids one or two hours before retiring, (2) use of a room humidifier in your bedroom, (3) controlled but forceful coughing and clearing of the chest before lying down, and (4) proper doses of a mild cough syrup (such as Robitussin, and Vicks Formula 44).

■ With guidance from a physical therapist or other health professional, establish a program of graded physical exercise that increases general physical fitness and improves breathing efficiency.

■ SORE THROAT

One of the most common health problems experienced by otherwise healthy adults is that of sore throat—a slightly painful, scratchy or raw feeling in the back of the throat (see figure 9). This is often accompanied by a runny or stuffy nose, low-grade fever (100°–102° F), chills, muscle aches, and a feeling of tiredness. These symptoms fade after three to five days. Additional symptoms of hoarseness and slight cough may appear as well, suggesting that the inflammation has also involved the upper airways.

Although extremely common and typically easy to manage, this sort of sore throat, or upper respiratory infection may cause considerable distress and has many possible complications.

WHAT CAUSES SORE THROAT?

Most acute bouts of sore throat are due to local infections. These infections generally result from invasion of the pharynx and the surrounding areas by one of more than a hundred different viral agents. Typically, the infecting virus spreads to the upper respiratory tract from another person, a cold "carrier," thus creating a small epidemic of upper respiratory illnesses. For reasons that are still unclear, common colds and sore throats occur most often during cold winter months. It may be that crowding and poor ventilation favor the spread of these diseases.

Perhaps a quarter of sore throats in adults are the result of bacterial, not viral, infection, and a majority of these involve the *streptococcus* agent. This bacterium, dreaded in prepenicillin days because of the complications of rheumatic fever and scarlet fever, is spread by direct contact and by airborne droplets produced by coughs and sneezes. Upper respiratory infections may occur in clustered outbreaks or as isolated cases.

On occasion, a sore throat is part of a general medical condition. Allergic drug reactions, certain tumors of the lymph glands, and diphtheria may create symptoms that closely resemble simple sore throat.

HOW CAN A SORE THROAT AFFECT YOU?

Most viral upper respiratory infections run an uncomplicated course. With or without treatment, the scratchy throat, stuffy nose, feverishness, and aching subside in three to five days. Hot gargles soothe the raw throat, mild sprays give relief to nasal congestion, and preparations containing aspirin or Tylenol help control fever and relieve the muscular aches.

A few persons develop bothersome or, on occasion, serious complications from sore throats. The viral agent or an associated bacterium may infect the lungs to cause pneumonia, usually accompanied by chills, high fever, and cough. Or, the upper respiratory infection may extend into the facial sinuses, with local pain and soreness over the eyes or cheeks. In these cases, prompt treatment with antibiotics is required.

Although the symptoms of bacterial (usually streptococcal) sore throat tend to be more dramatic than the symptoms caused by viral disease, it is often impossible to distinguish between the two on initial examination. If in doubt, many doctors will attempt to grow, or culture, the bacterial organism from throat secretions and if streptococcus is found, will prescribe a course of antibiotics (usually a penicillin preparation by mouth); some doctors will prescribe such a course of treatment based on the likelihood that the infection is streptococcus. Unlike bacteria, the viruses that cause sore throat do not respond to currently available antibiotics.

Consult Your Doctor Now <u>IF</u>

■ You have a severe sore throat that interferes with swallowing, speaking, or breathing.

■ You develop chills, high fever, chest pain, or pain and soreness over the eyes and cheeks during or after a typical sore throat.

Goals of Care

■ To minimize the local and general discomforts of an acute sore throat.

■ To prevent serious complications from an acute upper respiratory infection.

Self-Care Technique

■ If you experience the typical symptoms of a simple sore throat (and especially if others around you have had similar symptoms), do the following: (1) Avoid strenuous or prolonged exertion for two to three days; however, actual bed rest is usually neither necessary nor desirable. (2) Drink generous amounts of water and other fluids, since fever and mouth breathing cause excessive loss of body fluids. (3) Take medications containing aspirin or Tylenol, usually in doses of two tablets by mouth every four hours while you are awake. (4) Gargle with warm, salty water (one tablespoonful of salt per pint of water) every four hours to ease throat soreness. (5) If cough is bothersome, take a cough syrup (for example, Robitussin DM, one to two teaspoonfuls by mouth every four hours). Remember that many cough syrups of this type contain large amounts of alcohol and may cause drowsiness and/or react with other medications such as those used to treat hypertension and depression. (6) If stuffy nose is a problem, *cautiously* use nasal decongestant spray (for example, Neo-Synephrine, 0.25 percent, three times a day for three to four days). Prolonged use of decongestant sprays may lead to a "rebound" swelling and blockage of nasal passages.

The Heart and Circulatory System

■ HIGH BLOOD PRESSURE

As people age, blood pressure levels typically increase. For instance, men forty years of age have average blood pressure readings of 130/80, while those seventy-five years of age have levels of 160/90. This normal increase results from a gradual loss of elasticity and decreasing diameter of the small arteries throughout the body.

A condition of significant high blood pressure exists when either upper (systolic) pressure or lower (diastolic) pressure or both (combined) pressures are found to be consistently elevated beyond well-established "normal" levels for a particular age. Most experts consider systolic readings of 160 and above and diastolic readings of 95 and above abnormal for a person aged fifty years or older if these readings are shown on three or more separate examinations over a two-week period.

WHAT CAUSES HIGH BLOOD PRESSURE?

Most persons with significant elevations of blood pressure (approximately 30 percent of the elderly United States population) have what is called essential hypertension. The cause of essential hypertension is not known; however, it clearly runs in families. Some rare forms of hypertension develop as a result of kidney disease. However, essential hypertension is not so much a disease state as a risk factor. Hypertension is a problem known to be associated with future heart and brain disease and is clearly made worse by factors such as obesity, lack of exercise, smoking, and poor dietary habits (especially use of excess salt).

HOW CAN HIGH BLOOD PRESSURE AFFECT YOU?

Uncontrolled high blood pressure leads to accelerated narrowing and hardening of the arteries that supply blood to vital organs. These arterial changes may result in coronary heart disease, with angina, heart attack, or congestive heart failure; strokes; and early death. In a few people, these changes lead to kidney damage, poor circulation to the legs, or eye disease with failing vision.

There are no reliable symptoms of this major health problem! Although nervousness, headaches, and palpitations are commonly believed to be clues, even severe high blood pressure may exist for years with no symptoms at all. Therefore, *you should have your blood pressure taken at least once a year, and if an abnormal blood pressure reading is found and subsequent readings in a two-week period are also abnormal, you must consider this condition serious and follow the advice given by your doctor.*

Consult Your Doctor Now IF

- Your blood pressure is greater than 190/110, which can be dangerous.
- Irregular pulse or heartbeat is noted.
- Sudden loss of vision is noted.
- Chest pain or angina occurs (see pages 205–207).
- A severe or unusual headache occurs.
- You have bothersome anxiety or uncertainty about high blood pressure.

Goals of Care

- To reduce blood pressure levels to a normal range by means of a safe, comprehensive program.
- To maintain blood pressure in a safe range for years, relying on a program that produces minimum inconvenience, that results in no drug side effects, and that removes the hazards of heart, brain, and other blood vessel diseases.

Self-Care Techniques

- Establish a personalized blood pressure record or chart. Include dates, readings, pulse rate, and weight. (See Appendix C. page 294, for a blood pressure chart to use for your medical records.)

- Have your blood pressure taken regularly, at least twice every month. Accurate blood pressure readings are essential for proper diagnosis and safe management of hypertension.
- Master the technique of blood pressure measurement (see page 104) and follow a schedule.
- Follow a reasonable diet. This usually involves decreasing your salt intake, eating foods with low fat content, and cutting back on calories to reduce weight.
- Exercise regularly (see chapter 5).
- Stop smoking.
- Take prescribed medications *exactly* as directed. Missed doses may result in a dangerous rebound rise in pressure. Obtain a list of the most common side effects for which to watch. These often include weakness, dizziness on standing up, and difficulties with vision.
- Take alcohol only in moderation—no more than two drinks per day.
- Practice relaxing. Learn relaxation exercises (see Appendix B).

VARICOSE VEINS

A large network of thin-walled veins serves to return circulating blood from the legs upward toward the chest cavity and the heart. Unlike blood flow in arteries, where the pumping action of the heart moves blood rapidly, flow in veins is quite slow. Flow in the leg vein system is made especially sluggish by the upright posture of humans. Blood from the lower legs must move upward several feet against the force of gravity.

Leg veins often become weakened, dilated, and inefficient. When the veins appear as cordlike, bumpy, bluish lines under the skin of the calf and thigh, they are known as varicose, or dilated, veins.

Most adults have a few unsightly varicose veins, usually located in the calf region. Others, often women who have had several pregnancies, have more extensive varicosities. The venous network rarely becomes so badly weakened and inefficient that it develops large, bulging, uncomfortable varicose veins.

WHAT CAUSES VARICOSE VEINS?

A family, or hereditary, tendency for varicose veins is suggested by the fact that over 50 percent of individuals needing surgical treatment for this condition have close relatives with a similar problem.

Three factors act together to produce damage to the venous network: (1) Upright posture places the pull of gravity on the column of blood that extends from feet to legs to heart. (2) Abnormal pressure—such as from pregnancies, obesity, or lower abdominal tumors—in the large collecting veins in the abdomen may further dilate leg veins. (3) Direct injury to the legs, especially if it is complicated by inflammation (phlebitis), may cause blockage and local weakening of the walls of the delicate veins.

HOW CAN VARICOSE VEINS AFFECT YOU?

Small varicose veins of the calf or thigh are important only from a cosmetic standpoint. Elastic or dark-colored stockings usually support and conceal them. However, larger, bulging veins that extend along the calf and thigh are often accompanied by feelings of heaviness, achiness, and itchiness—symptoms that probably result from stretching of the veins and the surrounding skin. The poor circulation in very prominent varicosities, especially in older adults, may lead to skin damage followed by swelling, discoloration, and even ulcers of the lower legs. Although injury to a varicose vein may result in large bruises, actual rupture or tearing of the vein rarely occurs.

Varicose veins that are not effectively managed with elastic stockings may be treated by injection or surgical stripping. Small but bothersome veins can be injected with a special solution under local anesthesia. Most of these veins will then close down with little or no scarring. Larger veins, especially those that run from the lower calf into the thigh and cause pain or pressure, can be removed by stripping.

■ *Consult Your Doctor Now* **IF**

- You have significant pain, redness, or swelling around a varicose vein.

■ *Goal of Care*

- To manage varicose veins and prevent their progression and complications.

■ *Self-Care Techniques*

- Avoid wearing tight stockings or undergarments that block blood flow up from the legs.
- Avoid unnecessary and prolonged standing. Elevate your feet when sitting or lying down.

- Wear well-fitting elastic stockings (for example, support hose) or smoothly wrapped elastic binders (Ace binders) while up and about.

■ CHEST PAIN

All persons experience momentary, often unexplained aches and pains in the chest—"a stitch when I run," "a cramp when I turn." However, there are three types of chest pain of special importance to older adults: pain caused by angina; pain related to pleurisy; and the unique pain of shingles, herpes zoster infection.

Anginal pain, the result of poor circulation of blood and oxygen to the muscles of the heart (see figure 10), is often described as a sensation of pressure or a feeling of tightness across the upper chest or under the breastbone. Many individuals report vague feelings of squeezing or aching that run into the left chest, neck, or left shoulder and arm. Although frightening and uncomfortable, the distress of angina is not sharp or severe. Typically, anginal pain is brought on by situations that stress the heart and circulation; a heavy meal, sudden exertion, or emotional upset notoriously trigger the pain. An average anginal attack subsides within minutes to a half hour.

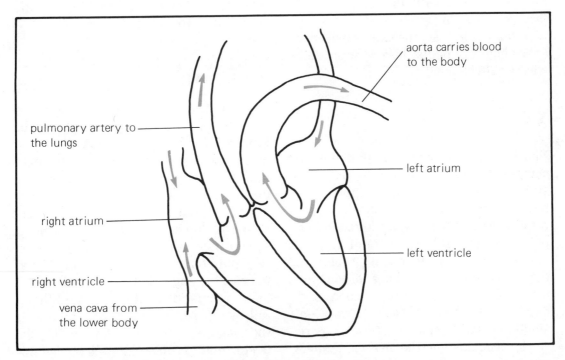

Figure 10. Circulation of blood through the chambers of the heart

Pleurisy, the pain caused by irritation of the lining of the lungs and chest cage, is usually sharp and knifelike and is felt along the chest wall. The pain is made worse by coughing or deep breathing and is accompanied by feelings of shortness of breath. (See page 192.) Unlike anginal pain, pleurisy pain is well localized over the area where either pneumonia or other lung damage is present. This type of chest pain tends to last for hours or even days, disappearing only when the underlying condition is resolved.

Shingles is the pain caused by infection of a major nerve in the chest wall by the herpes zoster virus. The remarkable chest pain of shingles occurs most often in older adults. Typically, sharp, burning pain develops like a band around one side of the chest. Then, within three to four days, clusters of painful red blisters arise along the path of the pain. Although the rash crusts and clears up within a week or so, the skin sensitivity and shooting pains may persist for weeks or even months.

WHAT CAUSES THESE TYPES OF CHEST PAIN?

The aching chest pain of *angina* may be compared to a leg cramp. In both instances, inadequate blood supply to a hardworking muscle produces temporary tissue damage that is signaled by a painful warning. In the case of angina, the most common underlying problem is the narrowing or blockage of one or more arteries that supply blood and oxygen to the heart muscle. Physical or emotional stress that places still more work demands on the heart's limited capacity and borderline blood supply precipitates the anginal attack.

The pleura, the thin transparent membranes that cover and lubricate the outer surfaces of the lungs, contain many sensitive nerve endings. Almost any irritation of these structures causes *pleurisy,* an area of inflammation in the lung. Common causes of pleurisy are pneumonia, a blood clot at the surface of the lung, or a rib fracture that damages the pleural surface.

For reasons that are not well understood, the herpes virus that causes chicken pox in children may reactivate and spread along a nerve pathway in an older person. Most often, this pathway is around the chest or upper abdomen, and the inflammation produces burning (neuritic) pain, redness, and skin blistering, or *shingles.* The condition seems most likely to develop in older adults who suffer from chronic diseases.

HOW CAN THESE CHEST PAINS AFFECT YOU?

Angina serves as a warning that the heart's circulation is overtaxed or stressed. In most cases, immediate rest and control of strain relieve the pain within minutes. In addition, the drug nitroglycerin, which is taken as a pill under the tongue, will typically interrupt and end an anginal attack. One of several new medications may be taken by mouth to prevent anginal pain. Nonetheless, the anginal attack indicates that heart circulation is abnormal and that a full-blown heart attack may follow. If the diagnosis of angina is in doubt, the doctor may recommend an exercise tolerance test, where the heart function is monitored by an electrocardiogram tracing during carefully graded exercise on a treadmill or stationary bicycle.

The pain of *pleurisy* most often points to pneumonia, an infection of the lungs. Although the pain itself may be sharp and quite disabling, the major problem relates to the treatment of the underlying lung condition. In some older persons, especially those recovering from operations, from medical problems like heart failure, or from any prolonged period of bed rest, the pain of pleurisy suggests that a blood clot has escaped from the veins of the leg and caused potentially serious circulatory slowing in the lungs. In this situation, "thinning" of the blood, or reducing the blood's tendency to clot, may be lifesaving.

Most adults recover from *shingles* in a matter of two to four weeks, though severe inflammation along the course of the body nerve may leave scattered scars behind. A few unfortunate individuals (between 10 and 25 percent) are left with a line of burning pain and skin tenderness that persists for weeks to months. Control of both the painful rash and the residual local pain requires careful use of drugs. No practical specific medical or surgical therapies are yet available for these problems.

■ **Consult Your Doctor Now IF**

- You experience one or more attacks that have the characteristics of angina.
- You develop chest pain that has the characteristics of pleurisy.
- You experience a sensitive and painful rash on your chest wall.

■ **Goal of Care**

- To recognize and manage the underlying causes of significant chest pain.

■ **Self-Care Technique**

- Use a chest pain chart that includes the following: the dates and times of attacks of chest pain; the location of the pain or distress (where it started, moved, or radiated); a description of the pain; any precipitating events; accompanying symptoms (sweating, anxiety, palpitations, shortness of breath, cough, and so on); and what relieved the pain (rest, medications, and so on). (See Appendix C, pages 322–323, for a chest pain chart to use for your medical records.)

■ **EDEMA**

Your tight wedding band makes your finger puffy and stiff. After a bus trip from New York City to Florida, your shoes seem tight, and both feet are swollen. Each morning, your aunt with heart trouble awakens to find her eyelids puffed almost shut. In each case, the local swelling represents a collection of fluid that is called edema. The swelling of edema is typically painless, temporary, and not accompanied by color changes of the skin. To be sure, there are other types of body swelling. For example, inflammations of the skin (dermatitis) or of the joints (arthritis) may cause puffiness. However, in these instances, the pain, redness, and special localization help distinguish the swelling from edema.

WHAT CAUSES EDEMA?

There are many causes of painless swelling, or edema. Localized edema occurs when any body tissue is damaged, causing blood (plasma) to leak out of the blood vessels into the surrounding structures. The swelling of your hand after too many games of tennis is an example of this injury-type edema.

Edema also occurs when the body's drainage channels, the veins or the lymph vessels, are blocked. The blockage produces abnormally high pressures within the channels, resulting in gradual leakage of plasma fluids out into nearby tissues. Examples of this sort of blocked drainage include the narrowing of varicose veins, with subsequent leg swelling (see pages 203–205), and lymph channel scarring in an area of breast surgery, with subsequent puffiness of the arm.

Certain types of heart disease and kidney failure cause the body to take on and retain abnormal amounts of salt and water. In such cases, the edema tends to appear in areas affected by the pull of gravity, for example, in the feet, after prolonged sitting, or in the face, after sleep.

HOW CAN EDEMA AFFECT YOU?

The slight swelling and tightness of feet and ankles experienced by many healthy people at the end of a long day are simply a nuisance. Elevation of the legs relieves this edema within a few hours.

More obvious leg (or other) swelling that remains after an overnight rest is abnormal and requires treatment. Although the edema itself causes little or no discomfort at first, the stretched skin eventually becomes irritated, itchy, and thickened. After specific treatment of the underlying cause (such as varicose veins), the edema can usually be relieved by elevation of the swollen part, use of fitted elastic binders (Ace binders), and moderate restriction of salt intake (to about one teaspoonful per day).

Persistent, or chronic, edema caused by various types of heart trouble is the result of salt and water overload of the body. As a result, gradual weight gain, feelings of heaviness, easy fatigue, and, in many instances, increasing shortness of breath are accompaniments of the edema. Fortunately, reduction of salt intake, regular use of drugs (diuretic agents) that promote salt loss and water loss through the kidneys, and, when indicated, the use of digitalis to improve heart function control these symptoms.

■■■ *Consult Your Doctor Now* **IF**

- You have unexplained ankle edema that remains after an overnight rest.
- You have facial swelling in the morning that disappears as you become active.

■ **Goals of Care**

■ To recognize the cause or causes of any edema.

■ To control the local swelling of edema and to prevent any of its long-term complications.

■ **Self-Care Techniques**

■ If you have local edema, such as the simple ankle swelling that may accompany varicose veins, do the following: (1) Avoid prolonged sitting or standing; run in place or contract your leg muscles when you are forced to remain inactive. (2) Elevate your legs whenever possible. (3) Put two- to three-inch blocks under the foot of your bed to promote drainage of edema fluid into your blood circulation at night. (4) Wear well-fitted (not constricting or loose) elastic stockings during the day.

■ If you have the more complicated "general" salt-and-water edema, keep a careful record (same time each morning) of your weight and follow the prescribed salt-restricted diet and medical program outlined by your doctor.

■ **CONGESTIVE HEART FAILURE**

The heart, a wonderfully efficient, muscular pump, is the vital power source for all blood circulation (see figure 10). Venous blood, returning from nourishing body organs such as the liver and the brain, is drawn into the two spaces (or chambers) of the right side of the heart. The chambers contract with each heartbeat, forcing this "used" blood through the lungs, where oxygen enriches, or "recharges," it. The oxygen-rich blood is then forced into the body's arteries by the contractions of the left-heart chambers, and flows on to bring oxygen and nutrients to all body tissues. Rhythmic nerve activity stimulates the pumping action of the heart to help maintain a critical balance between the blood expelled and the blood returned.

Any type of heart disease or damage may upset this balance, resulting in a backup, or pooling, of blood in the heart itself and in other organs. This unbalanced state is congestive heart failure (CHF). Weakness or other improper functioning of the left heart chambers causes congestion in the lungs, whereas weakness of the right heart chambers causes congestion and the pooling of fluid in the liver and other body organs. In many cases, damage to the left side of the heart produces lung congestion, which leads, in turn, to strain on the right side of the heart and liver congestion.

Sudden injury to the heart muscle, as in a heart attack, may trigger a single, brief episode of heart failure. Prolonged damage by the stress of untreated high blood pressure (see pages 202–203) may produce persistent heart failure.

WHAT CAUSES CONGESTIVE HEART FAILURE?

Any condition that interferes with the regular, smooth pumping action of the heart muscle may lead to congestive heart failure. Most often, blockage of one or more arteries that nourish the heart muscle (coronary artery disease) damages the muscle and reduces its contracting power. As a result, blood no longer flows efficiently into the arteries; rather, it backs up into the lungs and causes congestion.

Many persons have congestive heart failure as a result of damage to the heart valves—flexible, gatelike structures that help control the flow of blood through the heart's chambers. The inflammatory damage of rheumatic fever, a disease of childhood, may scar and deform heart valves, retard the flow of blood, and cause CHF. Other abnormalities of heart valves are congenital in origin—that is, present at birth—and produce CHF in infancy or childhood.

The extra work caused by uncontrolled high blood pressure (see pages 202–203) may eventually cause strain on and failure of the heart muscle. Excessively rapid (over 200 per minute), slow (less than 40 per minute), or irregular heart rates (arrhythmias) may slow blood circulation through the heart and cause congestion of the lungs and other organs.

Some individuals with mild forms or degrees of heart damage will develop congestive heart failure when additional stresses are placed on the body. For example, anemia, high fever (see pages 154–156), or certain medical conditions (thyroid trouble, for instance) may cause heart failure in a person with only mild heart disease.

HOW CAN CONGESTIVE HEART FAILURE AFFECT YOU?

Most often, weakness of the left-heart muscle leads to lung congestion and breathing difficulties. A person may breathe normally at rest but finds that slight exertion produces unusual, often crippling breathlessness—for example, climbing one flight of stairs may produce heavy breathing in someone who once raced up three flights of stairs. Breathlessness may appear after lying down, the result of "flooding" of the lungs by extra returning blood. Stretching of the lung tissue by congestion often produces a bothersome, hacking cough. All these symptoms subside promptly when the heart muscle recovers function or the body fluid is decreased by drugs that produce a loss of salt and water.

Prolonged strain of the left-heart muscle or damage to the right-heart muscle causes congestion of the liver and other organs. As these fluids accumulate, the body weight increases, the abdomen appears swollen and full, and the ankles swell (see pages 207–209). In addition, congestion of body tissues often causes general weakness, easy tiring, and poor appetite.

Prompt and specific treatment of the heart difficulties—whether heart attack, valve damage, or arrhythmia—is mandatory. Digitalislike drugs (for example, Digoxin) may make the heart muscle stronger and more efficient. Heart surgeons can replace many scarred heart valves with artificial ones. Drugs like Digoxin, quinidine, and propranolol (Inderal) may transform an irregular heart-beat to a regular, effective one.

Other measures are effective in controlling the congestion of heart failure. Salt may be restricted in the diet (see page 208) or removed from the body by the action of medications called diuretics, compounds that stimulate urine formation and flow. Such medications include Lasix, HydroDIURIL, and Dyazide. Extra water in the body is also removed by the action of these compounds. Correction of added stresses of conditions like anemia and thyroid disease is important in the heart-failure patient. Finally, regular periods of rest are an important part of general management.

Consult Your Doctor Now IF

- You experience increasing or unexplained shortness of breath on simple exertion or during sleep.
- You develop persistent overnight swelling of the lower legs.
- You experience bothersome pounding of the heart (palpitations).

Goals of Care

- To recognize and relieve symptoms of congestive heart failure.
- To correct the primary heart difficulties and associated stressful conditions that cause congestive heart failure.

Self-Care Techniques

- Review with your doctor the key elements in your heart condition and its management: the cause and nature of the heart disease itself, factors that may add stress to the body, the symptoms of congestive heart failure and how to recognize them, and the dietary and drug measures that are essential to health maintenance.

- Use a congestive heart failure chart. Items should include the date; your weight; your pulse—both the rate and regularity; any symptoms (for example, breathlessness on exertion, breathlessness on lying down, cough, increase in body weight, irregular heartbeat, abdominal pressure, or ankle swelling); diet (amount of salt, and approximate volumes of fluid); medication (digitalis, diuretics, and other); and probable side effects of drugs. (See Appendix C, pages 324–325, for a congestive heart failure chart to use for your medical records.)

- If you have a heart disease, join a support group such as Heart to Heart. Contact the American Heart Association (7320 Greenville Avenue, Dallas, TX 75231) for information on a local chapter or consult your local telephone directory.

The Digestive System

CONSTIPATION

Adults have established, regular patterns of bowel movements. Many have daily movements, and most have more than four each week. Like other bodily functions, such as eating and sleeping, bowel activity is individualized and is affected by many personal and environmental factors. Thus, slight "irregularity" is the rule.

Constipation may be defined as a decrease in the frequency of bowel movements below the "normal" (usually below three per week or one every three days) for a particular individual who is consuming an adequate diet. In addition, movements tend to become hard, dry, and painful to pass when they are infrequent.

WHAT CAUSES CONSTIPATION?

Constipation is a symptom; it is not a disease but is rather the result of some disease or body imbalance. It develops whenever the lower bowel, or colon, fails to propel and expel digested and nondigested food and waste regularly and efficiently (see figure 11).

Ordinarily, the colon's contents remain bulky and soft because the nondigestible plant fibers from vegetables, fruits, and bran hold small amounts of water in the bowel. Major causes of constipation may be either local (in the colon) or general (throughout the body). Blockage of the lower bowel by a tumor, the inflammation of diverticulitis, or a hernia or slowing of colon action by colitis are important local causes. General conditions that contribute to delayed emptying of the colon include drug use (especially antacids, strong pain medications, iron supplements, and medications for hypertension), metabolic illnesses (like diabetes and thyroid trouble), and conditions such as stroke and depression.

With few exceptions, factors such as emotional upsets, travel, and simple changes in the diet do not produce constipation.

HOW CAN CONSTIPATION AFFECT YOU?

Tradition has it that "sluggish bowels" lead to poor appetite, crankiness, and mental dullness. In actual fact, constipation usually produces only slight lower abdominal cramps and local pain with bowel movements. More prolonged constipation may result in bloating of the abdomen, nausea, and bleeding with bowel movements. There are two hazards of infrequent bowel movements—those related to the underlying cause and those produced by overenergetic attempts at corrective treatment with laxatives and enemas.

Consult Your Doctor Now IF

- Any change in bowel habits continues for more than two weeks.
- Sharp or severe abdominal pain or soreness occurs.
- Red or blackish blood appears with bowel movements.
- Loss of appetite, vomiting, or loss of weight develops.

Goals of Care

- To discover and understand the cause, or causes, of decreased colon activity.
- To establish a safe, comprehensive program that results in regular bowel movements.

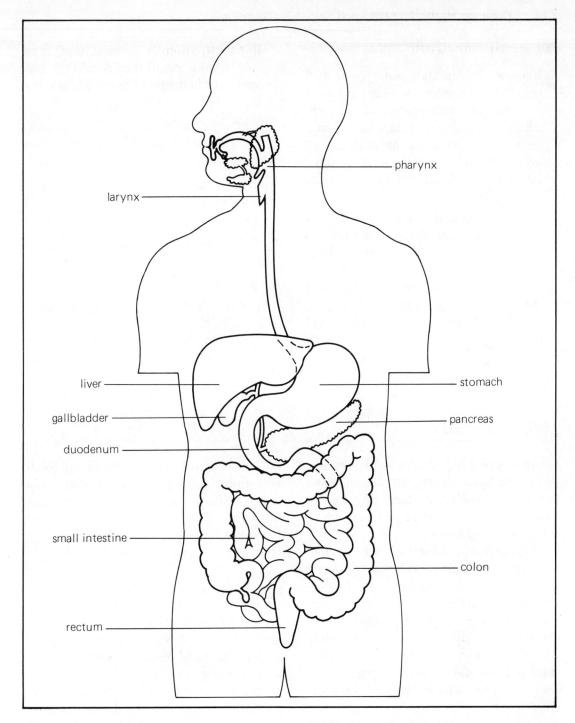

pharynx

larynx

liver

stomach

gallbladder

pancreas

duodenum

small intestine

colon

rectum

Figure 11. The digestive system

Self-Care Techniques

- Keep a constipation chart or record that indicates dates and times of bowel movements, appearance of movements, associated symptoms (such as cramps, pain, or bleeding), and your weight. (See Appendix C, page 321, for a constipation chart to use for your medical records.)

- Review personal events of the past month, searching for (1) the first noticeable change in your bowel habits; (2) any change in appetite; (3) any occurrence of abdominal pain; and (4) the use of *any* drug, especially in treating stomach ulcer, high blood pressure, depression, pain, diarrhea, or glaucoma.

- If constipation is present less than two weeks, or if this condition has been studied and diagnosed, start a high-fiber diet (see chapter 6).

- If a comfortable, "normal" bowel movement does not occur by day four, use one glycerin suppository as directed.

- If the suppository is ineffective after two days, administer a gentle Fleet (prepackaged) enema.

- If the enema is not effective, contact your doctor.

- *DO NOT*
  1. Take strong laxatives such as castor oil or Ex-Lax.
  2. Use any laxative for more than two weeks.

■ DIARRHEA

Most adults have a remarkably regular pattern of bowel movements. Some have two to three each day, others only two to three each week, but most have a predictable bowel habit.

Diarrhea is an increase in the frequency or volume of movements for a given individual. In most cases, the person with diarrhea has more frequent movements that are also watery and loose or poorly formed. In addition, any irritation of the bowels may produce painful abdominal cramps, nausea, and if severe, actual bleeding into the movements.

Episodes of diarrhea that last more than ten to fourteen days or diarrhea that occurs in repeated bouts—so-called *chronic diarrhea*—is usually due to medical conditions that require special study and treatment. *Acute diarrhea,* or spells of abnormally frequent and loose bowel movements that typically last less than ten days, is another matter.

WHAT CAUSES DIARRHEA?

Any process that irritates the bowel, stimulates its secretions, or increases the water content of material being digested may produce diarrhea.

Many cases of acute diarrhea (gastroenteritis) are caused by the actions of viruses and bacteria. Viruses, most of which are easily spread by contaminated food and water, may infect the wall of the bowel and, by producing local inflammation, cause "weeping" of fluids into bowel contents and high-volume diarrhea. Some bacterial organisms act in a similar manner. Germs (such as those causing typhoid fever) reach the intestine in poorly preserved meats, milk, or vegetables; infect the wall of the bowel; and stimulate fluid loss. Still other bacteria (such as those that cause some forms of traveler's diarrhea) cause gastroenteritis by releasing potent chemicals or toxins that damage the intestinal lining.

Many magnesium-containing laxatives (for example, milk of magnesia and Epsom salts) and antacids (for example, Gelusil and Maalox) may stimulate diarrhea if used in generous amounts. In fact, excessive use of any sort of laxative may lead to watery diarrhea. Many other types of drugs, from antibiotics to alcohol, can irritate the bowel and cause acute diarrhea.

Finally, individuals with the problem of irritable bowel may experience acute episodes of diarrhea. These persons' responses to emotional stress are thought to produce irritability of the bowel, which causes rapid movement of its contents.

HOW CAN DIARRHEA AFFECT YOU?

In most instances, acute diarrhea results in temporary loss of water and salt from the body in amounts that can be corrected by increasing fluid intake. If these losses are rapid and continue for several days, serious dehydration and loss of critical body elements may occur.

Contaminated meat or dairy products may produce two to three days of simple gastroenteritis: six to twelve loose, watery movements each day, with mild abdominal cramps and slight weakness. More severe attacks of food poisoning may include nausea and vomiting. As a rule, a light diet of clear fluids and the use of an absorbent medicine (like Pepto-Bismol and Donnagel) serve to control these symptoms.

Acute traveler's diarrhea may be disabling, especially in older persons. The explosive watery movements, severe cramps, weakness, dizziness, and slight fever may last four to five days. Only rarely does the fluid and salt loss caused by diarrhea lead to such serious dehydration that antibiotics and intravenous fluid treatment are necessary.

The acute diarrhea caused by direct infection of the intestine by typhoidlike bacteria may be quite severe, with watery, even bloody movements; abdominal pain; fever; and general discomfort. Full courses of antibiotics and intravenous fluids are often required for prompt and complete recovery.

Most diarrhea related directly to medications such as digitalis, antibiotics, and diuretics is mild and tapers off in two to three days after the drug treatment is stopped.

■■■ *Consult Your Doctor Now* **IF**

- You have acute diarrhea that has lasted more than three days.
- You have acute diarrhea and bloody bowel movements.
- You have acute diarrhea complicated

by chills, fever, vomiting, severe abdominal pain, or fainting.

Goals of Care

- To control the symptoms of acute diarrhea, or gastroenteritis.
- To prevent complications of acute diarrhea.

Self-Care Techniques

- Keep a diarrhea chart or record that indicates the date; the time of each bowel movement; the texture and color of each bowel movement (solid, loose, or liquid; tan, brown, black, or red); associated symptoms such as pain, cramps, nausea, vomiting, fever, chills, and rectal soreness; and treatment (time, type and volume of fluids, antidiarrheal medications, and other medications). (See Appendix C, pages 326–327, for a diarrhea chart to use for your medical records.)
- Force fluid intake to replace salt and water lost by diarrhea. Eight to ten glassfuls of water, fruit juice, or soup should replace the daily losses. Milk, milk products, and solid foods seem to prolong the diarrhea in some individuals.
- Take regular doses of a safe antidiarrheal agent until the symptoms have been controlled for one full day (for example, Pepto-Bismol, two tablespoonfuls by mouth four to eight times a day).

■ HEARTBURN

Under usual circumstances, fluids and well-chewed food move silently and smoothly from mouth to stomach, propelled by the muscular walls of the esophagus (see figure 12). Once the fluids and food are in the stomach, the chemicals and acids released by the stomach lining digest, or break down, the food particles. After digestion, the material moves down from the stomach to the bowel.

If stomach secretions back up into the lower end of the esophagus, a deep, burning pain or less severe discomfort may develop under the lower breastbone—this is heartburn. It occurs most often approximately one hour after meals, when lying down, or when foods like citrus juices are swallowed. In addition, some people with heartburn complain of food sticking in the lower breastbone area, of belching, and/or of regurgitating partly digested food.

About 10 percent of otherwise normal healthy adults experience heartburn on a daily basis; thus this is a common problem among adults.

WHAT CAUSES HEARTBURN?

In most cases, heartburn is caused by a combination of the following three factors: repeated reflux (or backup) of stomach secretions, slow emptying of

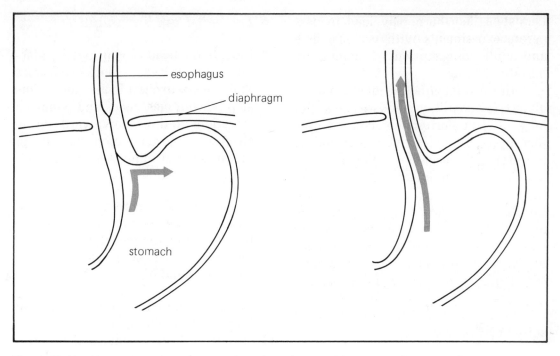

Figure 12. Heartburn occurs because a weakened esophagus sphincter muscle cannot close enough to stop the contents of the stomach from backing up into the esophagus.

the esophagus, and chemical irritation of the esophageal lining.

Reflux esophagitis often results from a weakness in the valvelike muscle that normally keeps the stomach contents moving downward. Increased abdominal pressure, like that produced by pregnancy or obesity, may force the muscle open. Also, many drugs (such as pain medications, certain sedatives, and asthma medications) seem to relax this muscle, causing a reflux of stomach secretions. Leaning over, straining, or lying flat puts more pressure on the weakened muscle. Foods like citrus juices often irritate the esophageal lining, so individuals with heartburn learn to avoid them. Cigarette smoking, alco-

hol, and fatty foods also increase heartburn in some instances.

Some people have heartburn as a result of a hiatus hernia, or bulging of part of the stomach into the chest cavity. Here, conservative treatment usually prevents bleeding and blockage. Still others may have underlying peptic ulcers (see pages 229–232) or a form of esophagitis related to alcohol abuse. Cancer of the esophagus occasionally causes heartburn.

HOW CAN HEARTBURN AFFECT YOU?

Heartburn is a burning discomfort in the chest, which causes distress and anxiety.

Persistent heartburn may lead to desperate experiments with various diets and with consumption of potentially harmful drugs.

Reflux esophagitis, the most common underlying condition, tends to be a lifelong problem. Fortunately, conservative therapy is often effective in controlling this type of heartburn. Weight loss, avoidance of fruit juices and fats, reduction in smoking and alcohol consumption, use of antacids, and elevation of the head of the bed relieve esophagitis and pain. Rarely, the inflammation causes ulceration, with subsequent bleeding, scarring, and narrowing of the esophageal opening. If this occurs, surgical treatment is required to ease any difficulty in swallowing.

▆ *Consult Your Doctor Now* <u>IF</u>

▪ You have unexplained heartburn that lasts for more than two weeks.

▪ You have heartburn that is associated with weight loss, difficulty in swallowing, or vomiting of blood.

▆ *Goals of Care*

▪ To control the symptoms of heartburn.

▪ To prevent the complications of reflux esophagitis.

▆ *Self-Care Techniques*

▪ Elevate the head of your bed by placing its upper legs on blocks or frames that are six to eight inches high. This step encourages food and stomach secretions to drain downward during sleep. It is more effective than sleeping on several pillows, since the pillows tend to slide.

▪ If your weight exceeds your "lean" weight at ages twenty to twenty-five by more than 10 percent, start a practical diet and exercise program (see chapters 5 and 6).

▪ Modify your diet by (1) decreasing fat intake, (2) avoiding citrus juices and chocolate, (3) omitting or decreasing alcoholic beverages, and (4) not eating food during the three to four hours before bedtime.

▪ Stop smoking cigarettes.

▪ Take two tablespoonfuls of an antacid preparation containing magnesium and aluminum (for example, Riopan or Maalox) one hour after each meal and at bedtime or chew two to four tablets of Gaviscon after meals and at bedtime.

▆ LOSS OF APPETITE, NAUSEA, AND VOMITING

Few bodily sensations are more disagreeable than nausea and vomiting, which in many cases are preceded by loss of appetite. Each symptom may occur by itself, but failing appetite may lead to nausea, and nausea to vomiting. The combination of symptoms may vary, depending on the cause.

Appetite, or a positive interest in food, is a complicated phenomenon, while *anorexia,* prolonged loss of appetite for normally attractive food, is even more difficult to understand. All persons experience temporary loss of appetite during times of stress and high emotion—such as from anxiety, fear, depression, or joy. But a disinterest in food may progress to an active feeling of revulsion, accompanied by vague but disagreeable feelings in the pit of the stomach—this is *nausea.* The nauseated person may feel weak and sweaty and oversecrete saliva. Intense or persistent nausea often leads to *vomiting.* Vomiting is forceful spasms of the abdominal muscles, which force stomach contents upward into the esophagus and throat, and from there to the outside, often with some relief of the nausea.

The anorexia-nausea-vomiting sequence seems to represent the complex outcome of a great number of psychological and physical reactions—some normal and protective, some abnormal and harmful. When the sequence of symptoms lasts more than a day or so, or when it recurs repeatedly, a significant disease often exists.

WHAT CAUSES LACK OF APPETITE, NAUSEA, AND VOMITING?

Appetite, lack of appetite, nausea, and vomiting are controlled by several nerve centers in the lower brain. Local chemical changes in these areas and nerve impulses arising from all parts of the body interact to trigger anorexia-nausea-vomiting events. Once the centers are stimulated, nerves in the abdomen and elsewhere coordinate a series of physical changes that lead to vomiting. Stomach contractions cease, and the lower outlet to the stomach closes; strong abdominal muscles then go into spasm, forcing stomach contents upward into the esophagus. Breathing stops momentarily as the food and secretions flow outward.

Many individuals with persistent nausea and vomiting have some type of *abdominal disease.* Partial or complete blockage of the stomach (by a peptic ulcer), intestine (by a tumor), or colon (by diverticulitis) leads to backup of digested food and vomiting. Inflammatory processes like gallbladder disease and hepatitis (viral infection of the liver) may be complicated by nausea and vomiting.

A common cause of poor appetite, nausea, and vomiting in adults is *drug effect.* Aspirin, antiarthritis pills, parkinsonism medications, and alcohol produce these symptoms by their direct action on the lining of the stomach. Digitalis, morphinelike painkillers, and certain asthma treatments (theophylline) seem to stimulate vomiting centers in the brain to cause poor appetite, nausea, and vomiting. Chemically induced vomiting may result from medical conditions such as kidney failure, uncontrolled diabetes mellitus, and advanced liver disease.

On occasion, *diseases of the nervous system* cause prolonged and disabling nausea and vomiting, Some stroke victims experience frequent vomiting; persons with brain tumors often experience nausea and vomiting; dizziness caused by ear damage (see page 179) may be accompanied by these symptoms.

Many people with intense pain (from a kidney stone, for example) feel nauseated and have no appetite. Finally, anorexia may be a prominent feature of depression and chronic anxiety.

HOW CAN LOSS OF APPETITE, NAUSEA, AND VOMITING AFFECT YOU?

If severe or persistent, loss of appetite, nausea, and vomiting lead to decreased intake and loss of body fluids and food. As a result, rapid, even dangerous loss of weight and strength may occur if the underlying medical condition is not corrected. Intense vomiting may become a medical emergency and require hospitalization for the administration of intravenous fluids and medications to replace lost nutrients (such as potassium and glucose), to control symptoms, and to treat the underlying problem.

When poor appetite and restricted food intake continue for weeks—as may occur with depression or cancer of the intestine—weight loss, muscle weakness, and fatigue may become problems in themselves.

Retching (dry heaves) and vomiting, if severe and uncontrolled, may cause irritation and even tearing of the lining of the esophagus and stomach, with dramatic and life-threatening bleeding.

■■■ *Consult Your Doctor Now IF*

- You have unexplained loss of appetite, nausea, and/or vomiting that lasts for more than two days.
- You have loss of appetite, nausea, and/or vomiting that prevents you from taking important medications for conditions such as diabetes mellitus, heart disease, parkinsonism, or high blood pressure.

- You have severe nausea and vomiting that are causing weakness, faintness, or stomach bleeding (red or black material in the vomit).

■■■ *Goals of Care*

- To control loss of appetite, nausea, and vomiting.
- To prevent the complications of nausea and vomiting such as excessive weight loss, malnutrition, and dangerous loss of fluids and salt.

■■■ *Self-Care Techniques*

- Use a vomiting chart that records such information as the date and time of vomiting; the nature (color and contents) and approximate volume of vomit; the food and fluid intake by mouth; all medications taken (for nausea and vomiting or for other conditions); associated symptoms (such as pain, diarrhea, faintness, or dizziness); and your body weight. (See Appendix C, pages 328–329, for a vomiting chart to use for your records.)
- If loss of appetite and nausea are due to temporary causes, (1) maintain fluid intake with sips or small glasses of cool drinks such as ginger ale, cola drinks, apple juice, and skim milk; (2) avoid fluids with strong smells (such as coffee and meat soups) or high fat content (like milk shakes); and (3) try taking balanced antacids (such as Mylanta-II or Maalox TC) one tablespoonful every four hours or so.

■ ABDOMINAL PAIN

All persons experience brief aches and pains in the abdomen, ranging from the hunger pains of an empty stomach to the dull cramp of a full bowel. Significant pain, that which demands attention and care, can usually be recognized by one or more of the following features: (1) It always occurs in one particular area. (2) It is quite severe or unpleasant. (3) It lasts for more than an hour, or it comes back repeatedly. (4) It is accompanied by other symptoms such as nausea, vomiting, or diarrhea. In adults, five conditions account for more than 90 percent of complaints of significant abdominal pain (or, as the British say, "dyspepsia"). These five conditions are duodenal ulcer, gastric ulcer, gallbladder disease, esophagitis, and functional distress.

Duodenal ulcer, an inflammation of the upper small intestine, often develops in early middle age and persists throughout life. The pain of an active ulcer is typically a burning or sharp pain. It is most often located deep in the pit of the stomach, just above the navel. Many ulcer patients have pain at night. The discomfort seems worse two to three hours after meals, and ingesting milk or food often relieves ulcer pain (see pages 229–232).

The distress caused by a *gastric ulcer,* an area of inflammation in the stomach itself, may be distinctive. This condition is more likely to arise in adults fifty to sixty years of age. The pain is persistent, often described as "dull" or "aching." It is most often located in the middle of the upper abdomen, and it may run through to the back. Gastric ulcers may not respond promptly to food and milk. They often cause nausea and vomiting, so weight loss may be an associated problem.

The pain of *gallbladder disease* tends to occur in attacks or spells. Starting at mid-life, the attacks begin suddenly, last for hours to a day or more, and then subside completely. The pain is steady, dull, and often quite severe, usually centered deep under the right ribs or above the navel. The ache may run into the back, and nausea and vomiting are quite common (see pages 225–228).

Esophagitis, irritation and spasm of the esophagus, produces a fairly characteristic form of abdominal pain. The major symptom is heartburn—burning pain, often occurring in waves, located behind the breastbone and often relieved in a few minutes by milk or antacids (see pages 216–218). In addition, sour material may be belched up, especially after large meals or at night. If the esophageal irritation is severe, mouthfuls of solid food may "stick" on swallowing, causing still more heartburn and pressure.

Many other people with years of bothersome abdominal pain who have no obvious medical disease are said to have *functional distress,* though the condition is given such labels as irritable colon syndrome, irritable bowel syndrome, spastic colon, functional bowel syndrome, and mucous colitis. Typically, the pains are vague in nature, occur in different areas of the abdomen, are not regularly related to meals, and are not complicated by vomiting. This condition may be difficult to diagnose and to treat effectively. These individuals often undergo repeated tests and X-ray studies to no avail.

WHAT CAUSES ABDOMINAL PAIN?

Any condition that irritates the hollow portions of the gastrointestinal tract will produce spasm and abdominal pain. In addition, inflammation of the surface of structures like the gallbladder gives rise to localized sharp pain and tenderness.

The exact cause, or causes, of *ulcers* of the duodenum (intestine) and stomach are still not known. Overproduction of stomach acid and digestive enzymes occurs in most patients with duodenal ulcers, and it may be that a weakness or other abnormality of the stomach lining permits stomach ulcers to develop. Many drugs, including alcohol, steroids, and aspirin and most other arthritis medications, predispose individuals to ulcers.

The pain of *gallbladder disease* results from a combination of blockage of bile flow by gallstones and inflammation of the outer surface of the gallbladder wall.

Most experts feel that *esophagitis* pain is triggered by the irritating action of stomach acid that backs up (refluxes) into the esophagus. This action generates spasm that produces pain and partial blockage of swallowed food.

Finally, the direct cause of *functional distress* is unclear, but it seems that a long-standing emotional disorder or some nervous abnormality of the stomach and upper intestine is at fault. Stress of any sort tends to activate the oversensitive system and leads to pain.

HOW CAN ABDOMINAL PAIN AFFECT YOU?

Abdominal pain is a two-edged sword. On the one hand, it may serve as a life-saving warning of active disease; on the other hand, it can produce misery, worry, and expense.

Significant pain should *always* be heeded and, in most instances, investigated thoroughly before being dismissed or treated with painkilling medications. Some types of distress, as noted earlier, are quite distinctive and point to a simple condition (the man with years of duodenal ulcer disease has little difficulty recognizing when the ulcer is again active). However, very similar pain may result from disease of the pancreas, a condition requiring very different treatment, so abdominal pain must always be treated with respect.

Prolonged or repeated pain can be demoralizing. It distracts the victim, makes sleep difficult or impossible, interferes with eating, and often leads to feelings of depression. Fortunately, most conditions that cause abdominal pain can be controlled, if not cured, by modern medical and surgical treatments.

■ *Consult Your Doctor Now* **IF**

- You have unexplained abdominal pain that lasts for more than an hour; is severe enough to keep you awake; is accompanied by nausea, vomiting, or other unpleasant symptoms; or makes you feel anxious.

- You have typical abdominal pain of an established condition (for example, ulcer) that has changed in severity, quality, or location.

Goals of Care

- To identify the nature and cause of any abdominal pain.
- To control or eliminate abdominal pain.

Self-Care Technique

- Fill in an abdominal pain chart that includes the dates; the onset times of the pain; any precipitating events; the location of the pain (use figure 11); the severity of the pain—1 to 4, with 4 being the most painful; the nature of the attacks—in spells or constant; any associated symptoms (nausea, vomiting, diarrhea, fever, and so on); and the method used to obtain pain relief (rest, food, medications, and so on). (See Appendix C, pages 330–331, for an abdominal pain chart to use for your medical records.)

■ DIVERTICULOSIS AND DIVERTICULITIS

The colon, or large bowel, is a hollow, tubelike organ that connects the small bowel and the rectum. About four feet in length, this muscle-lined passage absorbs water from digested food in the bowel, mixes the contents of the bowel, and transports waste materials for excretion (see figure 13).

As time and wear and tear weaken the walls of the colon, the pressure inside the colon pushes out small fingerlike pouches of the bowel lining. These pouches, or diverticula, are most common in the lower third of the colon. It is estimated that almost half the adults in the United States have diverticula—and, therefore, the condition known as *diverticulosis*—even though most have no illness or symptoms related to them.

On occasion, the very tip of a colonic diverticular pouch becomes inflamed and swollen. If this reaction continues and produces irritation of the actual colon wall and surrounding areas, *diverticu-litis* is present. The importance of diverticulitis as a medical disorder in adults has been compared to that of appendicitis. If the diverticulum bursts, contents from the colon may enter the general abdominal cavity, producing life-threatening infection, or peritonitis, and bloodstream contamination.

WHAT CAUSES DIVERTICULOSIS AND DIVERTICULITIS?

Two factors work together to produce diverticula in some older people—local weak spots in the colon wall and abnormal pressures inside the colon. The wall of this part of the bowel is made up of bands and sheets of muscle, with small, often weaker gaps in between. Pressure within the colon builds up when the muscle sheets contract to propel food along its course. Excessive pressure, which may result from a low-bulk diet and irritability of the colon, slowly bal-

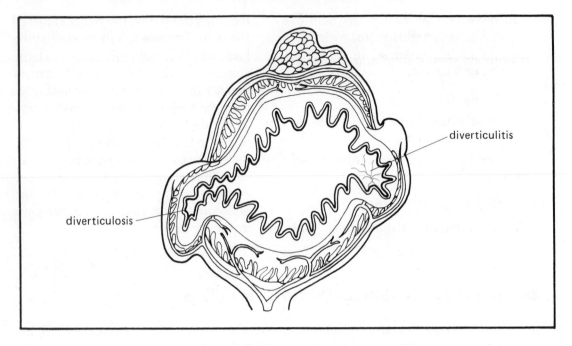

Figure 13. A cross section of the colon showing diverticulosis and diverticulitis

loons the lining of the colon through these weakened gaps, and diverticula result.

The actual cause of diverticulitis, or inflammation of these pouches, is not known. Once started, however, the process may spread to involve the surrounding colon wall. Severe inflammation may penetrate the wall of the bowel, leading to serious infection within the abdominal cavity.

HOW CAN DIVERTICULOSIS AND DIVERTICULITIS AFFECT YOU?

In most instances, diverticulosis of the colon causes no symptoms or illness. Some older people with diverticula will complain of occasional cramps in the left lower abdomen associated with bloating, gas, and constipation. Increasing the dietary intake of fiber with added bran, fresh vegetables, grains, and fruit often relieves the colon spasm.

Diverticulitis may produce increasing left lower abdominal pain and soreness, constipation, and fever—so-called left-sided appendicitis. A great majority of these attacks of diverticulitis subside on conservative treatment with a liquid diet, bed rest, and antibiotic therapy, but a few progress to a stage that requires an operation to remove the inflamed section of the bowel.

If an ulcer forms at the edge of a diverticular pouch, bleeding into the colon may result.

- You have persistent lower abdominal cramps or steady pain and soreness.
- You pass stools that are red or reddish black in color.

Goals of Care

- To prevent the development of any diverticula.
- To prevent the complications of diverticulosis, diverticulitis and bleeding.

Self-Care Techniques

- Avoid the use of drugs (such as painkillers, antidepressants, and iron salts) that slow down bowel action and cause high pressure in the colon.
- Avoid the use of drugs that irritate the colon (such as irritating laxatives like castor oil, and saline laxatives, like magnesium sulfate).
- Eat a diet high in vegetable fiber, or roughage. A daily intake of thirty to forty grams of fiber, which increases the water content and softness of bowel movements, can be accomplished by eating generous portions of wheat bran (in cereal and muffins or sprinkled on other foods), whole wheat bread, and leafy vegetables (see chapter 6). Also, you may supplement dietary fiber with a bulk laxative such as Metamucil.

GALLBLADDER DISEASE

The gallbladder is a small, pear-shaped, membranous sac attached to the liver. Bile, a vital digestive juice secreted by the liver, is stored in the gallbladder. From the gallbladder, bile flows along a narrow tube (the bile duct) on its way to the upper intestine, where it is first mixed with partly digested food. When this food leaves the stomach on its way to the intestines, the gallbladder squeezes out the stored-up volume of bile to accelerate digestion and the absorption of fats and other nutrients, which takes place in the intestines. Between meals, much of the bile is stored in the gallbladder.

If the chemicals contained in gallbladder bile become too concentrated, small crystals begin to form in the bile, much as ice crystals form in cold water. The crystals may then clump together in the shape of fine gravel or pebbles known as *gallstones*.

Most gallstones lie quietly in the gallbladder for years and cause little damage to the lining of the sac. When a stone is squeezed out of the gallbladder along with bile, however, it may become lodged in the narrow part (neck) of the gallbladder (see figure 14). If the stone blocks the flow of bile, the gallbladder swells up, and its walls become inflamed. This is *cholecystitis* (literally, "inflammation of the gallbladder").

Almost 20 percent of adults in the

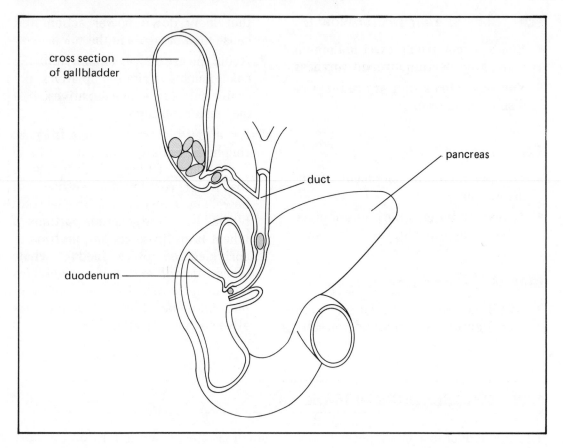

Figure 14. Gallstones

United States have or will develop gall-stones, and about half of these will eventually develop signs of cholecystitis.

WHAT CAUSES GALLBLADDER DISEASE?

Many body factors interact to produce critical changes in the chemical makeup of bile. First, some ethnic groups seem to have inherited abnormalities of bile for-mation. Southwest American Indians and certain northern European groups have remarkably high rates of gall-bladder disease. Second, certain female hormonal factors seem to affect bile formation, for gallbladder disease occurs three times more often in women than in men, especially in women who are over-weight or have had several pregnancies. Third, a few medical conditions seem to predispose individuals to the develop-ment of gallstones and other gallbladder diseases. Persons with diabetes mellitus and certain forms of anemia experience more of these problems than others. In the last analysis, however, almost any person, especially anyone over fifty, is a potential candidate for gallbladder disease.

HOW CAN GALLBLADDER DISEASE AFFECT YOU?

The majority of adults with gallstones never develop significant problems—their bile functions well, digestion is normal, and no treatment is required. In the absence of definite symptoms—many cases are discovered when X rays are taken for other conditions—most doctors prefer to treat the condition with weight reduction, low-fat diet, and careful observation.

However, about one-third of the people with gallstones do develop signs of gallbladder inflammation when a stone prevents the gallbladder from emptying completely. The gallbladder swells up, it becomes irritated, and its walls become inflamed. Pain, usually severe, is felt deep below the right rib cage, or in the right upper abdomen. The pain is often steady; lasts from one to twenty-four hours; and is accompanied by nausea, vomiting, and slight fever. Most often this acute attack subsides with medical treatment. Most experts recommend surgical removal of the gallbladder shortly after the episode ends.

A few persons with gallstones are less fortunate in that one or more stones from the gallbladder pass into the main bile duct, blocking all bile flow from the liver to the bowel. As a result, yellow bile pigment backs up into the blood and produces jaundice (yellow skin) accompanied by dark brown urine due to the escape of bile pigment through the kidneys, abdominal pain, vomiting, fever, and other signs of a serious medical illness. Operations to relieve this sort of blockage may be long and complicated.

Cancer very rarely develops in the stone-containing gallbladder. However, if it should develop, the condition is always serious, and recovery is often only temporary after surgical treatment.

■ *Consult Your Doctor Now IF*

■ You have one or more attacks of unexplained right upper abdominal pain and tenderness with gastrointestinal upset.

■ You have an unusual yellow tinge to your skin and dark brown urine.

■ *Goals of Care*

■ To relieve symptoms of gallbladder disease.

■ To prevent complications of gallbladder disease.

■ *Self-Care Techniques*

■ Maintain your body weight at or below 10 percent above your lean weight at age twenty to age twenty-five.

■ Be certain that any medical condition you have, such as diabetes mellitus, is under proper control.

■ Do not use drugs that lower blood cholesterol levels (for example, clofibrate or Atromid-S), for they tend to increase gallstone formation.

■ Consume a diet low in fat and cholesterol. As practical first steps, omit foods with high cholesterol and high saturated-fat content, for example, visibly fat meats, organ meats, eggs, butter, lobsters, oysters, shrimp, and clams; substitute soft margarine for butter, skim milk for whole milk, and egg whites for whole eggs; and eat more whole grains, fruits, and vegetables. Reduce your dietary fat intake to about 30 percent of your total calories; reduce your daily cholesterol intake to 100–150 mg per day (the U.S. average is about 500 mg per day). In addition, reduce your saturated fat intake to about 10 percent of your total calories. (See chapter 6.)

■ HEMORRHOIDS

Under normal conditions, the anus, a two-inch-long canal that represents the lowermost portion of the colon, is flattened and empty. The anus serves primarily as a valve, or clamp, that relaxes periodically to allow the passage of bowel movements. Its inner wall contains a large network of thin-walled veins that drain blood upward from the pelvis.

The irritation of hard bowel movements and the increasing pressure from above generated by coughing and straining may combine to dilate the veins within the anus. These dilated, or varicose, veins (see pages 203–205) of the anal canal are hemorrhoids, or piles.

Some of these soft, round swellings are located an inch or two inside the anal canal (internal hemorrhoids), whereas others occur as small purple tabs around the anal opening (external hemorrhoids).

More than half the adult population of the United States has hemorrhoids, but only a small number of people will develop local symptoms that require special care.

WHAT CAUSES HEMORRHOIDS?

As with varicose veins in the legs (see pages 203–205), the exact causes of hemorrhoids are still not known for certain. Some individuals seem to have lifelong weakness of the vein walls and thus develop bothersome hemorrhoids as young adults. Some studies show that women who have had several pregnancies are especially prone to this problem, suggesting that the enlarged womb has put pressure on the vein system. Piles are uncommon in countries where high-fiber diets are consumed. Therefore, it may be that constipation and hard bowel movements contribute to weakness and dilatation of the veins.

HOW CAN HEMORRHOIDS AFFECT YOU?

Most people with hemorrhoids have no symptoms at all or have occasional drops of red blood on the toilet paper or on the surface of the bowel movements. If blood is present, it is important to have a careful rectal examination, including a sigmoidoscopy (direct inspection of the inside of the anus and rectum through a slender, lighted tube), to be certain that no tumor or other condition is present. Mild itching of local skin may occur, but it is usually caused by dermatitis and not by the hemorrhoids.

Large hemorrhoids that have been present for many years may slide through the anal opening during a bowel movement—a so-called prolapse. If they become trapped or locked in this location, pain and bleeding may occur, making sitting and bowel movements exquisitely painful. Bed rest, local warm compresses, and mild pain medication usually relieve the acute episode, but surgical removal of the offending tabs is often desirable.

Some individuals experience sudden clotting of blood in an external hemorrhoid. This usually occurs while lifting heavy objects or straining during bowel movements. The blocked hemorrhoid becomes very painful and tender. The condition, however, usually subsides in five to seven days with rest, local warm soaks or baths, and use of soothing lotions to decrease local irritation.

Hemorrhoids do not progress into polyps or tumors, but it is always dangerous to assume that all anal bleeding is due to simple hemorrhoids.

Consult Your Doctor Now IF

■ You develop unexplained bleeding from your anal canal.

■ You experience severe or repeated anal pain with bowel movements or straining.

Goals of Care

■ To prevent acute symptoms of hemorrhoids.

■ To prevent complications (such as bleeding, prolapse, or clotting) of hemorrhoids.

Self-Care Techniques

■ Design and follow a high-fiber diet. You can have softer movements that cause less local irritation of hemorrhoids by adding bran (three tablespoonfuls a day) to your meals, eating generous portions of fresh vegetables and fruits, and using whole wheat bread.

■ Develop the habit of regular and prompt bowel movements. "Schedule" a movement thirty to sixty minutes after breakfast or another meal. Always move your bowels promptly when you feel the urge, thereby avoiding straining and undue pressure.

■ For minor hemorrhoidal bleeding or itching, apply cold compresses to the anal area three to four times a day. Keep the skin soft and moist with creams or salves (for example, Aquaphor, Lubriderm, or plain Vaseline). Note: Pain-reducing agents may produce even more itchiness and skin irritation.

■ For painful or tender hemorrhoids, (1) rest in bed until the pain decreases; (2) take hot, soapy sit-down baths twice a day and apply hot, wet compresses to the anal area every two to three hours; and (3) keep the area soft by using bland creams or salves.

■ PEPTIC ULCER DISEASE

The normal stomach is a magnificent digestive machine. It holds, mixes, partially digests, and propels food downward with remarkable efficiency. The act of eating starts the gastric juices of the stomach flowing. The acid and pepsin (the chemical that digests proteins) secretions act together to begin the complex process of splitting foods into smaller units. As swallowed foods fill the stomach, even more juices are released, and the gentle kneading action of the stomach walls mixes the contents of the stomach effectively. Then, within a few minutes, the valvelike lower end of the stomach relaxes, and the contents of the stomach pass into the intestine for the next step in digestion (see figure 15).

Normally, the rate of acid and pepsin release is carefully controlled—the amounts released just meet the needs for digestion. In addition, the normal stomach wall is protected from the action of these chemicals by a thin film of mucus secretions. When the secretion rate is increased and/or the protective mucus barrier is abnormal, the lining of the stomach or of the upper intestine is eroded, or eaten away, in small patches, resulting in sores, or lesions, known as ulcers. The stomach lesions are called gastric ulcers, while the intestinal sores are known as duodenal ulcers. Both gastric and duodenal ulcers are called peptic ulcer disease.

Although the incidence of peptic ulcer disease in the United States seems to be decreasing in recent years, some studies suggest that as many as 10 percent of adults will have an ulcer at some time in their lives.

WHAT CAUSES PEPTIC ULCER DISEASE?

Peptic ulcers are caused by the actions of stomach acid and pepsin on the inner

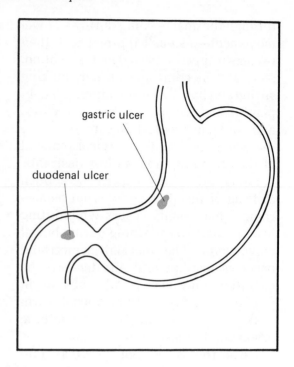

gastric ulcer

duodenal ulcer

Figure 15. Duodenal and gastric ulcers

linings of the stomach and duodenum (upper intestine). In the case of gastric ulcers, in general, the protective mucus barrier seems to be abnormal. As a result, the highly irritating digestive juices attack the stomach lining, which dissolves and leaves shallow, round holes in the stomach wall. Studies of persons with duodenal ulcers suggest that the victims overproduce acid and pepsin secretions. For example, when persons with duodenal ulcers eat, the secretion response is excessive, and at night the stomach juices formed are abnormally rich in acid and pepsin. As a result, the stomach and intestine of these individuals are constantly bombarded by powerfully erosive digestive juices—and ulcers form. Some persons, therefore, develop both duodenal and gastric ulcers.

Just why certain people develop one or more ulcers and why the ulcers tend to recur throughout life is not clear. Duodenal ulcers seem to run in families and are much more common than gastric ulcers. Gastric ulcers tend to occur in older persons; many develop in persons past sixty. Gastric ulcers seem especially prone to reappear after initial treatment.

The notion that certain personality types—for example, the hard-driving executive—are prone to develop ulcer disease is not valid; however, emotional stress probably does make ulcer symptoms worse. Certain drugs, most notably aspirin and the new drugs used against arthritis, may irritate the stomach and activate ulcers. In addition, smoking, alcohol, and caffeine stimulate stomach secretions.

HOW CAN PEPTIC ULCER DISEASE AFFECT YOU?

When peptic ulcers are active—that is, when they are most raw and inflamed— pain is the problem. Most often, ulcer pain is felt as a steady aching or burning pain deep in the middle of the upper abdomen. Food or milk typically gives relief, but then the pain returns in an hour or so. Duodenal ulcer pain is especially prone to recur in the early morning hours. Nausea and vomiting may accompany the pain and are especially associated with active gastric ulcers. With careful dietary and medical management, most persons with peptic ulcer disease maintain full and active lives.

However, three serious complications may occur: bleeding; perforation, or rupture; and obstruction. If the ulcer extends deep into the lining of the duodenum or stomach, the digestive juices may weaken large blood vessels and produce hemorrhage. Sudden loss of large volumes of blood leads to vomiting of red material, whereas slower leakage produces anemia and black stools. Deeper erosion, especially of the thin-walled duodenum, may break through the intestine, flooding the abdominal cavity with irritating secretions and producing severe pain and shock. Patients with brisk bleeding or perforation require immediate surgical treatment. Progressive nausea, vomiting, and sensations of abdominal fullness suggest obstruction of the duodenum, which may occur when a chronic ulcer produces scarring and narrowing of the passage from the stomach to the intestine. Some patients with obstruction recover with stomach suction, but others require an operation to relieve the mechanical blockage and to decrease the stomach secretions.

▬ *Consult Your Doctor Now IF*

- You have repeated or persistent (lasting more than two weeks) unexplained upper abdominal pain that seems to be relieved by meals or that awakens you at night.
- You notice signs of gastrointestinal bleeding (vomiting of red or brownish material or passing of black or reddish black bowel movements).

▬ *Goals of Care*

- To relieve the symptoms of peptic ulcer disease.

- To promote healing and prevent complications of peptic ulcer disease.

Self-Care Techniques

- With the advice and approval of your doctor, design and follow a diet that will buffer or reduce the effects of stomach secretions on the ulcer. Such a diet should include three regular meals each day, with no eating after the evening meal and the exclusion of coffee and any other foods or substances that seem to cause abdominal pain.
- Avoid smoking and alcohol.
- Design a program of antacid therapy. Antacids are liquid and solid mixtures of magnesium, calcium, or aluminum compounds. Antacids neutralize gastric acid, thereby relieving pain and hastening ulcer healing. No particular medication or schedule is clearly superior, but the following rules apply: (1) Take the antacid by mouth one hour after each meal and at bedtime; some doctors advise extra doses three hours after each meal if the symptoms are severe. (2) Select an antacid that gives relief without producing diarrhea or constipation. In general, medications containing aluminum alone (for example, Amphojel and Basaljel) or aluminum with a balance of magnesium (for example, Maalox and Gelusil) do not cause diarrhea. (3) Avoid antacids that contain excessive calcium (which may cause kidney damage) or that consist of sodium bicarbonate (which may add large quantities of sodium, a substance to be avoided if hypertension or heart disease is present). (4) Choose an antacid that is potent enough to be effective in small volumes (for example, Maalox TC or Gelusil-II are effective in doses of one tablespoonful) yet is not too expensive (that is, it should cost less than $2.50 per day when properly used).
- If it is prescribed, use one of a new group of antiulcer drugs that block the stomach's response to stimulation and favor ulcer healing. Both Tagamet and Zantac seem to offer effective relief to persons with peptic ulcer disease.

The Urinary Tract

■ URINARY TRACT INFECTIONS

The urinary tract (see figure 16) consists of the kidneys, ureters, bladder, and urethra. The kidneys filter waste products from the blood and form urine. The paired ureters are small tubes that carry the urine from the kidneys to the bladder. The bladder stores urine until it is emptied through the urethra. The urethra is the short passage to the outside of the body. In healthy persons, the linings of

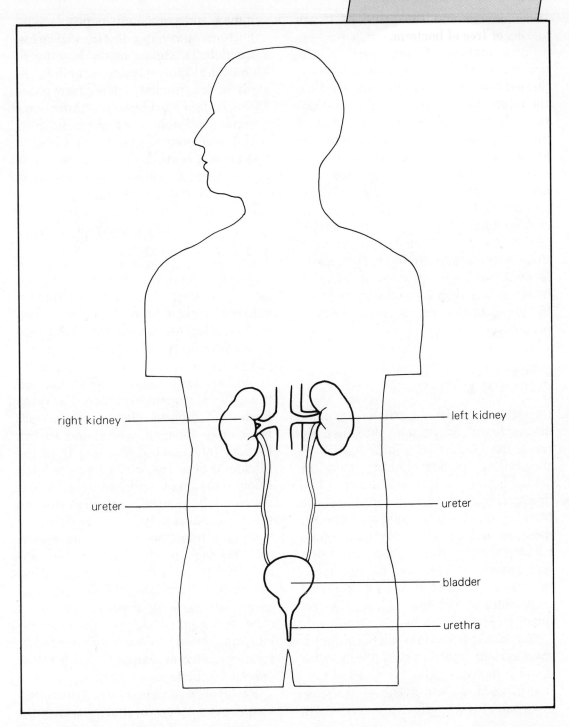

Figure 16. The urinary tract

these organs and the urine itself are sterile, o

Inf of the uri nts is t rethri- hral r

w

urinary tract are con- rection in one organ often s to the other organs.

A majority of urinary tract infections occur in women, though symptoms of these infections are similar in both sexes. Isolated or single episodes of infection do occur, but older individuals are likely to have chronic or recurrent urinary problems.

WHAT CAUSES URINARY TRACT INFECTIONS?

Bacterial organisms, which are commonly found on normal skin, usually reach the bladder by contamination of the urethral opening; clothing, hands, or sexual activity may infect the sensitive lining. Once lodged in the urethra and bladder, the bacteria multiply if body defenses fail to inactivate them, soon causing local inflammation—urethritis and cystitis. In response to this irritation, the muscles of the bladder contract to produce symptoms such as the frequent and painful passage of urine.

If invading bacteria reach the kidneys, more serious infection may follow, with damage to vital tissue, blockage of normal urine flow, and eventual scarring. Urinary tract infections are more common and persistent in people with conditions that block the flow of urine. Birth defects, stones in the bladder or kidney, multiple pregnancies, or enlargement of the prostate gland (see pages 268–270) favor urinary tract infections. General conditions like diabetes mellitus may lower body resistance and lead to this and other types of infection. People having these conditions are more prone to have repeated infections.

HOW CAN A URINARY TRACT INFECTION AFFECT YOU?

Some men and women experience no symptoms despite having bacterial organisms in their urine. However, when true bladder infection occurs, most people do develop symptoms. The symptoms produced by urethritis and cystitis include burning or pain on urination and urgent and frequent urination. The urine itself may appear cloudy. Chills and fever may develop with more severe bladder infections. If bleeding from the bladder occurs, the urine turns a reddish color. Treatment with antibiotics and generous fluid intake usually controls these infections in two to three days.

Kidney infection is much more serious. Damage to the kidneys' delicate filtering system can lead to high blood pressure or even kidney failure. Chills, fever, low back pain, and generalized ache accompany kidney involvement. Hospitalization is often recommended to treat the infection correctly with intravenous antibiotics.

Recurrence of urinary tract infection should prompt careful studies of all parts of the urinary tract, since partial blockage of urine flow at any level will permit bacteria to reinfect the trapped urine.

Consult Your Doctor Now IF

- You have burning or pain on passing urine and an unusually high frequency of urination.

- You pass red or reddish brown urine.

- You develop chills and fever with pain in your back or side.

Goals of Care

- To detect and treat promptly any urinary tract infection.
- To prevent progressive damage to the kidneys by repeated urinary tract infections.

Self-Care Technique

- Drink ten or more glasses of liquid each day to keep your urine dilute when you have an active infection.

The Nervous System

HEADACHES

Most structures that surround and protect the brain are sensitive to pain. The skin, the scalp, the muscles, some skull bones, and the large blood vessels respond to injury with painful sensations. The brain itself does not have pain nerve endings; thus most brain injuries are not painful by themselves.

Headaches may be caused, therefore, by almost any condition that irritates or injures the many tissues around the skull. Most bothersome headaches are classified as either *acute,* occurring suddenly and tending not to recur, or *chronic,* occurring repeatedly or lasting for long periods of time, often over a matter of months or years.

Mild acute headaches may accompany many viral infections, fatigue, or emotional upsets. Severe "blinding" headaches accompanied by pain in the neck, vomiting, and mental changes are caused most often by serious bleeding (subarachnoid hemorrhage) or infection (meningitis) in and around the brain. Temporal arteritis, a condition found almost exclusively in older people (see pages 259–260), is accompanied by one-sided pain and tenderness in the temporal area.

Chronic types of headache, which may plague the victim for years, are most often one of two types: migraine headaches or tension, or muscular, headaches. Migraine headaches characteristically begin suddenly, are preceded by sensations of flashing lights, produce severe throbbing pain in one side of the head, and are accompanied by gastrointestinal upset. In contrast, tension, or muscular, headaches tend to be dull and nagging, are located in the forehead or in the back of the upper neck, hang on for weeks or even months, and are associated with muscle spasms in the scalp and neck.

WHAT CAUSES HEADACHES?

The mild, rather vague headache of infections and various types of stress probably results from unusual tension or spasm in the muscles of the forehead, scalp, and neck. Sinus infections, which may complicate or follow head colds, irritate the lining of the sinuses in the forehead, resulting in deep aching pain in that area.

Bleeding or bacterial infection in the spaces or linings of the brain stretch the structures of the involved blood vessels to produce severe headache and stiffness of the neck (see figure 17). Inflammation of the temporal (temple) artery causes local swelling, tenderness, and sharp pain, often making pressure on the scalp (for example, a hatband) uncomfortable.

Migraine headaches, which tend to run in families, seem to result from spasm, or narrowing, of the scalp and brain arteries followed by sudden stretching. As a result, the increased blood flow seems to "pound" the sensitive walls of the arteries and surrounding structures.

Emotional stress, fatigue, and many other factors combine to cause prolonged muscle spasm in the scalp and neck, which gives rise to still more tension and muscle pain.

Conditions such as head injury, tumors of the brain, and morning hangovers cause other types of headache.

HOW CAN HEADACHES AFFECT YOU?

Some headaches represent fairly specific diseases (migraine headaches, for example), but most are actually symptoms of another underlying condition. For this reason, the effects of this symptom depend largely on the basic disease process. Most people with mild or moderate headaches are distracted, irritable, and slightly nauseated.

The severe, incapacitating headaches caused by bleeding or infection within the brain space require emergency hospital care for treatment of both the major disease and the headache symptom. Although the one-sided pain and tenderness of temporal arteritis may be tolerable, the threat of permanent damage to vision argues for prompt diagnosis and treatment.

Victims of migraines often seem to be "slaves" to the periods of frequent headaches, finding the sharp and pounding pain, nausea, and secondary fatigue just bearable if they retire to a dark, quiet room.

Almost any stress increases the headache distress. The prolonged aching and pressure of tension headaches leave persons discouraged and tired, and many become dependent on prescribed and nonprescription drugs.

■ *Consult Your Doctor Now* <u>IF</u>

- You have an acute headache accompanied by any mental changes, fever, or stiffness of the neck.
- You have an acute headache on one side of your head along with tenderness or swelling of the scalp.

■ *Goals of Care*

- To recognize and treat promptly headaches that may be caused by life-threatening conditions—for example, bleeding or infection around the brain.
- To control the distress of chronic headaches.

■ *Self-Care Techniques*

- Keep a record of your headaches for one week. Include information on the following: date and time of the onset and relief of each headache; special events that preceded the onset of the headache—for example, injury, physical stress, or emotional stress; location of the headache; nature (steady, throbbing, burning, or dull) of the pain; severity (mild, moderate, or severe) of the headache; any associated symptoms such as visual changes, local tenderness, nausea, vomiting, mental changes, or muscle spasms; the treatment used; and the effects of the treatment. (See Appendix C, pages 332–333, for a headache chart to use for your medical records.)
- For mild to moderate acute headaches, (1) apply cold compresses to the area for fifteen to twenty minutes three times a day and (2) take two aspirin or Tylenol by mouth with juice or water every four hours.

■ **STROKE**

The brain—that fragile, uniquely organized, and infinitely complicated mass of nerve cells and fibers—requires a constant supply of oxygen and nutrients. Major arteries from the heart carry large volumes of blood over four sets of vessels to all areas of the brain—areas controlling sensation, or feeling; movement; consciousness; pain; vision; and hearing (see figure 17).

Any interruption of the blood flow produces instant damage in that particular area of the brain deprived of its supply of oxygen and nutrients. If the area of the brain that controls arm movement is affected, paralysis follows; if the deprived area is concerned with controlling sensation in the face, numbness and loss of sensation result; if the blood-deprived area maintains consciousness, a coma will follow. Sudden interruption of any of the brain's arterial blood flow with resultant loss of bodily functions is termed a *stroke,* or *cerebrovascular accident.*

WHAT CAUSES A STROKE?

The immediate, or direct, cause of a stroke is blockage or bursting of one

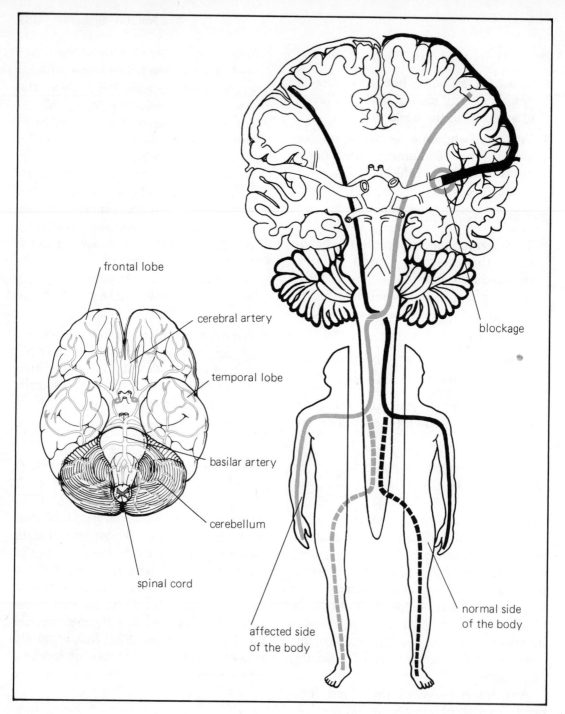

frontal lobe

cerebral artery

temporal lobe

basilar artery

cerebellum

spinal cord

blockage

normal side
of the body

affected side
of the body

Figure 17. When a person suffers a stroke, the flow of blood as well as the nerve impulses
to the affected side of the body are blocked.

of the arteries of the brain. Most strokes are caused by the narrowing of a brain artery (arteriosclerosis) and/or by a blood clot (cerebral thrombosis). Approximately 15 percent of strokes are caused by blood clots that have formed on the lining of the heart. Small fragments of these clots break loose and are swept into a brain artery, where they wedge and block circulation to vital nerve centers. Most of the remaining strokes result from actual hemorrhage, or bleeding, into the brain after rupture of a blood vessel.

Many conditions lead to stroke. Regardless of the immediate cause of a cerebrovascular accident, six chronic yet *potentially manageable* conditions contribute heavily to the chances of experiencing a crippling stroke: hypertension, diabetes mellitus, cigarette smoking, heart disease, obesity, and elevation of fat levels in the blood. Some of these factors, known as risk factors, can be modified to prevent a stroke.

Hypertension, or high blood pressure, is the most powerful predictor of stroke. The higher the pressure, systolic or diastolic, the greater the chances of a cerebrovascular accident. Recognition and careful control of high blood pressure are now the best forms of stroke prevention (see pages 202–203).

Diabetes mellitus, especially if poorly managed, increases artery damage and thus the likelihood of developing a stroke. Diabetics in general are about three times as likely to experience strokes than are nondiabetics of comparable age (see pages 245–246).

Cigarette smoking, especially among heavy smokers (more than one pack per day), adds to the risk of stroke. Strong evidence exists for the role of *heart disease* in arterial brain disease; a history of heart attack, heart failure, or abnormalities in the electrocardiogram (ECG) increase the risk of stroke. Finally, *obesity* and the *elevation of fat levels in the blood* seem to be minor but real risk factors for stroke.

The 30 to 40 percent decline in stroke mortality during the last thirty years can be attributed, in part, to control of these critical risk factors.

HOW CAN A STROKE AFFECT YOU?

The effects, both immediate and long-term, of an acute stroke depend on such factors as the location of the arterial vessel damage, the location and size of the brain injury, the age of the victim, and the presence of other medical conditions.

The most minor stroke is the *transient ischemic attack* (TIA), an abrupt loss of some bodily function as a result of a blockage of one small blood vessel. A TIA often precedes the appearance of a full-blown, larger stroke. Transient ischemic attacks can last for minutes or up to twenty-four hours and result in weakness in an arm, blindness of one eye, or difficulty in speaking.

A *stroke in progress* is a vascular accident that begins abruptly and worsens over a period of hours to days. Weakness of one side of the body, often accompanied by numbness, may progress to a total paralysis of that area.

The *completed stroke,* which accounts for a majority of cerebrovascular accidents, represents the final, or permanent, stage of brain damage. Paralysis of one side of the body, slurred speech, loss of vision of one side, or many other combinations of abnormalities often remain with little change for years after the initial episode. If the brain damage involves vital centers, such as those that control breathing or circulation, death may occur in as many as 10 to 15 percent of victims of completed strokes.

Bleeding into the brain, or *cerebral hemorrhage,* is a dramatic, life-threatening event. The symptoms include sudden headache, collapse, disturbed consciousness, and profound paralysis.

The moral of the stroke story is clear: Prevention of cerebrovascular accidents by vigorous management of high blood pressure, diabetes mellitus, smoking, and other risk factors is the first order of business!

New approaches to care and rehabilitation now offer realistic hope to stroke victims and their families. Well-planned medical treatments may prevent or correct deformity and dependence. Physiatrists, specialists in rehabilitation, can plan and conduct an overall approach to restoring function. Physical therapists and orthopedic surgeons can often restore effective walking skills. Occupational therapists can help restore hand function and the ability to perform the ordinary tasks of daily living. Speech therapists are now able to analyze and correct some stroke-related language problems, and many victims of stroke thought to have mental deficits have been shown to have simple language difficulties. Team approaches to economic recovery may provide spectacular successes; psychologists, social workers, vocational rehabilitation experts, and concerned employers often help return the well-motivated individual to his or her previous level of performance.

Consult Your Doctor Now *IF*

- You have poorly controlled hypertension, diabetes mellitus, or heart trouble.
- You experience sudden blindness, speech difficulties, or weakness or numbness of an arm or leg.

Goal of Care

- To control the risk factors that increase the threat of stroke.

Self-Care Techniques

- Consult your doctor and design a diet that will let you reach and maintain your proper body weight. In addition, restrict your fat intake to less than 30 percent of your total daily calories; less than 10 percent of these calories should come from animal fats. (See chapter 6.)
- If you smoke, start a campaign to quit.
- If you have diabetes mellitus or heart disease, work with your doctor to establish proper control of the disease.
- If you have high blood pressure (defined as systolic reading higher than 160 or a diastolic reading higher than 95), begin a program to control your pressure.

- If you have had a stroke, join a support group such as Stroke Clubs. For further information, write Stroke Clubs, American Heart Association, 7320 Greenville Avenue, Dallas, TX 75231.

■ DEMENTIA AND ALZHEIMER'S DISEASE

Normal intellectual, or mental, function is remarkably rich and complicated. Learning, memory, and orientation (the understanding of your location in time and place) are essential to daily living. Skills like judgment, calculation, and use of language reflect the higher intelligence that makes humans unique. All these functions and skills depend on an adequate number of normal brain cells and nerve circuits.

Progressive loss of most or all of these aspects of mental function is called dementia. Difficulty with only one mental function, most often memory, should not be confused with true dementia. (See pages 147–149.)

The progress of the dementia may be measured in months or years, depending on the cause of the dementia. Typically, decline in intellectual function begins as forgetfulness and simple confusion. As time passes, however, the victim and those around him or her become aware of frequent errors in judgment (for example, opening the door of a moving car), problems with calculation (for example, overdrawing the checking account), and difficulties with language (a watch becomes "that time thing").

The person with advanced dementia is typically lost, unable to care for himself or herself, and often unable to communicate. The victim becomes easy prey for injuries and infections.

WHAT CAUSES DEMENTIA AND ALZHEIMER'S DISEASE?

True dementia, or progressive mental deterioration, is a gradual loss of functioning in the brain areas most concerned with higher intellectual processes. About three-quarters of dementia victims have a unique pattern of brain cell damage, Alzheimer's disease, whose cause is still unknown.

A few stroke patients develop dementia. Small blood clots destroy critical brain centers in a stepwise fashion, producing progressive loss of mental functions as well as paralysis and difficulty with speech.

Some adults with severe depression (see pages 139–141) become forgetful, withdrawn, and confused—in a state of pseudodementia. Such symptoms can be corrected if recognized and treated vigorously. Many types of drug therapy (sleep medications, alcohol, and pain therapy) and medical conditions (thyroid deficiency and certain vitamin deficiencies) may be complicated by a dementialike state that improves when the drug is discontinued or the condition treated.

HOW CAN DEMENTIA AND ALZHEIMER'S DISEASE AFFECT YOU?

While a few types of dementia progress from slight memory loss to advanced mental deterioration in a few months, most forms advance over a period of two to ten years.

Early in the course of Alzheimer's disease, for example, confusion is the major problem. Familiar names and objects are forgotten, passages in books and newspapers are read and reread, travel in new towns is difficult, and work effectiveness decreases. Language skills are lost in most victims, even though some individuals still have the capacity to think clearly and understand events. In many cases, the person is only partly aware of these problems.

Later, the mental difficulties become obvious. Important people and dates are forgotten, calculations and decisions are difficult or impossible for the individual to make, and the person must rely on others for home supervision and safe transportation.

Advanced dementia and Alzheimer's disease rob the victims of both identity and independence. Family members are not recognized, assistance is needed with personal care, and willpower is lost.

With few exceptions, the dementia process may slow down or even appear to stop at points in its course.

Consult Your Doctor Now IF

- You have *total loss* of memory for any event.
- You are experiencing significant difficulties because of forgetfulness, confusion, or poor judgment.
- You or your loved ones are worried about your apparent loss of some mental functions.

Goal of Care

- To recognize and correct any condition that causes reversible loss of intellectual functions.

Self-Care Techniques

- If forgetfulness or simple confusion are problems to you, review your medical conditions and all drug therapy in detail with your doctor. Almost any disease and any drug may contribute to mental dysfunction!
- Review the section "Forgetfulness," pages 147–149.

PARKINSONISM

Parkinsonism (named after James Parkinson, who first described the condition more than 150 years ago) is a chronic, progressive disorder of the brain that most often affects adults fifty years of age and older. Degeneration of specific brain tissue produces four major types of problems that characterize this disease: (1) All bodily movements are awkward and slow. (2) A peculiar shaking movement (tremor) affects the hands, head, and other parts of the body. (3) Muscles of the face and extremities become stiff or contracted. (4) The nerve reflexes concerned with body posture or position are abnormal. In addition, some persons with parkinsonism suffer from severe constipation, bladder difficulties, low blood pressure, or partial decline in mental function.

Parkinsonism is a relatively common condition, and some experts suggest that as many as 1 percent of people seventy years and older will have some form of it. Most individuals with this disorder develop the early signs in their late fifties, and their difficulties progress slowly for many years. Slight stiffness of one arm or hand may be present for years before the patient and his or her family notice the tremor, the lack of spontaneous movements (like blinking or arm movements during walking), and a tendency to fall. Modern therapy can relieve many of these symptoms, but the average life span is decreased somewhat in parkinsonism victims.

WHAT CAUSES PARKINSONISM?

In a majority of parkinsonism cases, the cause is not known. Nerve cells in a critical area of the brain simply degenerate or die over a period of years. As a result, a critical "messenger" chemical (dopamine) is lost, and thus control over body movements becomes defective. No proof exists that viral infections, inherited chemical abnormalities, or hardening of the brain arteries causes parkinsonism.

The specific cause is known in a few cases. In some persons treated with drugs (such as Compazine and Haldol) for dementia or depression, a reversible form of this condition develops. Individuals exposed to certain toxic materials such as manganese or carbon monoxide may be left with the chronic movement disorder. Finally, several rare, usually fatal degenerative and hereditary brain diseases may produce many of the features of parkinsonism.

HOW CAN PARKINSONISM AFFECT YOU?

In its earliest stages, parkinsonism produces few symptoms—generally stiffness or weakness of a hand, which may make writing difficult or tying a shoestring a slow process; slight hand tremor, which may be noticeable only when the person is tired and nervous; or a "flat" facial expression, which is often apparent only to someone who has not seen the person for many months. Treatment at this stage usually consists of counseling and reassurance.

Within three to four years, most people with parkinsonism develop problems. Their speech becomes soft, slow, and slurred; walking seems awkward and slow, with some shuffling; body movements such as turning in bed and arising from a chair are difficult; and fine motor skills such as the use of a steak knife are limited. Treatment at this stage usually consists of mild prescription medications (such as Artane and Symmetrel) for control of the tremor and stiffness. As the condition advances, more serious difficulties appear. Walking is difficult, and falls may lead to fracture of the hip or wrist; writing is slow and frustrating; work and travel become tedious and hazardous; and depression is often a major concern. At this stage, usually reached after eight or ten years, stronger drugs (such as levodopa and Sinemet) are used to maintain mobility and independent daily activities.

Although parkinsonism is typically a slowly progressive condition that may be complicated by infections and injuries, it does not cause death. Many of the difficulties experienced by both patient and doctor relate to the effects of drug therapy rather than to the disease itself.

Consult Your Doctor Now IF

- You have stiffness or awkwardness, balance difficulties, changes in your speech, or any symptoms that lead you to suspect parkinsonism.
- Your parkinsonism is being poorly controlled by your current medical program.

Goals of Care

- To control the symptoms of parkinsonism.
- To prevent the complications of parkinsonism, such as falls, loss of mobility, and social isolation.

Self-Care Techniques

- Use a daily activities chart. Select three to four commonplace chores you perform each day (such as shaving, tying shoes, getting up from a particular chair, or walking up a flight of stairs) and chart the degree of difficulty you experience with each; this will give you an index, or guide, to follow. Also include on the chart the frequency and ease of bowel movements, all medications used for the condition and for other conditions, and any side effects from medication. (See Appendix C, pages 334–335, for a daily activities chart to use for your medical records.)
- Remain physically active and physically fit. Participate in outdoor activities that require walking and total body movement. Follow the exercise program outlined in the pamphlet *Home Exercises for Patients with Parkinson's Disease* available from the American Parkinson Disease Association, 116 John Street, New York, NY 10038.
- Eat a balanced, high-fiber diet (see chapter 6) that keeps your weight at about 10 percent greater than your lean weight at ages twenty to twenty-five.
- Recognize and deal with depression. If you feel sad, frustrated, and dependent, express your feelings and seek psychological aid.
- Become familiar with the many resources available to you, both personal and professional. Obtain a copy of *A Manual for Patients with Parkinson's Disease* from the American Parkinson Disease Association, 116 John Street, New York, NY 10038.

Metabolism and Glands

■ DIABETES MELLITUS

All bodily reactions require energy, and the final source of almost all energy for human cells is the simple sugar glucose. Derived from many foodstuffs, glucose circulates in the bloodstream to reach all cells and tissues, from skin to skeleton. To be available for fueling life processes, however, glucose must enter each cell. This step of entrance and activation requires the presence of still another potent chemical messenger, a hormonal agent called insulin, which is produced normally by the pancreas gland.

When insulin is unable to help in the transfer of glucose into the cells, *diabetes mellitus* occurs. Diabetes mellitus can be traced to the lack of insulin effect on sugar metabolism. While some children and young people suffer from an actual lack of body insulin (so-called juvenile-onset, or Type I, diabetes), a vast majority of adult diabetics seem to produce adequate insulin that simply fails to transfer glucose (so-called maturity-onset, or Type II, diabetes).

Prolonged and untreated lack of sugar-dependent energy may drive the body to a series of dramatic responses: (1) Extra glucose is released into the blood, flooding the body with sugar, which "spills" into the urine. (2) Other body tissues release protein and fat fuels, literally burning up the body reserves and certain vital substances. (3) Abnormal fats accumulate in blood vessels, with eventual development of arteriosclerosis (hardening of the arteries) and cardiovascular disease. (4) Certain bacterial and other types of infectious agents may invade the body, with the production of frequent skin, urinary, and lung infections.

WHAT CAUSES DIABETES MELLITUS?

About 90 percent of adults with diabetes suffer from the maturity-onset, non-insulin-dependent form of diabetes. These individuals produce enough pancreatic insulin but cannot transport glucose to its normal site of action. Some of these diabetics have a strong family history of the disease, suggesting an inherited trait. A majority of the patients are overweight when the condition is discovered, so experts feel obesity somehow contributes to abnormal insulin-glucose action. At any rate, dietary treatment and weight loss are the cornerstones of treatment. A sedentary lifestyle certainly increases the risk of developing diabetes and its complications. Many adults can avoid using insulin and other medications by following regular exercise programs. Many drugs used by older persons stress the glucose-insulin system and increase the likelihood of diabetes. Notorious for this effect are thiazide diuretics (used in hypertension and fluid retention), estrogen hormones (used for the treatment of osteoporosis and menopausal symptoms), and glucocorticoids (used in arthritis treatment).

HOW CAN DIABETES MELLITUS AFFECT YOU?

Many adults with maturity-onset diabetes have no complaints except obesity, and the diagnosis is made when an abnormal blood or urine test is reported. Although these asymptomatic individuals seem well, uncontrolled diabetes is a major risk factor for arteriosclerosis and its complications of heart attack, stroke, and kidney disease.

In other diabetics, the diagnosis is made when the blood sugar problem and body-wasting tendency are dramatic, with unexplained weight loss, severe thirst, and frequent urination. Repeated or persistent infections of the skin or urinary tract (see pages 160–162 and 232–235) may lead to the discovery of abnormal blood glucose levels.

Finally, a few diabetics experience serious, even life-threatening complications when their glucose-insulin balance is severely disturbed. In addition, infection or heart attack may upset the already delicate balance, causing a rise in blood sugar, vomiting, failure of mental functions, and the possible occurrence of circulatory shock (ketosis). In these circumstances, immediate hospitalization and vigorous therapy are mandatory.

Consult Your Doctor Now **IF**

- You have symptoms suggesting the presence of diabetes—unusual thirst, frequent passage of large volumes of urine, unexplained weight loss, or repeated infections.

Goals of Care

- To prevent the development of diabetes mellitus in susceptible persons.
- To control diabetes and prevent its numerous complications—heart attack, stroke, kidney disease, and infection.

Self-Care Techniques

- Reach and maintain your proper body weight by following a professionally prescribed low-calorie, low-fat, high-fiber diet.
- Follow a practical, well-designed exercise program that is safe for you (see chapter 5).
- Quit smoking.
- Limit alcohol intake to a minimum or moderate level.
- Be certain all other medical conditions are well controlled and properly monitored, especially conditions such as hypertension, heart disease, and any infection.
- Review *all* drug treatments with your doctor or pharmacist for their possible effects on diabetes and its drug treatment.
- Have all your immediate relatives (brothers, sisters, and children) screened for early or asymptomatic diabetes mellitus.
- Join a support group. Contact the American Diabetes Association, Two Park Avenue, New York, NY 10016, for information on a local group, or check your telephone directory.

■ OBESITY

In this affluent, fitness-fixated society, the term *obese* would seem to apply to anyone who *looks* fat, *feels* fat, or is *judged* by some standard to be fat! The fact is that the terms *fat, overweight,* and *obese* are not well defined or widely accepted.

Following the lead of life insurance companies, some experts define *obese,* or obesity, in terms of excessive weight for a given height and body build in persons of a particular age. Accordingly, if you exceed this "ideal" weight by a significant amount (for example, 10 to 20 percent), your risk of dying prematurely increases. Other individuals prefer direct measurement of body fat. For example, if a "pinch" of the skin on your upper arm is greater than one inch, you are obese. Still others rely on the traditional rule that says your best weight after middle age is your leanest weight when you were twenty to twenty-five years old; anything above that figure is considered excess weight. In point of fact, all three definitions have some merit. One expert in the field of aging and diet suggests that the best or healthiest adult weight lies between 2 and 10 percent above the individual's lean weight at age twenty.

However defined, obesity, or being significantly overweight, is risky. Early death rates increase in proportion to the level of obesity. Disability and death from diabetes (see pages 245–246), hypertension (see pages 202–203), coronary heart disease, gallbladder disease (see pages 225–228), and kidney failure are greater in overweight persons. In addi-tion, there are obvious psychological and social disadvantages to being obese in the United States.

WHAT CAUSES OBESITY?

People gain and hold extra body weight only when the calories (energy) they consume exceed the calories (energy) they burn by activity and basic body operation (see chapter 6).

A few adults are obese as a result of biological or chemical imbalances in the body. Family traits, rare brain disorders, and a few glandular conditions may cause excessive weight gain, usually in early life.

The body normally becomes fatter after ages twenty-five to thirty as the water and mineral contents decrease. By age seventy-five, the proportion of fat almost doubles. There is increasing evidence that some of the shift to fat can be prevented by sustained physical fitness. Many medical conditions such as heart disease, arthritis, and stroke, to name a few, cause those afflicted to restrict physical activities, which in turn may cause them to gain weight. Dietary habits often change with advancing age. People tend to consume more fatty and starchy foods, which cost less than protein-rich foods.

Psychological factors loom large in obesity. Some investigators have shown that early childhood abnormalities of hunger-feeding behaviors are critical in the evolution of fatness. Others point to the disturbed body image held by many overweight persons ("I am too fat to be loved") as a major force in the development and maintenance of the overweight state.

In summary, obesity is the result of many complicated and interactive biological, sociological, and psychological forces. Rarely can an individual change only one of the three forces and expect to achieve early success with weight loss. *Prevention is paramount!*

HOW CAN OBESITY AFFECT YOU?

At a personal level, obesity is an unhappy, self-perpetuating phenomenon. Increasing weight means decreasing mobility, which means more time for overeating and less incentive to move about. Only by early interruption of this unfortunate cycle can truly disabling obesity be prevented.

There is abundant evidence that obesity is hazardous. Conditions like diabetes mellitus, coronary heart disease, hypertension, gallbladder disorders, and osteoarthritis are more common and complicated in overweight individuals. In addition, falls and crippling are more common, and most surgical operations carry higher risks in the obese person.

Depression is often a serious problem in fat people, many of whom become discouraged and poorly motivated to fight for weight control. Predictably, social isolation may become increasingly frustrating and defeating as physical movement is curtailed and feelings of failure grow.

▰ *Consult Your Doctor Now* __IF__

- You have finally reached a firm decision to control your weight.

▰ *Goals of Care*

- To achieve and maintain your desirable or ideal weight.
- To prevent the physical and psychological complications of obesity.

▰ *Self-Care Techniques*

- Use a weight chart or record that includes the following: the date; the time weighed (always weigh in at the same time in the morning before breakfast); your weight (in underclothes); how you feel (happy, sad, hungry, frustrated, and so on); and any special event that happened the previous day (such as a party, a visit, or an illness). (See Appendix C, page 336, for a weight chart to use for your medical records.)
- Check your daily food intake by maintaining a diet log (see pages 79–81 and Appendix C, pages 338–339).
- With the advice of a dietician or other expert, draw up a *practical* dietary plan that (1) contains a balanced mixture of essential nutrients; (2) contains a reasonable baseline of calories (for example, 1,000–1,200 calories for women, 1,200–1,400 calories for men) plus a caloric allowance for any level of activity (for example, 20 percent extra calories if performing sedentary tasks, 40 percent if doing household or office work); and (3) follows the pattern of your usual eating habits (mealtimes, snacks, and eating out).
- Design a practical exercise program that will assist you to burn about 400 to 500 calories per day (see chapter 5).
- Explore the possibility and desirability of joining Weight Watchers or some similar organization.

Muscles and Bones

▬ LOW BACK PAIN

In humans, the spine (vertical column, or backbone) is an architectural wonder as well as a mechanical nightmare. The twenty-four spoollike blocks, or vertebrae, are balanced in a vertical column, each separated by discs of elastic cartilage. The entire spinal column is held in line by strong ligaments and muscles (see figure 18). The constant pull of gravity and endless twisting motions—as well as diseases of the bones, joints, and nerves—combine to produce an endless array of painful conditions. The lower third of the spine seems especially

vulnerable to disease and injury. Fifty to 70 percent of adults will experience significant low back pain at one time or another. The most common causes of low back pain are lumbosacral sprain, herniated disc, and vertebral compression fracture.

Lumbosacral sprain often occurs after lifting heavy objects, after prolonged standing, or after sudden twisting of the body. These stresses apparently tear the leathery supporting spinal ligaments and bruise the muscles that provide strength and mobility to the lower spine. These

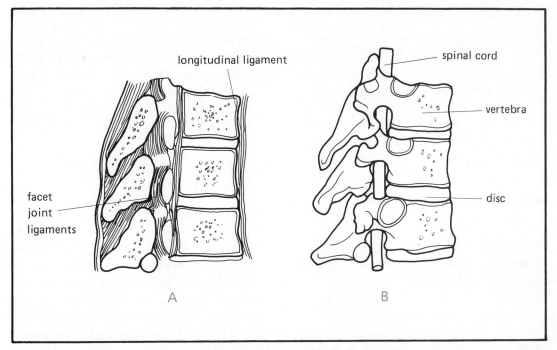

longitudinal ligament

spinal cord

facet joint ligaments

vertebra

disc

A

B

Figure 18. Two views of the spinal cord: **A** shows the ligaments of the spinal cord and **B** shows the relationship between the vertebrae and the spinal column itself.

injuries then produce aching pain deep in one side or along the middle of the lower spine, and any movement of the spine increases the discomfort.

Comfort and flexibility in the lower (lumbosacral) spine require maximum cushioning and elasticity of the discs (best regarded as washers between spools), which are held in place by a circular band. After years of stretching and twisting, the disc band may tear. The weight of the body then forces the central disc ball out of alignment, and a *herniated disc* is the result. The disc presses against sensitive nerves and ligaments. The resulting pain is both local, over the disc itself, and referred, into the leg along the course of an irritated nerve.

A vertebral *compression fracture* most often complicates osteoporosis (see pages 257–259), one of several conditions that soften and weaken the vertebrae. Over the years, as the calcium-containing bone minerals "leech out," the vertebral blocks crumble and collapse under the constant pounding of daily activities. Finally, a routine activity like bending over may be enough to crush the lower vertebrae, which gives rise to sudden back pain that is increased by sitting, standing, or coughing.

WHAT CAUSES LOW BACK PAIN?

Unusually rapid or awkward movements of the lower body may stretch or even tear some of the tendons, ligaments, or muscle bands that support the spine, causing low back pain. In addition, the muscles around the damaged structure often go into spasm, which increases the

pain and lameness. Repeated bouts of *lumbosacral sprain* occur when the supporting ligaments and muscles have been permanently weakened.

The low back pain caused by a *herniated disc* occurs most often in middle-aged people. This is probably due to the combination of age-related weakening and back injury that finally tears the ligaments covering the disc. This lets the disc, which acts like a cushion between the vertebrae, push out against nerve fibers that run into the legs. As a result, severe local pain and tenderness (much like that of lumbosacral sprain) is accompanied by sharp, knifelike pain that radiates down into the thigh, knee, or lower leg and foot. If the disc presses on nerves that control movement, weakness of the leg or foot may be present.

A *vertebral compression fracture* occurs when bending, lifting, or a minor fall crushes a weakened vertebral bone. This sudden deformity puts pressure on sensitive ligaments, causing sharp pain, muscle spasm, and stiffness. Standing and walking increase the pressure and therefore the discomfort, whereas lying down typically gives considerable relief.

HOW CAN LOW PACK PAIN AFFECT YOU?

Severe low back pain of any sort may be crippling. Standing is often uncomfortable, walking may be impossible because of pain and spasm, and most types of work are prohibited. In most cases prompt conservative treatment speeds recovery. Bed rest helps reduce pain. Pain medications and antiarthritis drugs, hot compresses, and careful exercises for

Low Back Pain

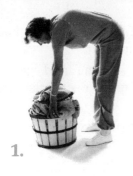

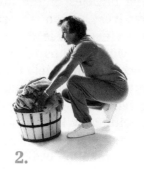

1. Incorrect way to lift, by bending the back.

2. Correct way to lift, by bending the knees.

1.

2.

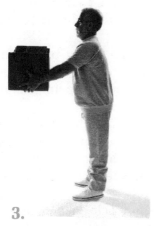

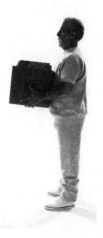

3. Incorrect way to hold object; places strain on back.

4. Correct way to hold object; reduces strain on back.

3.

4.

5.

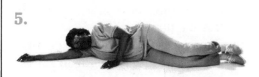

6.

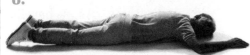

5. Resting on the side with the knees bent is a correct position for persons with back pain, as the spine is straightened in this position.

6. Persons with back pain should avoid sleeping on the stomach, as this arches the back.

7.

7. Lying on the back with the feet slightly raised or the knees slightly bent is a correct position. The foot of the mattress is raised six to eight inches.

Figure 19

the muscles of the lower back hasten recovery. Even so, return to simple activities may lead to a recurrence.

Most victims of *lumbosacral sprain* recover completely and learn to prevent attacks by practicing proper posture, strengthening their back muscles, and avoiding awkward bending and lifting. A majority of persons with *herniated discs* function well with similar medical therapy, but about 10 percent eventually need surgery to remove the displaced disc. Finally, conservative treatment of the attack of back pain plus specific treatment of the condition causing bone softening (for example, osteoporosis) lead to recovery from *vertebral compression fractures*.

Consult Your Doctor Now IF

- You have sudden, severe, and unexplained low back pain.

- You have low back pain along with pain that runs into one or both legs.

Goals of Care

- To relieve low back pain promptly and completely.

- To prevent recurrence of low back pain.

Self-Care Techniques

- Work to maintain your "ideal" body weight (see chapter 6).

- Maintain muscle tone and general flexibility by regular exercise (see chapter 5).

- Practice proper posture while sitting, standing, lying, and lifting heavy objects (see figure 19).

- During a spell of acute low back pain, with guidance from your doctor, follow a program that includes the following:

  1. Bed rest. Using a low pillow and firm mattress, remain on strict bed rest until the acute pain has decreased significantly.

  2. Hot packs. Using a heating pad or hot-water bottle, apply local heat carefully to the painful area for thirty minutes three to four times a day.

  3. Massage. If muscle spasm and tenderness are present, have a family member or friend massage the involved muscle bands three to four times a day.

  4. Exercise. When pain has decreased a bit, cautiously begin to do exercises that will help strengthen the spinal muscles.

  5. Pain medications. As a baseline, take two to three aspirin or Tylenol tablets every four hours.

■ FOOT PAIN

The lifelong punishment dealt to the many delicate bones and joints of the feet causes many disabling foot problems. Four painful conditions are especially important to older people: anterior metatarsalgia, hallux valgus, corns, and calluses.

Anterior metatarsalgia (literally, "pain in the front of the foot") is a burning pain and sensitivity to pressure felt along the ball (the central part of the sole) of the foot (see figure 20). Typically, this disability develops in overweight women who have flat feet. Flat feet is a condition in which the normal longitudinal (front to back) arch of the foot is lost. With advancing years and wear-and-tear effects of walking in high-heeled shoes, the already relaxed ligaments of the flat foot are sprained and slack. Stretching produces tenderness and painful swelling of the joints and bones

of the ball of the foot on standing and walking.

The term *hallux valgus* refers to a combination of abnormalities of the foot that commonly produces foot deformity and pain (see figure 20). Usually a late complication of flat feet, these changes include (1) angulation, or twisting, of the great toe toward the outside margin of the foot; (2) swelling and soreness of the base of the great toe, or a bunion; and, in many cases, (3) inflammation and degenerative arthritis of the involved toe. These changes may produce no symptoms for years, but then irritation of tight shoes eventually leads to redness, tenderness, and local pain in the bunion.

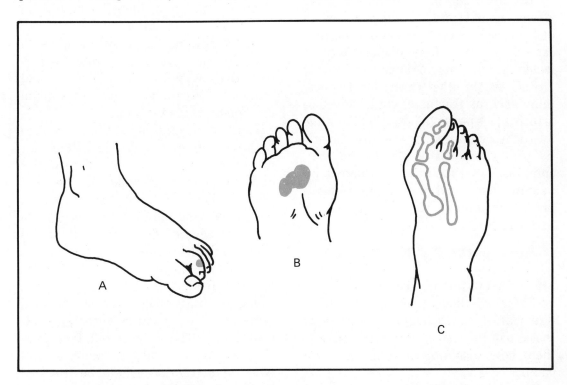

Figure 20. Common foot problems include **A** hammertoes, **B** anterior metatarsalgia, and **C** hallux valgus.

Corns and *calluses* are areas of hard, thickened skin produced by pressure and friction of the skin over prominent bones and joints. Most often, prolonged irritation of the skin over the little toe and great toe by tight shoes produces small patches of thick, leathery skin. Pressure on the corn (usually less than one-half inch in size) or callus (usually larger than one-half inch in size) drives the corn or callus against the underlying tissues, with subsequent production of pain and lameness.

WHAT CAUSES FOOT PAIN?

Most deformities and pains in the feet are the end results of chronic mechanical failure—the slow breakdown of joints, supporting ligaments, and bony parts after years of stress and vigorous use. In many cases, structural abnormalities, especially flat feet, predispose the affected individuals to later mechanical difficulties. In other cases, local conditions such as fractures, gout, or osteoarthritis (see pages 255–257) set the stage for further damage. Degenerative arthritis of the smaller joints of the foot, compression of the bases of the toes by narrow shoes, and loss of the front-to-back arch interact to give rise to pain and deformity.

HOW CAN FOOT PAIN AFFECT YOU?

Many persons literally live on their feet— standing, walking, and running from dawn till dusk. Development of any of these painful foot conditions reminds them how disabling even a tiny corn can be!

The sharp burning pain of *metatarsalgia* will persist until the downward weight of the body is distributed away from the base of the toes. A wide, comfortably fitting shoe is essential to accomplish this. Then a felt or rubber pad (metatarsal pad) may be inserted into the shoe and fixed to the sole just behind the painful bony ridge. Some foot experts (podiatrists) recommend special outside plates (metatarsal bars) that also decrease pressure on the base of sore toes. Weight reduction and regular foot exercises help provide relief.

The mechanical changes of *hallux valgus* that cause painful bunions and degenerative arthritis are more difficult to correct. A wide, specially shaped shoe that decreases pressure on the deformed great toe often helps relieve acute pain. Regular soaking of the inflamed bunion and protection by a soft felt ring may help. Many individuals with severe pain and lameness are helped only by surgical therapy, which usually consists of removal of excess bone under the bunion and repair of the toe joint.

Corns and *calluses* may be controlled by local treatment, but they will appear or recur as long as bony deformities and pressure irritations of the foot persist. The pain and tenderness on weight bearing may be decreased for a time by several maneuvers. First, all shoes should be carefully fitted, and a program should be designed to provide gradual weight loss when indicated. Then, careful abrasion and/or chemical removal of the sensitive corns and calluses should be carried out (see page 255). Finally, special foot exercises and walking instructions should be provided by a podiatrist; if followed, improvement occurs in most individuals.

■ Consult Your Doctor Now IF

■ You have foot pain along with *any* change in color or skin breakdown in any part of the foot.

■ Goals of Care

■ To manage foot abnormalities such as flat feet in order to prevent the complications of pain, deformity, and disability.

■ To control pain caused by disease in the feet.

■ Self-Care Techniques

■ Inspect your feet for possible problems, including (1) any discolorations, ulcers, local swellings, or tenderness; (2) early corns or calluses; (3) crack-ing of the skin between the toes; or (4) redness or infection around or beneath the toenails.

■ For temporary relief from corns and calluses, (1) soak your foot in warm water for fifteen minutes; (2) using an emery board or pumice stone, carefully rub down and thin out the hard part of the painful area; (3) cut out a piece of 40 percent salicylic acid plaster slightly larger than the corn, apply it to the skin with the sticky side down, and surround this with a thin felt pad cut to cover the area; (4) leave this plaster and pad on overnight, changing it the next evening; and (5) repeat this procedure until the skin is thin and less sensitive.

■ Consult your doctor, nurse, or podiatrist for treatment of persistent or complicated foot problems.

■ ARTHRITIS

Three types of arthritis, or inflammatory damage of the joints, are especially common in older adults: osteoarthritis, rheumatoid arthritis, and gout. *Osteoarthritis,* also called degenerative or wear-and-tear arthritis, is by far the most common, as it affects more than 40 million persons living in the United States. This condition, which increases in frequency among the aging, tends to involve large weight-bearing joints like the hip and knee.

Rheumatoid arthritis, the classical "rheumatism," most often begins in young people. Rheumatoid arthritis develops slowly and involves inflammation of the lining of small joints of the hands, wrists, and feet. Its chronic and persistent nature means that more and more persons have the disease in old age.

Gout, classically a disease of "rich-living" men, appears in middle or late life as a sudden inflammation of one joint, usually the great toe, though any joint may be attacked. An attack may subside completely only to occur again in future years, for the underlying chemical cause, high body levels of uric acid, is present throughout life.

WHAT CAUSES ARTHRITIS?

Many aspects of osteoarthritis resemble simple age-related alterations seen in healthy adults. However, weakening and splitting of joint cartilage caused by a lifetime of pressures and injuries to the joints, accelerates degeneration. At some point, the cartilage damage leads to thickening and roughness of surrounding bones, and arthritic symptoms appear.

The precise cause of rheumatoid arthritis is still unknown, but prolonged inflammation of the joint lining eventually damages cartilage and bones. If not controlled, rheumatoid arthritis leads to deformity, weakness, and limited movement in hands, feet, and other joints.

Abnormally high blood concentrations of a body chemical called uric acid lead to the acute joint inflammation of gout. Tiny crystals of uric acid form inside joints and act like foreign bodies, producing painfully red and swollen toes, feet, or knees. Some of the extra uric acid is derived from the diet from foods such as liver, sweetbreads, and sardines. Alcohol ingestion may also trigger an acute attack of gout.

HOW CAN ARTHRITIS AFFECT YOU?

Only about 20 percent of individuals with osteoarthritis have significant symptoms. Hip involvement produces pain, stiffness, and lameness in the groin or buttocks. The distress typically worsens when one is standing or walking. Degenerative joint disease of the knee is often very disabling, creating pain on standing, swelling, and joint instability. Low backache and stiffness at the end of the day result from osteoarthritis of the spine. Aspirin and other anti-inflammatory drugs, exercise, and avoidance of further injury may control symptoms of osteoarthritis. Surgical repair, however, is required in advanced cases of hip disease.

Persons with active rheumatoid arthritis often complain of general weakness and tiredness. In this condition, small joints of the fingers, hands, and feet are red, swollen, and tender, and morning stiffness is a prominent feature. Rest, heat, and large doses of aspirin during active attacks usually control symptoms. Several new anti-inflammatory drugs are now available to relieve symptoms and help prevent permanent deformity.

Over 90 percent of people with gout are men. Attacks of gouty arthritis typically begin suddenly, with severe pain, tenderness, and redness of the great toe. Other small joints may become inflamed during an attack. The attack typically subsides in a matter of days if treatment is begun promptly. Uric acid kidney stones may complicate gout in some people.

■■■ *Consult Your Doctor Now* <u>*IF*</u>

■ You have unexplained pain, swelling, or redness in *any* joint.

▄ *Goals of Care*

- To control pain, swelling, and other symptoms of active arthritis.
- To prevent permanent joint changes and disability.

▄ *Self-Care Techniques*

- If you are overweight, establish a safe and sane diet and exercise program (see chapters 5 and 6) to lessen the stress on your joints.
- Work with your doctor to establish an exercise program that keeps arthritic joints flexible and muscles strong (see chapter 5).
- If you have active osteoarthritis or rheumatoid arthritis, work out a daily schedule of heat treatments and aspirin therapy. Most regimens recommend that you do the following: (1) Apply moist heat to affected joints two or three times a day for twenty to thirty minutes. (2) Massage the sore muscles after heat treatment. (3) Take three tablets of aspirin by mouth every four hours while awake. Tablets may be crushed and swallowed in applesauce or other soft food, *or* you can take buffered/coated aspirin (for example, Ascriptin, Bufferin, or Ecotrin).
- Use a cane for balance and lessening of stress on sore, inflamed joints.
- Join a support group. Check your local telephone directory for a listing, or write to the Arthritis Foundation, 3400 Peachtree Road, NE, Atlanta, GA 30326.

▄ OSTEOPOROSIS

The human skeleton is a marvelously strong and dynamic structure. The bones of the skeleton grow slowly but steadily in size and strength during childhood. During the teen years, the bones grow so rapidly that the rocklike mineral portion takes another ten years to crystallize fully. Even then, most bones maintain their strength and shape by a balance of forces. These forces include the addition of calcium and other building blocks in the diet to bone surfaces and the loss of equal amounts of bone by biological action.

During the fifth decade of life, bone substance begins to decrease, especially in the backbone and in the long bones of the arms and legs. In twenty or thirty years, when persons are in their sixties or seventies, as much as 50 percent of the skeletal mass and strength may be lost, creating the very real hazard of painful and disabling fractures from minor injuries. Excessive loss of bone may lead to osteoporosis—literally, "soft bone."

Osteoporosis itself causes no symptoms, and it is usually recognized only after X rays are taken of a suspected fracture. Typically, an elderly woman develops low back pain, hip pain, or painful swelling of her wrist after a trivial fall, and X rays show a break in the thin, "washed-out" bone.

WHAT CAUSES OSTEOPOROSIS?

Both women and men experience thinning of most parts of the skeleton after age forty, so some loss of skeletal strength is part of normal aging. Women, however, appear to be more at risk than men for developing osteoporosis.

Bone loss becomes much greater in women after the menopause (see pages 261–262). The dramatic decrease in estrogen production that characterizes this event seems to speed up the course of osteoporosis, with the result that fractures of the hip, spine, and wrist occur with increasing frequency after age sixty-five. Skeletal loss in men and premenopausal women is about 0.5 percent each year at age forty; with the menopause, this loss may increase to 2 or 3 percent per year in women. The severity of this bone loss and the risk of bone fractures depend on the following factors: exercise, dietary intake of calcium, and absorption of vitamin D.

Inactivity leads rapidly to loss of bone substance, so individuals disabled by arthritis and other medical conditions are especially prone to developing osteoporosis. Many diseases seem to increase the likelihood of osteoporosis, among them thyroid conditions, liver diseases, and alcoholism.

Since many women consume diets low in calcium, eating only small amounts of dairy foods and vegetables, bone mineral is not replaced at normal rates. Poor diets and lack of exposure to sunshine combine to produce a lack of vitamin D, which is essential for normal calcium absorption and use.

HOW CAN OSTEOPOROSIS AFFECT YOU?

In its early stages, osteoporosis produces no discomfort or disability—if high blood pressure is the silent killer, osteoporosis is the silent thief! In women most at risk, however, the progressive loss of bone often leads to fractures of the spine and limbs.

Most often, bending over or a minor fall results in collapse or fracture of a vertebral bone in the lower back. Sharp local pain, muscle spasm, and lameness on sitting and walking appear suddenly and last for two to three weeks.

In other cases, a fall puts sudden stress on the osteoporotic thigh bone, breaking it at a point just below the hip joint. Hip pain, weakness of the leg, and general body shock may follow, and most orthopedic surgeons recommend an operation for the correction of the fracture within twenty-four to forty-eight hours.

Still other types of fractures occur in older people with osteoporosis. Treatment is usually successful, though repeated spine fractures eventually lead to loss of body height and rounding of the shoulders.

Experts generally agree that proper exercise, high-calcium diets, and supplements of vitamin D can slow the progress of osteoporosis. Debate continues about the usefulness and safety of giving estrogen replacement therapy.

▬ *Consult Your Doctor Now* __IF__

- You experience sudden, severe middle or lower back pain.

■ You underwent a total hysterectomy (surgical removal of the uterus and ovaries) or other procedure that included removal of the ovaries before age fifty.

▨ Goals of Care

■ To prevent the further progression of osteoporosis.

■ To prevent the fractures and disability that may complicate osteoporosis.

▨ Self-Care Techniques

■ Establish a regular program of weight-bearing exercise, such as walking or bowling (see chapter 5). A brisk thirty-minute walk and a carefully designed set of aerobic exercises three times a week will suffice.

■ Women should consume at least one gram of calcium daily (see chapter 6). Review your diet, using the diet log (pages 338–339). If you consume less than one gram of calcium each day, plan dietary changes that increase your calcium intake. For example, each eight-ounce glass of skim milk contains about 200 mg (one-fifth of a gram) of calcium, and five slices of American cheese contain about 600 mg (three-fifths of a gram) of calcium. *Or,* your doctor and you may agree that you should use calcium supplements. Several forms of tablets are available. Six hundred fifty (650) mg tablets of calcium carbonate provide 260 mg of calcium, 650 mg tablets of calcium gluconate provide 60 mg of calcium, and one tablet of Os-Cal provides 250 mg of calcium and 125 IU (international units) of vitamin D. In addition, maintain a high fluid intake.

■ If your doctor agrees, take a pure vitamin D preparation or a multivitamin capsule that supplies the recommended 800 IU of the vitamin each day. Maintain a high fluid intake.

▨ POLYMYALGIA RHEUMATICA

The scientific name tells the story: *Poly-* means "many," *myo-* means "muscle," *-algia* means "ache or pain," and *rheumatica* refers to rheumatism, or inflammation of the musculoskeletal system. Polymyalgia rheumatica, or PMR, is a unique inflammatory condition of older adults that causes pain and stiffness of muscle groups around the neck, shoulders, and back. It is one of those rare conditions that almost never occurs before age fifty and only rarely before age sixty-five.

Although the condition is relatively uncommon, it is of considerable importance to older adults because it is somehow related to another condition, temporal arteritis, which may produce permanent blindness.

Temporal arteritis may develop as an isolated condition, or it may appear as part of PMR. Twenty to 50 percent of patients with PMR will have some evidence of associated temporal arteritis, a fact that is critical in planning treatment. Temporal arteritis consists of inflammation of one or both arteries in the temples. The process may narrow or even block the blood vessel to the temple. It may also involve other blood vessels that supply the eye, the brain, or the heart—resulting in grim consequences such as blindness, stroke, or heart attack.

WHAT CAUSES POLYMYALGIA RHEUMATICA?

No specific cause is known for polymyalgia rheumatica. However, some experts feel that PMR and temporal arteritis are immune or allergic disorders. PMR is typically a disease of white people and affects women twice as often as it affects men.

HOW CAN POLYMYALGIA RHEUMATICA AFFECT YOU?

Most often, PMR begins gradually, with vague feelings of tiredness and weakness and loss of weight. In a matter of weeks, the muscles of the neck, shoulders, and back become painful, stiff, and weak. Typically, movements like lifting or shrugging the shoulders are painful and awkward. Muscle pain may disturb sleep. The stiffness is most severe in the morning or after sitting still.

Proper diagnosis is often delayed because early features of PMR are not dramatic, nor are they much different from other types of arthritis (see pages 255-257) and rheumatism. Once recognized, however, PMR can be treated promptly and effectively with steroid drugs.

Individuals with PMR should be alert to the possible complication of temporal arteritis. Inflammation of the temporal artery produces severe, localized headaches, with tenderness along the scalp. When the process involves deeper arteries, blurring of vision or double vision may be warning signs that blockage of small vessels to the eye is imminent. Permanent blindness can occur suddenly in this condition. Diagnosis can usually be made by removing and studying a small segment of artery. Therapy with steroid drugs is quite effective. The PMR disease itself typically lasts a year or so and then subsides spontaneously.

Consult Your Doctor Now IF

- You develop new, one-sided headaches.
- You have new or unexplained blurring of vision, double vision, or spotty loss of vision.

Goals of Care

- To relieve the symptoms of polymyalgia rheumatica.
- To prevent loss of vision caused by temporal arteritis.

Self-Care Technique

- If you are receiving steroid treatment for polymyalgia rheumatica or temporal arteritis, do not omit the medication on your own, since the condition may flare up and eye damage can follow.

Special Problems of Older Women

■ MENOPAUSE

Throughout the reproductive years, the female hormones (mainly estrogens), chemicals produced primarily by the ovaries, control monthly menstrual cycles, help support pregnancies, and supply stimulation to the breast tissues and to the genital organs. In addition, these powerful hormones help maintain the structure of many other tissues, most notably bones and skin.

After age forty-five, the output of estrogen hormones by the ovaries begins to decrease. Eventually the estrogen output drops so low that cyclic menstrual bleeding stops completely—this is the menopause. This event (or nonevent) occurs at about age fifty, though occasional spotting may continue for a few more months. The termination of all menstrual cycle activity, plus twelve months for good measure, means the end of childbearing.

It also means many other things, for a loss of estrogen hormones is felt throughout most body systems. Three-fourths of all postmenopausal women experience hot flashes—uncomfortable waves of warmth, redness, and sweating that sweep over the chest, neck, and face without warning. In most cases these disappear without treatment within four to five years. Shrinkage of gland tissue in the breasts and decrease in elasticity of the supporting ligaments may cause change in breast size and shape. Postmenopausal estrogen lack seems to accelerate normal skin aging (see pages 165–167), and the surfaces of the vagina and lower bladder often show similar thinning.

Finally, and perhaps most important, loss of the effects of estrogen leads to slow, steady weakening of bones and can lead to a condition known as osteoporosis (see pages 257–259), which leaves the bones susceptible to fractures.

WHAT CAUSES MENOPAUSE?

The major features of the menopause result from loss of estrogen hormones. Just why the ovaries undergo slow but progressive shrinkage and loss of glandular activity at this stage of life is still a mystery.

Surgical removal of the uterus and ovaries (total hysterectomy) leads to early and immediate estrogen withdrawal and an artificial menopause, with all the usual features.

Debate still rages over the effectiveness and wisdom of giving estrogen therapy to replace the hormones lost at the time of menopause. Careful estrogen replacement begun at or soon after menopause will reestablish menstrual periods (which are infertile), slow down bone loss, and delay certain skin changes.

There is some evidence, however, that this treatment predisposes the individual to the development of cancer of the uterus. Therefore, most experts reserve estrogen replacement for young women who have undergone hysterectomies.

HOW CAN MENOPAUSE AFFECT YOU?

Although a majority of women experience hot flashes before or at the time of menopause, most of these troublesome spells disappear in four to five years. Some women complain of tiredness and irritability, but these symptoms are usually more related to psychological factors than to hormonal changes themselves.

Most menopausal women have no serious long-term problems related to decrease in estrogen secretion, but bone loss does predispose victims to fractures of the vertebral, wrist, and hip bones. In addition, changes in vaginal and bladder tissues may lead to bothersome dryness, irritation, and infection. One study suggests that continued normal sexual activity decreases the frequency and severity of these complications.

Several surveys indicate that the menopause alters female sexual behavior in different ways. About one-third of women questioned reported increased sexual activity and satisfaction ("No more hassle with birth control!"), whereas one-third felt less interested in sex. There is currently no proof that hormone levels solely determine sexual interest and performance.

▬ *Consult Your Doctor Now* <u>IF</u>

- You have spotting or vaginal bleeding after more than six months following the onset of menopause.

- You have hot flashes that are distressing or that interfere with your personal or professional life.

▬ *Goals of Care*

- To anticipate the symptoms that may accompany normal menopause.

- To control unpleasant and hazardous consequences of the menopause.

▬ *Self-Care Techniques*

- If you are over forty-five and suspect that you are beginning menopause, keep a chart that records the dates of the beginning and end of each menstrual period, the average heaviness of the menstrual flow, and any associated symptoms such as hot flashes or cramps. (See Appendix C, page 337, for a menstrual chart to use for your medical records.)

- Arrange for annual breast examinations and for internal pelvic examinations with Pap smears every one to two years. The incidence of cancer in these areas of the body increases following menopause. (Women who have undergone complete surgical removal of the uterus need not have Pap smears, for the high-risk tissues have been removed.)

■ BREAST CANCER

In early adolescence, female breasts undergo dramatic internal changes. Milk glands increase in size and number, supporting ligaments become stronger, and the surrounding protective fat increases. The milk glands and their drainage ducts then undergo cycles of change with each menstrual period and are greatly transformed with each pregnancy and period of nursing. By the time of the menopause, or change of life (around age fifty), almost all normal breasts have become slightly irregular, or lumpy, because of the many changes in glands, ducts, supporting tissues, and fat.

For reasons that are still not clear, around the time of menopause, a single gland cell may change appearance, divide abnormally and rapidly, and give rise to clumps of abnormal cells that spread into surrounding supporting ligaments and fat. Some of these tiny clumps of abnormal cells—a tumor, or cancer—may be destroyed by body defenses. However, in about 10 percent of women, the tumor continues to grow and spread. If not detected early and treated properly, the enlarging tumor invades normal tissue, grows into small blood vessels and lymph channels, and eventually spreads to the lymph glands in the neck and shoulder. Islands of cancer tissue, called metastases, may grow in bones, lungs, and liver and cause serious disease and death.

WHAT CAUSES BREAST CANCER?

The actual cause, or causes, of human breast cancer is still unknown, though scientists have shown that inheritance, viral infections, and certain chemical exposures are important factors in the development of cancer in laboratory animals. At present *all* women of all ages must be considered at risk.

Breast cancer is mainly a disease of older women. More than two-thirds of the breast cancers occur in women fifty years of age and older. Certain characteristics of women (called risk factors) do increase the chance of developing breast cancer. These are worth knowing and are as follows:

1. Heredity. Women whose mothers or sisters had cancer of the breast have two to three times the usual chance of developing this tumor.

2. Menstrual history. Those women whose periods began early (before age twelve) or ended late (after age fifty) are more prone to develop breast tumors.

3. Childbirth. Those women who had no children or who had their first child after age thirty seem more likely to develop breast cancer.

4. Other factors. Obesity (more than 10 percent overweight), daily alcohol consumption, and a history of earlier

breast disease of any sort seem to increase the chances of breast cancer. Debate continues, but currently there is no real proof that injury to the breast, low-dose X rays (such as chest films), diet, or use of birth control medications predisposes women to this disease.

It should be reemphasized that the cause of this cancer is still unknown.

HOW CAN BREAST CANCER AFFECT YOU?

At first, when the tumor lump is still very small and located deep in the breast tissue, no signs or symptoms are present. Later, usually in a matter of weeks to months, the cancer cells grow to form a ball, or mass, one-half to one inch in diameter, which may be felt as a hard, painless, slightly movable lump in the breast tissue. If the lump is ignored or missed, the tumor may eventually grow to the surface of the skin, producing a swelling that later ulcerates.

Of great importance is the fact that the clumps of tumor that spread to lymph glands in the armpit or neck enlarge to produce swelling that is usually painless. The clumps of tumor that escape into the general circulation may lodge in various bones and cause pain or fracture, lodge in the lungs to produce a condition like pneumonia, or lodge in the liver and cause pain and swelling of the abdomen.

Advanced and widespread cancer of the breast produces death by general wasting and destruction of vital organs.

▨ *Consult Your Doctor Now* __IF__

■ You feel a lump in your breast—any size or shape, whether firm or hard.

■ You have any unexplained discharge or drainage from a nipple.

■ You have a sore on a nipple or breast that does not heal in two weeks.

■ You have personal concerns or risk factors that make you anxious about cancer of the breast.

▨ *Goals of Care*

■ To master the techniques of breast self-examination.

■ To detect any abnormality of the breast in its earliest stages.

■ To obtain prompt medical care when an abnormality is detected.

▨ *Self-Care Techniques*

■ Master the technique of breast self-examination: (1) Study the outline provided in Appendix D on pages 342–343. (2) Try the visual and manual examinations, making note of any uncertainties or questions you may have. (3) Visit your doctor or his or her associate and ask the health professional to review and explain the technique. Most important, have the person coach you about normal breast appearance and feel. Keep in mind that 75 percent of breast tumors are found by the woman herself.

■ Using the calendar, establish a regular routine for monthly breast self-examination. If not past menopause, you should examine your breasts ten days after the onset of the menstrual period. If you are experiencing the menopause or have completed the menopause, the examination should be scheduled regularly for the first day of each calendar month.

■ If you find a change in your breast that you cannot explain, if you feel a definite lump of any size, or if you discover nipple discharge, consult your doctor promptly. But be aware that most masses you find are not cancers, and, in general, the smaller the lump, the more curable the tumor.

■ After age forty, arrange with your doctor to have an annual breast examination. The doctor may detect small lumps you have missed or have accepted as normal tissue.

■ Discuss the proper role of mammography in your care with your doctor. Mammograms are rapid, safe, and sensitive X rays of each breast that detect tumors and other abnormalities with about 90 percent accuracy. This accuracy is well beyond the range of other examinations. All women should have baseline mammograms at age forty, with repeat examinations every one to three years thereafter, depending on risk factors. While some experts argue that *all* women fifty years of age should have annual mammograms to detect early cancers, others suggest repeat studies every two years past fifty unless indicated differently.

■ PELVIC PROBLEMS

The pelvic, or lower abdominal, organs are suspended in a complicated "sling" of muscles and ligaments. In women, the urinary bladder, the uterus (womb), the vagina, and the rectum (lower bowel) enter the floor of the pelvis within a very small space (see figure 21). As a result, weakness or displacement of one of these organs often leads to secondary displacement or abnormal function in another.

Three abnormalities of the pelvic organs are especially common among older women: prolapse of the uterus, rectocele, and cystocele. *Prolapse of the uterus* refers to a falling, or sagging, of the womb downward through the base of the pelvis into the vagina (see figure 21). Normally the uterus is suspended above the vagina by supporting ligaments, and it tilts slightly forward in the pelvis. When these ligaments and surrounding muscles are stretched or weakened, the uterus descends into the vagina. A mild prolapse is present when the uterus rests in the upper part of the vagina; a severe, or complete, prolapse is present when the uterus bulges through the vagina.

A *rectocele* is a type of pelvic hernia (see figure 21). Here the wall of the lower bowel bulges forward into the weakened wall of the vaginal tube, producing pressure in the vagina and narrowing of the bowel. In a similar fashion, a *cystocele* consists of a bulging of the wall of the urinary bladder backward into the vagina (see figure 21). As a result of this pelvic weakness, the vagina is compressed by the bladder, which may itself become deformed and irritated.

Although each problem may exist alone, most women with rectocele or cystocele also have uterine prolapse.

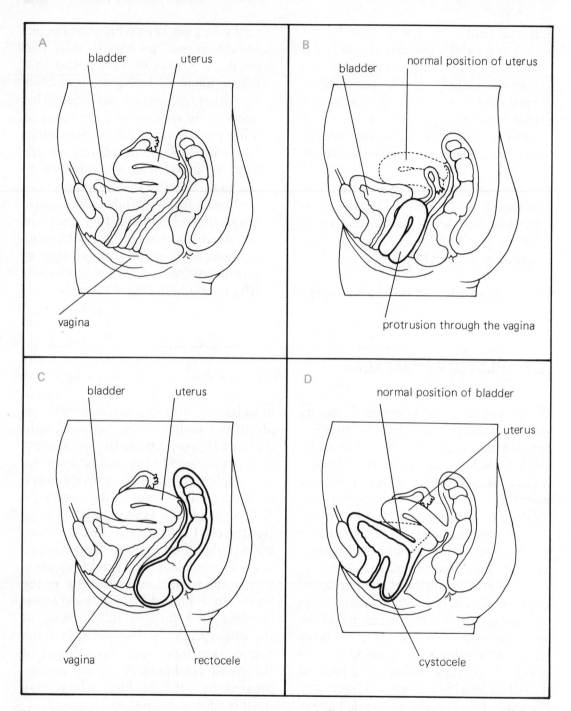

Figure 21. The normal pelvis and several pelvic problems: **A** shows the normal pelvis, **B** shows a prolapse or "fallen womb," **C** shows a rectocele, and **D** a cystocele.

WHAT CAUSES PELVIC PROBLEMS?

All three of these pelvic abnormalities are the result of weakness or relaxation of the ligaments and muscles that make up the base of the pelvic cavity. In turn, three factors seem to act together to weaken these structures: (1) Some women have poorly supported pelvic organs from the time of birth and readily develop uterine prolapse and other difficulties as adults. (2) Most women with one or more of these conditions have a history of delivering several children, often after prolonged or difficult labor. Experience suggests, therefore, that childbirth processes stretch and displace the critical structures that support the uterus, bladder, and lower bowel. (3) Finally, since these disorders are most common in later life, it seems that hormone changes of the menopause cause the support tissues to weaken—much as skin tends to sag and wrinkle.

Other factors also influence the development of these pelvic problems. Abnormal pressures in the pelvic cavity, such as may occur with tumors or extreme obesity, predispose individuals to the development of uterine prolapse. Vigorous coughing or sneezing may make any of these weaknesses or hernias obvious. Constipation and straining during bowel movements tend to enlarge a rectocele.

HOW CAN PELVIC PROBLEMS AFFECT YOU?

Prevention is still the best answer to all such pelvic problems, and there is no substitute for expert obstetrical care and postdelivery pelvic muscle exercises (Kegel exercises).

Many otherwise healthy women have small uterine prolapses, with or without associated cystocele or rectocele, that cause no symptoms at all. Since the uterus is a slightly movable organ, some tipping or falling is best regarded as normal and requires no treatment.

Once the prolapsed uterus or displaced urinary bladder or rectum begins to compress the vaginal space, most women experience feelings of fullness in this region and notice local pressure on sitting. The uterus that is prolapsed deep into the vagina may produce low backache and may bleed from local irritation. In time, an enlarging cystocele may interfere with bladder function; some women experience difficulty in emptying the bladder, and others have accidental loss of urine (incontinence) on coughing or straining. Although a moderate-sized rectocele may cause little or no difficulty, constipation and feelings of incomplete evacuation are fairly common.

Since these pelvic difficulties are basically mechanical in nature, spontaneous permanent correction should not be expected. Still, loss of excess weight and treatment of chronic cough may afford some relief. Considerable temporary decrease of pressure and other symptoms of these conditions can be obtained by use of a well-fitted vaginal pessary. This is a small, specially shaped device that presses against the walls of the vagina to support the surrounding organs. In time, however, the pessary becomes an irritant, so surgical repair of the hernia or weakened tissues is usually recommended, especially if several pelvic defects exist together.

■ To prevent complications of these pelvic problems.

Consult Your Doctor Now IF

- You develop unexplained vaginal bleeding.
- You experience urinary incontinence or feel that you cannot empty your bladder completely.
- You notice a fullness or bulging in your vagina.

Goals of Care

- To control the symptoms of mechanical pelvic problems (uterine prolapse, cystocele, and rectocele).

Self-Care Techniques

- If you are overweight (more than 10 percent above your ideal weight at ages twenty to twenty-five), work with a health professional to design a safe reducing diet.
- If you have a condition that produces a persistent cough, take steps to treat it.
- If your physician agrees, go through a trial of treatment with a vaginal pessary to obtain symptomatic relief.

Special Problems of Older Men

■ DISORDERS OF THE PROSTATE GLAND

The adult male's prostate gland is the size of a golf ball and is located just below the urinary bladder (see figure 22). Small and unimportant in children, the gland enlarges at puberty, and its secretions make up part of the male sexual fluid. After the fifth decade of life, the prostate undergoes further enlargement and internal change in response to male sex hormones. The central portion of the prostate gland typically enlarges in middle-aged men. The urethra, the tube that carries urine from the bladder to the outside, runs through the gland, so changes in prostate size or shape may interfere with emptying of the bladder. If

prostate enlargement begins to block urine flow or affect bladder function, the condition of benign (harmless) prostatic hypertrophy (enlargement), so-called BPH, exists. Also the incidence rate of cancer of the prostate increases steadily starting at about age fifty. In fact, 50 percent of men aged eighty will have developed some sort of prostate cancer.

The importance of prostate disease cannot be overemphasized. Surgical operations for BPH are the most common operations in men, and cancer of the prostate is the second most common cancer in men in the United States.

WHAT CAUSES PROSTATE PROBLEMS?

It is clear that male hormones somehow control normal prostate growth, stimulate the overgrowth in BPH, and strongly influence the abnormal growth of cancer cells. Just why certain older men develop troublesome BPH and others develop cancer is still not known.

BPH produces two types of problems—interference with urination and kidney damage. If the enlarging gland presses on the bladder outlet and narrows the urethral tube, urine passage becomes slow, and the bladder fails to empty rapidly and completely. In time, the bladder itself is damaged. Thus serious infection may occur in both the bladder and the kidneys.

Cancer of the prostate, if not treated early, grows steadily and silently, often invading the bladder and areas around the prostate gland. In addition, this malignant tumor, more than most others, tends to spread by way of the bloodstream into the bones throughout the body. As a result, long after cure is possible, cancer of the prostate causes bone pain, easy fractures, and disability.

HOW CAN PROSTATE PROBLEMS AFFECT YOU?

Benign prostatic hypertrophy probably develops to some extent in all men over fifty years of age. However, relatively

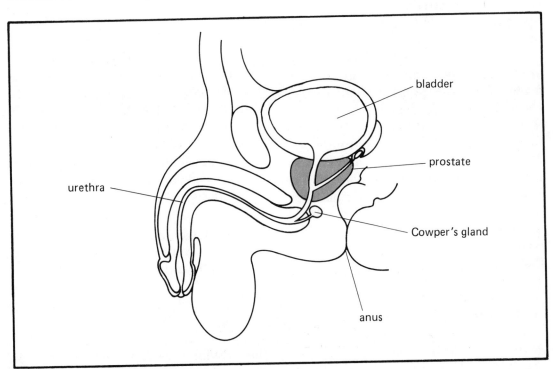

Figure 22. The prostate gland

few notice the early symptoms of bladder and urine blockage. At first, it is difficult to start urination, and urine flow is slow and halting. If the bladder outlet is partly blocked, emptying of the bladder is not complete, and urine must be passed frequently in small amounts throughout the night and day. Urine flow may be completely blocked, with sudden abdominal discomfort and general illness, when certain drugs further weaken the bladder function. Antidepressants, alcohol, and many nonprescription decongestants can precipitate this emergency. If infection develops in the bladder or kidneys, fever, chills, abdominal pain, and burning pain on urination may appear. The glandular enlargement can be relieved in most cases by a relatively simple and safe operation, one that usually preserves male sexual function.

Prostate cancer is rightly considered a special menace, for small, easily curable growths cause no symptoms. As a result, early diagnosis is usually made by a doctor's rectal examination or "accidentally" at the time of an operation for BPH. If the tumor grows through the gland and into the lower part of the bladder, partial blockage of urine flow may produce symptoms much like those of BPH. Wider spread to bones and other tissues is a life-theatening process, one that may respond to X-ray treatment or special drug programs. *Early detection remains the cornerstone of care!*

▬▬ Consult Your Doctor Now IF

- You pass red or bloody urine.
- You have increasing difficulty starting urination or passing urine.
- You have burning pain when you pass urine.

▬▬ Goals of Care

- To detect benign prostatic hypertrophy before bladder or kidney complications occur.
- To detect prostate cancer at its earliest stage.

▬▬ Self-Care Techniques

- After the age of fifty, schedule periodic health assessments, at least one every two years, and make certain that a careful rectal examination is performed. (The prostate gland is located just inside the rectum, or terminal colon, so a skilled doctor can readily determine its size, shape, and firmness.)
- If you have known or probable BPH, be very cautious in using antidepressants, nonprescription decongestants, and antiparkinsonism medications.

▬▬ IMPOTENCE

Sexual activities in men typically peak before age thirty, gradually declining thereafter in patterns that are unique to the individual. Several scientific studies have shown conclusively that these changes in sexual activity are *not* caused by failure of hormonal or glandular function. It follows that most sexual problems or dysfunctions in older men result either from true disease or from psychological or social difficulties.

Far and away the most common problem is that of impotence—the inability to have or to maintain a full erection. Almost every healthy man has experienced some difficulty with impotence in early years. In fact, isolated bouts of sexual dysfunction are normal occurrences. Impotence becomes more frequent and frustrating in later life, with more than one-quarter of the male population aged sixty-five reporting significant problems with erection and sexual functioning.

WHAT CAUSES IMPOTENCE?

Few human activities are more complicated than sexual behavior. Numerous medical, psychological, and social factors influence how people conduct this very personal part of their lives. Thus, the "cause" of impotence is often impossible to establish. All stages of male sexual activity—arousal, orgasm, and resolution—are less spontaneous and take a longer time to reach with advancing age. With mutual understanding, affection, and patience, however, most couples can expect to enjoy continuing closeness and rewarding sexual relations throughout their life together.

In only 10 to 15 percent of the men who complain of impotence are organic or disease-based problems the direct cause. A few people with long-standing diabetes mellitus develop nerve and blood vessel changes that interfere with sexual function. In addition, almost any hormonal imbalance (thyroid or adrenal)

may be associated with impotence. Local diseases that alter bladder or prostate gland function may lead to sexual difficulties. Severe heart, lung, or kidney disorders often result in a loss of sexual drive and impaired activity. Finally, perhaps most important, dozens of different drugs have been shown to interfere with sexual potency. Certain antidepressants, most antihypertensive medications, and sedatives, and *alcohol* may produce temporary impotence.

Emotional or psychological factors account for about 90 percent of problems with sexual performance in men. Many older men who complain of impotence have experienced similar problems in their youth, a pattern often attributed to lingering childhood conflicts. Most often, however, the appearance of adult sexual dysfunction relates to personal emotions. Guilt about a recent domestic strife, fear of being impotent, depression over the death of a friend, or self-concern about ill health may make sexual intercourse impossible. Typically, having experienced the frustration and embarrassment of impotence, the individual begins to avoid further encounters and simply adds anxiety to an already stressful situation. In fact, the term *widower's syndrome* has been used to describe a special, rather common example of this psychological crisis—an elderly man, who has recently nursed his wife through a long and demanding fatal illness, finally ends the period of mourning and seeks sexual activity with a new partner, only to experience impotence.

The stress of physical fatigue, loss of sleep, pain, or overindulgence in alcohol often causes temporary impotence.

HOW CAN IMPOTENCE AFFECT YOU?

A distinct loss in sexual potency typically produces immediate frustration and anxiety, which further interfere with normal expression and fulfillment. Fortunately, since most instances of failure of erection are related to obvious emotional stresses or other personal problems, a thoughtful and caring couple can usually resolve the tensions and expect a return to their usual level of sexual activity.

Sexual dysfunctions that relate to deeper emotional difficulties may require expert counseling for both persons involved. As the psychological problems are addressed, understanding of some basic principles of human sexuality will emerge. The couple will learn that (1) sexual dysfunction is extremely common at all ages and does not often indicate major pathology; (2) there is no place for blame in dealing with these problems, which involve two caring people; and (3) most sexual dysfunction can be corrected, even if the exact cause is not diagnosed.

When impotence develops gradually and full erections do not occur either spontaneously or on stimulation, the possibility of an underlying medical condition must be considered. Quite often a careful history review, a physical examination, and special laboratory studies will uncover the presence of a disease such as diabetes or adverse drug effects. In many such cases correction of the condition will restore sexual potency, often after a period of two to three months.

If impotence continues to be a problem, doctors will often recommend consultation with a urologist, an expert in disorders of the urogenital tract. Special tests may show that a narrowed blood vessel or damaged nerve is at fault. In many such cases, a skilled urological surgeon can implant two slender plastic tubes in the body of the penis, producing a flexible but erect organ. Even more satisfactory is a pair of inflatable tubes that can be controlled by a tiny pump sewn in place under nearby skin. As one expert said, "We can recommend these procedures with every confidence of a happy result."

Consult Your Doctor Now IF

- You experience distressing sexual impotence.

Goals of Care

- To maintain your sexual abilities and activities in a fashion satisfactory to you and your sexual partner.
- To recognize and correct any physical or psychological difficulties that may interfere with sexual performance.

Self-Care Technique

- Take stock.
  1. How often have you experienced impotence in the past month as compared to five years ago?
  2. Is there an irregular pattern to the impotence, or is the impotence a constant problem?
  3. Did the problem start abruptly, or has it developed gradually over months or years?

4. Have you had physical difficulties—such as pain, insomnia, or fatigue—that might influence your sexual functioning?
5. Have you had emotional or psychological problems—such as special anxieties, self-concern, depression, or feelings of guilt—that could contribute to impotence?
6. Do you have medical conditions—such as drug therapy, diabetes, heart disease, or hormonal imbalance (thyroid or adrenal)—that may influence your sexual functioning?

Fitness Exercises

Flexibility: Low Intensity

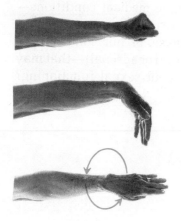

Hand Exercises. Raise your arms to a T position—extended to the sides, at shoulder height. Make fists with your hands. Tighten and then relax your fists. Do this five times. Let the hands flop down, relaxed; then raise them. Do this five times. Finally, describe circles with your hands at the wrists, five times in each direction, to loosen your wrists.

Head Roll. Slowly roll your head around in a circle, through its entire range of motion. Start by dropping it toward your chest. Then rotate it toward your shoulder, then toward your back, then toward the opposite shoulder, and finally forward again. Go in a clockwise direction five times and then in a counterclockwise direction five times to relax your neck muscles. As your head revolves, close your eyes and try to simultaneously relax those neck muscles, as well as the muscles in your shoulders.

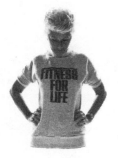
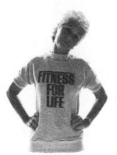
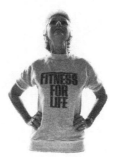
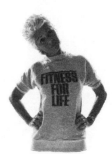

Flutter Kick. On your back on a mat or carpet, kick your legs in a flutter. Make sure your legs are up and your knees are bent so as to protect your back. If you have access to a pool, hold on to the sides of the pool with both hands behind you so that your back is in the water, your front is facing up, and your head is out of the water, facing your toes. (Do not do on land if you have a bad back.) On land or in the water, do this five times to limber your legs and feet and strengthen your abdominal muscles.

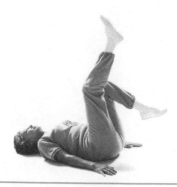

Arm Circle.   Raise your arms to a T position—extended to the sides, at shoulder height. Make fists with your hands. Tighten the elbows and muscles of your arms and make small circular motions, keeping your arms rigid. Make five rotations in one direction, five in the opposite direction. *Then* relax your hands and elbow, and make large circles with your arms still extended. Rotate five times in one direction and five times in the opposite direction to loosen your shoulders and elbows.

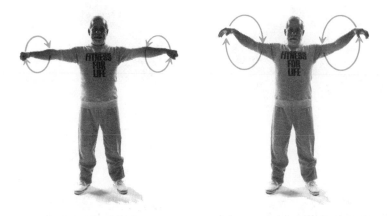

Seated Triangle.   As you sit in a chair, your hips facing forward, raise your arms to a T position. Inhale deeply. Now exhale, and as you do so, slowly move the right hand down to the toes of your left foot. Remember to keep the T so that as you rotate your trunk, your left arm follows the movement and rotates until it is pointing to the ceiling. Turn your head to the left so that you can look at the left thumb. Hold that position for five seconds. Inhale and come back to the original upright T position. Alternate five left and five right toe touches to loosen your trunk.

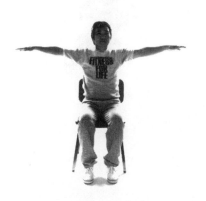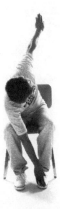

Front Slump.   Sitting so that your buttocks are firmly against the back of a hard chair, slump your shoulders and head, and let your arms drop to the sides. Now let your upper body slump down, bending slowly at the waist so that your chest is in your lap and your fingers are touching the floor. Hold for a few seconds; then s-l-o-w-l-y raise yourself to the upright sitting position. Tighten your abdominal muscles as you do so. Do this five times to limber the long muscles that run down your spine.

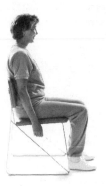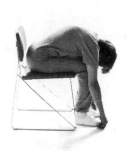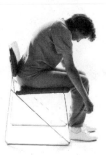

Sitting Stretch.   Sit on a carpet or mat, with your hands balancing you at your sides and slightly behind you. Spread your legs. Slowly stretch forward at the waist, and extend your arms forward as far as you can. Hold for three seconds or so. Return to a full sitting position. Repeat five times.

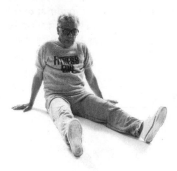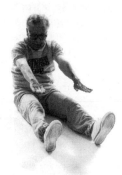

Flexibility: Medium Intensity

Wing Stretcher. Standing, legs apart, arms straight out to the sides at T position, bend at the elbow to bring your hands to your chest, palms down, with your fingertips touching. This is a four-count exercise. On each count of 1-2-3, pull your elbows back as far as you can. Keep your arms at shoulder height as you pull back three times; then, on count 4, swing your hands all the way, straight out to the sides, turning your palms up. Return to the starting fingertip position. Do this five times every day for a week. In the second week, increase to ten to limber and strengthen your upper back, shoulders, arms, and chest and to improve your posture.

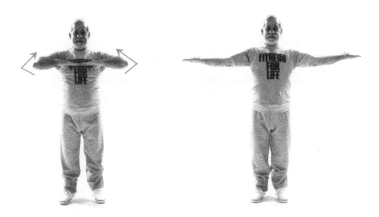

Knee-up. Lying on your back, stretch your legs straight, feet together. Bring your knees up as tight to your chest as you can. With your knees up, gently swing your ankles to the left and then to the right; then stretch out. Exhale as you bring your knees up; inhale as you stretch out. Repeat five times every other day this week and ten times every other day next week to tone your abdomen, hips, and thighs. On days when the pool is handy, do this with your arms spread behind you, holding on to the edge.

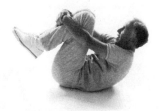

Flexibility: High Intensity

Alternate Floor Touch. Stand, legs far apart, arms out at shoulder height in a T position. A four-count exercise: (1) bend forward at the waist as you rotate your trunk to position your right hand (arms still straight) to touch your left toes; (2) return to a standing position; (3) bend down, this time rotating your body so that your left hand touches your right toes; (4) stand straight. Do ten times to limber your arms, back, and trunk and the backs of your legs. Exhale on the stretch; inhale on the return. Do five times for cool-down. (This exercise is most effective when you keep the knees straight; but if you have a lower-back problem, bending the knees a bit is OK. Not quite touching your toes is OK, too.)

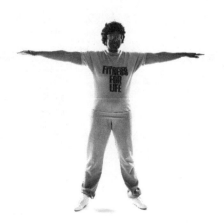
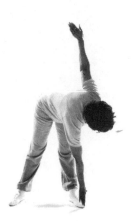

Knee Raise and Hug. Lying on your back, legs extended, feet together, arms at sides, raise your left leg about a foot off the floor. Hold it for a count of five; then bend the knee and pull it toward your chest. Clasp the knee with both hands, and pull it gently toward your chest as far as possible. Count to five; then return the knee to its original position. Exhale as you lift the leg and knee; inhale as you lower them. Then do the right leg and knee. Do ten to improve the flexibility of your knees and hip joints and to strengthen your abdominal muscles. Do five for cool-down.

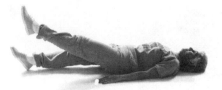
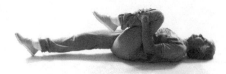

Sitting Stretch.   Sitting on the floor, back straight, legs straight and spread in front of you, hands resting on knees, bend forward from the waist. Extend your hands as far forward as you can. If you can touch your ankles, fine; if you can touch your toes, better; if you can touch the floor beyond your toes, best. Feel the s-t-r-e-t-c-h, but not to the point of pain. Hold it for five seconds; then return to the sitting position. Every day try to stretch a little beyond the previous day's limit. Exhale on the stretch; inhale on the return. Do ten to stretch the muscles of your arms, back, and the backs of your legs. Do five for cool-down.

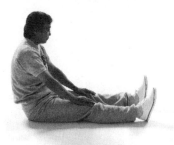 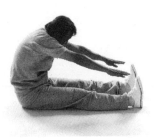

Strength: Low Intensity

Side Leg Raise.   Lie on your left side, with your head resting on your left arm, which is extended past your head, and your right hand on the floor in front of your abdomen to balance you. Lift your right leg sideward as high as you can. Hold it for a count of two. Repeat five times; then roll over and raise the left leg five times to help tone your hip muscles and trunk muscles.

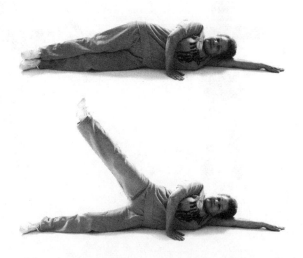

Leg Extension. Sitting, lift your left leg off the floor, and extend it fully in front of you. Hold it for the count of five; then slowly lower it. Do the same with the right leg. Do five of each leg to tone the thigh muscles.

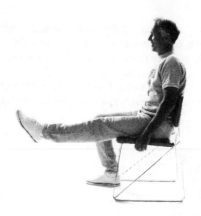

Arm Circle. Standing, legs apart, raise both arms at shoulder height to a T position. Make fists with your hands, and tighten the elbows. Then make small circles, keeping your arms rigid. Revolve five times in forward circles, then five times in backward circles. After that, relax your hands and elbows and make large circles with your still-extended arms. Revolve five times in big forward circles and five times in big back circles to limber your shoulders and arms. After doing this daily for a week, increase to ten times each set. After two weeks, increase to fifteen times each set, and keep the repetitions at that level daily.

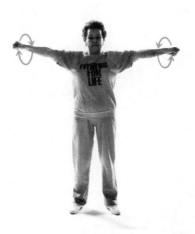
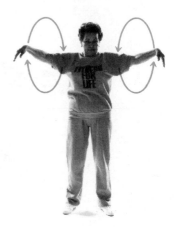

Tummy Tightener.   This can be done from the sitting position at any time. Do it whenever you think about it—when you are on the phone, when you are driving and are stopped at a traffic light, when you are sitting down to a cup of coffee. Sitting in a chair, contract your abdominal muscles as hard as you can. Try to hold this for about half a minute. Relax; let your tummy come forward by itself; then push it forward and hold. Do this five times. Strengthening those sagging abdominal muscles will not only firm them but will help your back as well.

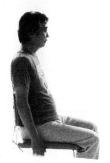 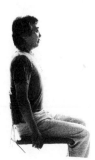

Thigh Strengthener.   Arms hanging loosely at your sides, slowly lift yourself from a sitting position to a standing position. After a count of five, slowly lower yourself back to a sitting position, keeping your back as straight as you can. As you do so, hold your loose-hanging hands slightly behind you so that you can feel the seat of the chair behind you to assure that you do not miss it as you sit.

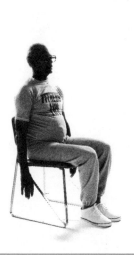 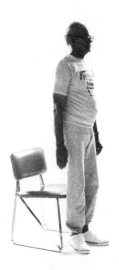 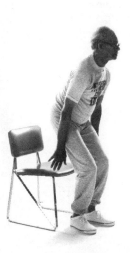

Rear Leg Raise. Feet together, stand behind your chair, facing it. Grasp the back. Lift your left leg back, and raise it as high as you can. Try to keep your knee straight. Slowly lower your leg back down to the floor. Do the same with your right leg. Repeat five times to help firm your buttocks, strengthen the lower back, and limber your hips and legs.

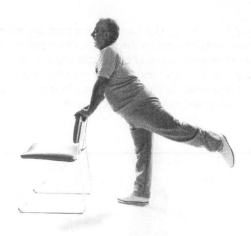

Strength: Medium Intensity

Chest Press-Pull. Standing, feet apart, bring your arms to shoulder height, and bend them at the elbows so that your hands are in front of your chest. Inhale deeply. Exhale as you p-u-s-h your palms against each other. Keep pushing for the count of five. Stop, separate your hands, rotate them in opposite directions, and hook the fingers of one hand to the fingers of the other. Inhale deeply. Exhale as you try to p-u-l-l them apart. Keep pulling for a count of five. Do ten sets of pushes and pulls every other day for the first month, twenty for the second, to strengthen arm, shoulder, and chest muscles.

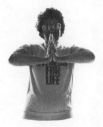 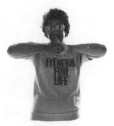

Head Curl.   Lying on your back on a carpet or mat, stretch out your legs, and hold them together. Tuck your hands, palms down, into the arch at the small of your back. Lift your head and shoulders, and elbows, off the floor. Hold for a count of five. You should feel a good tightness in your abdomen from the muscles holding up your head. Lower your head and shoulders, and elbows, back to the floor. Breathe deeply. Exhale on rising; inhale on relaxing. Do five every day the first week, ten every day the second week, and fifteen every day the third week. If you can build to twenty every day after that, all the better, since this is the best tummy-firming exercise.

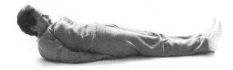

Wing Stretcher.   Standing, legs apart, arms straight out to the sides at T position, bend at the elbow to bring your hands to your chest, palms down, with your fingertips touching. This is a four-count exercise. On counts of 1-2-3, pull your elbows back as far as you can. Keep your arms at shoulder height as you pull back three times; then, on count 4, swing your hands all the way, straight out to the sides, turning your palms up. Return to the starting fingertip position. Do this ten times every day for a week. In the second week, increase to twenty times daily to limber and strengthen your upper back, shoulders, arms, and chest and to improve your posture. Exhale on 1-2-3; inhale on 4.

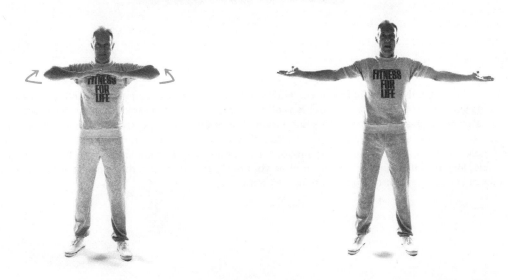

Leg Lift.   Lying on your back on a carpet or mat, stretch out your legs, and hold them together. Place your hands under your hips, palms down. Raise your left leg, knee straight, off the floor. Hold it for a count of five. Then lower it back to the floor. Inhale deeply. Exhale as you raise the straightened right leg and hold for a count of five. Repeat fifteen times to strengthen the abdominal and front thigh muscles. After doing this every other day for a month, try holding each leg up for a count of ten. (Do *not* try this with both legs at once, as this will place too much stress on the lower back.)

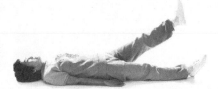

Side Leg Raise.   Lying on your right side on a carpet or mat, extend your straightened right arm in line with your body. Rest your head on the arm. Your left arm in front of you, palm on floor, helps balance you. Start with your legs together. Raise the straightened left leg as high as you can; then slowly lower it back to its original position. Do that ten times. Then roll over to your left side, and raise the right leg ten times. During the second week, raise each leg twenty times, and in the third week, thirty times. Done daily, this exercise strengthens hip and outer thigh muscles and slims down your flanks.

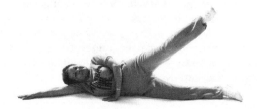

Strength: High Intensity

Flutter Kick.   On the floor, lie facedown, and tuck your hands under your thighs. Arch your back so as to bring your head off the floor and your legs off the floor, toes pointed. Hold this position as you slightly separate your legs and kick them in a continuous flutter for a minute. The legs should kick from the hips, with the knees only slightly bent. This can also be done in the swimming pool. Lie on your front, and hold on to the side of the pool. Point your toes, and kick in a whip action, with knees and ankles flexible, for a minute to limber and strengthen your back, your buttocks, the back of your neck, and the backs of your thighs. For cooling down, do half a minute.

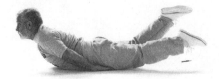

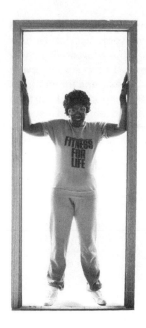

Samson Door Press. Stand in an open doorway with your feet apart. Lift your bent arms to about shoulder height (if the door opening allows), and place your hands on opposite jambs of the door frame. Push out a la Samson pushing over the pillars in ancient Israel. Exhale as you push. Hold for a count of ten. Relax, and inhale. Repeat ten times to build strength in your upper arms, shoulders, and upper back.

Arm Extension. In your left hand, hold an object that weighs two to three pounds, such as a two-pound or three-pound can of coffee (in a plastic bag if your hands are small), a book, or a dumbbell. Lift that hand and weight overhead; then slowly bend your arm until the hand holding the weight is behind your head. Slowly lift the weight until your arm is fully extended. Do ten times; then switch the weight to the right hand and do ten with that arm. After a month, go to five pounds, and work up to fifteen repetitions. After two months, go to ten pounds to strengthen your shoulders, upper arms, and hands.

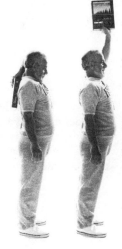

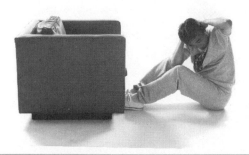

Sit-up. Lie on your back, hands folded behind your head, knees bent, feet on the floor. Have someone sit on your feet, or hook your feet under a heavy piece of furniture. Exhale as you curl your body upward. As you reach the sitting position, twist your body so that your right elbow touches your left knee (or comes close to it). The next time up, touch your left elbow to your right knee. Keep your lower back as straight as possible. Every other day during the first month, do ten, the second month twenty-five, the third month forty, to strengthen your abdominal muscles.

Chest Fly. With a book, can, or small dumbbell weighing two or three pounds in each hand, lie on your back on a bench or on the floor, knees bent. Hold your arms straight above your chest, and inhale deeply as you spread your arms to the sides with your elbows slightly bent. Exhale forcefully as you bring your arms (and weights) back to their starting position above your chest. At each session every other day, do five times the first two weeks, ten times for the third and fourth weeks, and fifteen times for the fifth and sixth weeks. On the seventh week, increase the weight to five pounds, and start the same cycle of five, ten, and fifteen repetitions for the seventh and eighth, ninth and tenth, and eleventh and twelfth weeks, to strengthen your chest muscles and improve shoulder motion in the lateral direction.

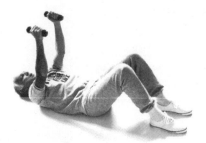 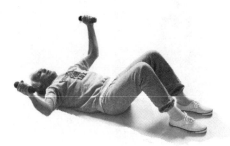

Squat. Standing, legs slightly apart, extend your arms straight ahead of you. This is a two-count exercise: (1) exhale as you lower your body to a nearly sitting position so that your thighs are parallel to the floor or until your buttocks just about touch the seat of a chair; (2) inhale as you *slowly* rise and return to the standing position. Move smoothly, keep your back straight, and breathe deeply. Do six squats every other day the first month, twelve every other day the second month, and twenty every other day the third month, to strengthen your thigh muscles.

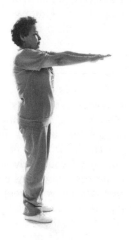 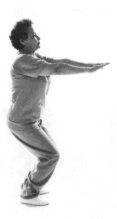

Relaxation Exercises ━━━━ *Appendix B*

DEEP-BREATHING EXERCISE

Smooth, slow breathing can help control anger or other strong feelings. It is important to breathe from the diaphragm. If your stomach goes up and down when you breathe, you are breathing properly. Breathing shallowly through the mouth increases tension.

The steps involved in this deep-breathing exercise are as follows:

1. Sit down and take smooth, slow breaths through your nose. Breathe out slowly until you are taking twice as long to breathe out as you are to breathe in.

2. Count to three as you breathe in. Count to six as you breathe out.

3. Clear your mind of thoughts and concentrate on your breathing. Breathe slowly through your nose, drawing deep breaths from your diaphragm. As you breathe out, say a word or sound to yourself, such as "relax."

4. Continue breathing in this manner for a few seconds or minutes until you feel the tension begin to leave your body.

PROGRESSIVE MUSCLE RELAXATION (PMR) EXERCISES

Progressive muscle relaxation uses a sequence of tensing various muscle groups to produce a reflex relaxation. It is a particularly useful technique when muscles are tense. The added benefit is that it highlights the difference between feeling tense and feeling relaxed. The sequence of muscles that are used can be abbreviated with practice and often can involve only those muscle groups that typically respond to tension.

1. Begin by finding a quiet spot. Sit comfortably or lie on your back. Uncross your arms and legs. Close your eyes. Begin taking some deep, slow breaths. Breathing with your stomach muscles, breathe in relaxation and breathe out tension. Try to keep out any intruding thoughts, reminding yourself that this is your time out. As any intruding thoughts enter, try repeating the word *relax* to yourself.

2. Relax your muscles. Remember to tense each muscle group first and then relax it. Here is the sequence of muscle groups that you will be relaxing.

Fists, Forearms, and Biceps

Focus on your left arm and hand. Put them in your lap. Think about how they feel. Tense your left arm and hand by clenching your fist tightly and pressing your arm against your lap. Hold the tension. Be aware of how it feels. Hold for three to five seconds and relax completely, all at once. Notice the difference between the tension and relaxation. Allow your arm to go limp. It may feel heavy. Feel a warm sensation in your fingertips as you get deeply relaxed.

■ Pause and repeat the exercise.

Now, tense your right arm and hand by clenching your fist tightly and pressing your arm against your lap. Hold the tension. Be aware of how it feels. Hold for approximately three to five seconds and relax completely, all at once. Notice the difference between the tension and relaxation. Allow your arm to go limp. It may feel heavy. Feel a warm sensation in your fingertips as you get deeply relaxed.

■ Pause and repeat the exercise.

Focus on your breathing again. Make it slow and comfortable and remind yourself that this is your time out from thoughts.

Neck and Shoulders

Focus on your neck and shoulders. Think about how they feel. Tense your neck and shoulders by shrugging your shoulders and pressing your chin toward your chest. Hold the tension. Be aware of how it feels. Hold for three to five seconds and relax completely, all at once. Try to notice the difference in feeling. Allow your shoulders to drop down comfortably and your neck to relax.

■ Pause and repeat this exercise.

Face

Focus on your facial muscles. Think about how they feel. Tense your face by clenching your jaw, wrinkling your brow, and squeezing your eyes tight. Hold the tension. Be aware of how

it feels. Hold for three to five seconds and relax completely, all at once. Notice the difference in feeling. Feel your jaw more slack, your brow smooth, and your eyelids relaxed.

■ Pause and repeat this exercise.

Chest, Back, and Stomach

While sitting in a chair, focus on your chest, back, and stomach muscles. Think about how they feel. Tense your chest, stomach, and back by tightening your stomach, pressing your back into the chair, and tightening your buttocks. Hold the tension. Be aware of how it feels. Hold for three to five seconds and relax completely, all at once. Notice the difference in feeling. Let yourself sink back comfortably into the chair.

■ Pause and repeat this exercise.

Thighs, Calves, and Feet

Focus on your left leg and foot. Think about how they feel. Tense your left leg and foot by raising both slightly off the floor and pointing your toe toward your head. Hold the tension. Be aware of how it feels. Hold for three to five seconds and relax completely, all at once. Notice the difference in feeling. Let your thigh and calf muscles unwind. Feel your toes get warm and comfortable.

■ Pause and repeat this exercise.

Focus now on your right leg and foot. Think about how they feel. Tense your right leg and foot by raising them slightly off the floor and pointing your toe toward your head. Hold the tension. Be aware of how it feels. Hold for three to five seconds and relax completely, all at once. Notice the difference in feeling. Let your thigh and calf muscles go slack. Feel your toes get warm and comfortable.

■ Pause and repeat this exercise.

Now take the next few minutes to make a mental check across your body. Think about where there is remaining tension, and as you breathe outward, release the tension. Remember, this is your time out.

■ Check across your arms and hands. Let them relax and feel warm and heavy.
■ Check across your neck and shoulders. Feel them relax.
■ Let go of any remaining tension in your face. Let your face feel smooth and relaxed.
■ Release any tension from your back and stomach. Feel a wave of warm relaxation travel all the way down to your legs and feet.
■ Allow both legs and both feet to relax and feel heavy and warm.
■ Close your eyes. Count backward from

five to one. At three you can open your eyes. At one you can stretch, Five, four, three, open your eyes, two, one, stretch.

Practice these exercises a minimum of twice a day, preferably not after eating.

IMAGERY RELAXATION EXERCISE

1. Find a quiet spot. Sit comfortably, or lie on your back. Uncross your arms and legs. Close your eyes. Begin taking some deep, slow breaths.
2. Picture a calm scene in your mind, such as lying on the beach, being warmed by the sun, or anything that is pleasing to you.
3. Imagine this calm scene in the greatest detail possible. Your muscles will relax as you concentrate.

It is essential to practice relaxation under "ideal conditions"—not under stress and in an uninterrupted environment—first in order to learn the skill. Once the skill has been learned, it can be applied under more stressful conditions.

Medical Records Charts

Basic Facts

Name: _____
         Last   First   Middle

Address: _____
        Street   City   State   Zip Code

Phone Number: _____ **Social Security Number:** _____

Date of Birth: _____ **Place of Birth:** _____

Height: _____ **Weight:** _____ **Marital Status:** _____

Health Insurance: Medicare _____
                    Identification Number   Effective Date

               Medicaid _____
                    Identification Number   Effective Date

               Other: _____
                    Company Name   Address

                    _____
                    Group Number   Certificate Number   Subscriber's Name

Main Doctor: _____
           Name   Specialty

           _____
           Address   Phone Number

Other Doctor: _____
           Name   Specialty

           _____
           Address   Phone Number

Allergies: _____

Drug Reactions: _____

Blood Type: _____

Notify in Case of Emergency: _____
                    Name   Relationship

                    _____
                    Address   Phone Number

Emergency Phone Numbers

Main Doctor:	_____	Police:	_____
Emergency Room:	_____	Fire:	_____
Hospital:	_____	Poison Control Center:	_____
Ambulance:	_____	Other:	_____

290

Name: _____

Health Problems

Problem	Date Problem Started	Current Treatment

Name: _____

Medications [Medicines Prescribed by Doctor]

Name of Drug, Place Purchased, and Prescription Number	Reason for Taking Drug	Date Started Taking Drug	Date Stopped Taking Drug

[Medicines Taken Without Prescription]

Name of Drug	Reason for Taking Drug	Date Started Taking Drug	Date Stopped Taking Drug

Dosage and Schedule	Results or Side Effects	Cost of Drug

Dosage and Schedule	Results or Side Effects	Cost of Drug

Name: _____

Blood Pressure and Weight				
Date	Systolic Blood Pressure	Diastolic Blood Pressure	Pulse	Weight

Name: _____

Chronic Problem Chart				

Name: _____

Health Maintenance		

History Check (✓) appropriate column.	**Yes**	**No**
Have you had major surgery in the last 5 years?		
Have you had a weight problem in the last 5 years?		
Do you take any prescription drugs?		
Do you smoke?		
Do you have any allergies?		
Do you suffer from a chronic illness?		
Does a member of your immediate family suffer from cancer, diabetes, chronic lung disease, or chronic heart disease?		
Do you eat a balanced diet?		
Do you exercise regularly?		
Do you have regular dental checkups?		
Do you give yourself a monthly breast self-examination (women)?		
Have you had any serious health problems in the last 6 months? If so, list: _____ _____		

Physical Examination Record Values in Shaded Box or Check (✓) If Normal	Date Checked				Laboratory Tests Record Values in Shaded Box or Check (✓) If Normal	Date Checked			
MEASURES					Cholesterol (circle if fasting)				
Height					Blood glucose (circle if fasting)				
Weight					Hemoglobin (Hgb) or Hematocrit (Hct)				
Blood pressure	/	/	/	/	Stool occult blood				
Other _____					Mammography (women)				
_____					Pap smear (women)				
_____					EKG				
_____					Other _____				
					_____				
					_____				
					_____				

SCREENING EXAMS	Date Checked				Immunizations Check (✓) If Done	Date			
Hearing					Tetanus				
Breast (women)					Influenza				
Rectal					Pneumococcal (high risk)				
Vision					Other _____				
Other _____					_____				
_____					_____				
_____					_____				

Name: _____

Hospital Stays

Name, Address, and Phone Number of Hospital	Date Admitted	Date Discharged	Reason for Stay

Medications and Dosages Prescribed	Diet Instructions	Follow-up Services Needed at Home

Name and Specialty of Main Doctor	Names and Specialties of Other Doctors	Major Tests and/or Treatment and/or Operation Performed

Physician Follow-up Appointments	Cost of Stay	Insurance Payment

Name: _____

Medical Visits			
Name, Address, and Phone Number of Doctor or Other Health Professional	**Reason for Visit**	**Date and Time of Appointment**	**Specialty of Doctor or Other Health Professional**

Questions to Ask Doctor or Other Health Professional	Health Problem	Recommended Treatment Plan	Needed Follow-up	Cost of Visit	Insurance Payment

Name: _____

Health Providers

Type of Doctor or Other Health Professional	Name, Address, and Phone Number of Health Provider	Date of Visit

Reason for Visit	Health Provider's Recommendations	Cost of Visit	Insurance Payment

Name: _____

Family History						

Blood Relatives	If Deceased . . .		Selected Diseases and Conditions Linked to Family Background*			
	Year of Death	Cause of Death	Alcoholism	Allergy	Cancer	Depression
Parents						
Grandparents						
Uncles and Aunts						
Brothers and Sisters						
Children						

*Check the box if any of your relatives had one of these medical problems.

iabetes	Gout	Heart Disease	Hypertension	Mental Disorder	Stroke	Ulcers	Suicide	Other

Name: _____

Major Illnesses, Injuries, and Surgeries

Illness, Injury, or Surgery	Age at Occurrence	Place of Treatment

Major Complications	Long-Term Impact on Health	Comments

Name: _____

Exposures to X Rays or Occupational Hazards

X-Ray Exposure or Hazard	Place of Exposure	Age at Exposure	Treatment Received

Place of Treatment	Long-Term Impact on Health	Comments

Name: _____

Sleep Chart						
Date	Amount of Time Taken to Fall Asleep	Number of Awakenings During the Night	Number of Hours Slept	Quality of Rest 0–5 (0=Not Rested at All 5=Very Well Rested)	Time Slept During the Day	All Medications Taken

Name: _____

Weight-Loss Chart			
Date	**Weight**	**Complaints** (Loss of appetite, nausea, vomiting, diarrhea, pain, weakness, and so on)	**All Medications Taken** (Prescription and over-the-counter)

Name: _____

Dizziness Chart			

	Duration of Episode		Situation at Occurrence (Moving, standing up, bending over, walking, and so on)
Date	Time Began	Time Ended	

Accompanying Symptoms (Ringing in ears, headache, nausea, vomiting, sweating, falling, and so on)	A Spinning or Turning Sensation		All Medications Taken
	Yes	No	

Name: _____

Fever Chart					
Date	**Times Temperature Taken**	**Oral Reading**	**Temperature or**	**Rectal Reading**	**Pulse Rate**

Accompanying Symptoms (Chills, sweating, pain, or nausea)	**All Medication Taken** (Names, times taken, and dosages)

Name: _____

Dental Chart	
Date of Dental Visit	**Examination and Treatments Performed** (X rays, cleaning, fillings, and so on)

Symptoms of Periodontal and Other Dental Problems (Bleeding gums, toothache, dry mouth, loose teeth, poorly fitted dentures, sores in mouth, and so on)	**Home Treatments** (Flossing, rinsing the mouth, and so on)

Name: _____

Asthma Chart						

Date	Time of Day Attack Occurred	Duration of Attack	Attack Developed			
			Rapidly	or	Slowly	With Exposure to Known Irritants / or / Without Exposure to Known Irritants

With Specific Treatment	or	Without Specific Treatment	Treatments Used	Effects of Treatments Effective or Ineffective		Complications, If Any

Name: _____

Influenza Vaccination Chart	
Date of Vaccination	**Type of Influenza Vaccination**

Name: _____

Constipation Chart			
Date and Time of Bowel Movement	**Appearance of Bowel Movement**	**Associated Symptoms** (Cramps, pain, bleeding, and so on)	**Body Weight**

Name: _____

Chest Pain Chart

Date of Chest Pain	Time(s) of Chest Pain	Location of Pain	Description of Pain

Precipitating Events	Accompanying Symptoms (Sweating, anxiety, palpitations, shortness of breath, cough, and so on)	What Relieved the Pain, If Anything (Rest, medications, and so on)

Name: _____

Congestive Heart Failure Chart

| Date | Weight | Pulse | | Accompanying Symptoms (Breathlessness on exertion, breathlessness on lying down, cough, increase in body weight, irregular heartbeat, abdominal pressure, or ankle swelling) |
		Rate	Regularity	

	Diet	All Medications Taken	Side Effects of Drugs
lt	Fluid Intake		

Name: _____

Diarrhea Chart		

Date	Time of Each Bowel Movement	Texture and Color of Each Bowel Movement (Loose, liquid, solid; tan, brown, black, red, and so on)

Associated Symptoms (Pain, cramps, nausea, vomiting, fever, chills, rectal soreness, and so on)	**Treatment** (Time, type of fluids, volume of fluids, and all medications taken)

Name: _____

Vomiting Chart

Date and Time When Vomiting Occurred	Nature of Vomit (Color and contents)	Volume of Vomit	Food and Fluid Intake by Mouth

All Medications Taken	Associated Symptoms (Pain, diarrhea, faintness, or dizziness)	Body Weight

Name: _____

Abdominal Pain Chart				
Date	**Onset Time of Pain**	**Precipitating Events**	**Location of Pain**	**Severity of Pain 1–4** (1 = Mild Pain 4 = Severe Pain)

Nature of Attack (In spells or constant)	Associated Symptoms (Nausea, vomiting, diarrhea, fever, and so on)	Method of Pain Relief (Rest, food, medications, and so on)

Name: _____

Headache Chart

Date	Duration		Events Preceding Onset of Headache (Injury, physical stress, emotional stress, and so on)	Location of Headache	Nature of Head (Steady, throbbi burning, dull, and so on)
	Time Began	Time Ended			

everity of Headache (ild, moderate, severe)	**Associated Symptoms** (Visual changes, local tenderness, nausea, vomiting, mental changes, muscle spasms, and so on)	**Treatment Used**	**Effects of Treatment**

Name: _____

Daily Activities Chart		
Date	**Test Tasks** (Shaving, tying shoes, getting up from chair, walking up stairs, and so on)	**Degree of Difficulty for Each Task 1-5** (1 = Least Difficult 5 = Most Difficult)

Frequency and Ease of Bowel Movements	All Medications Used	Side Effects of Medications, If Any

Name: _____

Weight Chart				
Date	**Time Weighed** (Same time before breakfast each day)	**Weight** (in underclothes)	**Feelings** (Happy, sad, hungry, frustrated, and so on)	**Special Events of Previous Day** (Party, visit, illness, and so on)

Name: _____

Menstrual Chart

Beginning Date of Menstrual Period	Ending Date of Menstrual Period	Average Heaviness of Flow	Associated Symptoms (Hot flashes, cramps, and so on)

Name: _____

Diet Log

When	Meat Group and Meat Substitutes	Dairy Products	Fruits and Vegetables
Breakfast			
Morning Snacks			
Lunch or Dinner			
Afternoon Snacks			
Dinner or Supper			
Evening Snacks			
Nighttime Snacks			
Total Number Servings			

Grains and Cereals	Fats and Oils	Sweets	Alcohol	Water

Self-Care Skills

DETERMINING YOUR BODY TEMPERATURE

It is important for you to know what your normal body temperature is.

You need to compare your normal body temperature with the temperature you have when you are not feeling well to determine whether you have a fever. In addition, taking and recording the body temperature at certain hours over a period of time can help determine the course of an illness and whether the illness is getting better or worse (see pages 154–156)

To determine your normal body temperature, you should take your temperature when you are not ill. You should do this over a period of three days at several specified times each day after resting for at least ten minutes each time. To do this, you need a good glass thermometer (which can be purchased at any drugstore for about two dollars). There are three types of glass thermometers—oral, rectal, and universal, which can be used both orally and rectally. (A rectal thermometer is used for children under six and for people who cannot keep an oral thermometer in their mouths or who may bite the end.) An oral, rectal, or universal thermometer may be used to take an axillary temperature (a temperature taken by placing the thermometer in the armpit and pressing the arm against the body). The digital thermometer shown below is a universal one.

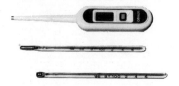

Temperature can be taken in three ways:

Oral Temperature

The glass oral thermometer has a long, slender silver tip. Place this cleaned tip well under your tongue and rest the thermometer at the side of the mouth for about three minutes for an accurate reading, though, when possible, it is preferable to leave it in for seven minutes. The normal temperature by mouth is between 97.6° F and 99.6° F. When you take your temperature orally, make certain you do not eat, drink, or smoke for a half-hour before.

Rectal Temperature

While a rectal temperature is considered the most accurate, it is difficult to take your own temperature this way. If, for some reason, it is essential that you obtain a rectal reading, be certain that the person taking your temperature is aware of the following: The glass rectal thermometer has a fat or bulb-shaped, blunt silver tip. A water-soluble lubricant, such as K-Y Jelly, is put on the tip, and the thermometer is inserted into the anus (the opening of the rectum) for a distance of about one inch. It is left in place for two to four minutes. Normal rectal temperature is between 98.6° F and 100.6° F. A rectal or axillary temperature is always taken when there is any interference with a person's ability to breathe, or when a person is confused, unconscious, or nauseated. When used for an older person, a rectal thermometer should always be inserted and held during the entire time it is in place. Insert the thermometer gently—never force it—and rotate it or change the direction of the insertion if resistance is met. *Do not continue to insert the thermometer if the insertion causes any pain.* Do not take a rectal temperature if the person has diarrhea or has had recent rectal surgery or an infection.

Axillary Temperature

You may use an oral, universal, or rectal thermometer to take an axillary temperature. Place the silver tip well inside the armpit, and hold the arm snugly against the body. Leave the thermometer in place for ten minutes. Normal axillary temperature is one degree below an oral temperature, or between 96.6° F and 98.6° F. Take an axillary temperature if you are unable to take your temperature orally and cannot have it taken for you rectally (for example, if you cannot close your mouth and you have painful hemorrhoids or diarrhea).

Procedures for Taking a Temperature

1. Before and after you use a thermometer, wash your hands with soap and water thoroughly. Do this twice.

2. Wash the thermometer with a small cotton ball or tissue, using soap and cool water—never wash a thermometer in hot water. Hold the thermometer at the top and use a twisting motion as you bring the cotton ball or tissue down over the bulb end. Make certain you clean the grooves around the bulb. Rinse the thermometer in cool, running water.

Repeat this procedure a second time with soap and a clean cotton ball or tissue. Then dry the thermometer with a clean cotton ball or tissue; once again, use a twisting motion. The silver tip will go into your mouth, so do not touch this end after washing.

3. Grasp the high-number end of the thermometer and shake the thermometer until the silver fluid (mercury) falls below 95° F. Shake it down by holding the glass end tightly and flicking only your wrist. When shaking a thermometer, stand clear of nearby objects.

4. Place the bulb end under your tongue. Close your mouth and breathe through the nose. Leave the thermometer in position for three to five minutes.

5. Remove the thermometer and read it in a good light (with the light behind you).

6. Hold the glass tip of the thermometer with your thumb and first two fingers. Bring it to eye level.

7. Rotate the tnermometer slowly between your fingers until you clearly see the silver line of mercury.

8. Read the long line immediately to the left of where the silver mercury stops. This gives you the full degree.

9. Count the short lines after the full degree. Each short line stands for two-tenths of a degree. Adding the long and short lines gives you a complete reading in degrees Fahrenheit. Reading a thermometer takes practice. If your eyesight is poor, find a thermometer with large figures or get a digital one.

Average Normal Oral Temperature Range:
97.6° F to 99.6° F
(36.5° C to 37.5° C)
Average Normal Rectal Temperature Range:
98.6° F to 100.6° F
(37° C to 38.1° C)
Average Normal Axillary Temperature Range:
96.6° F to 98.6° F
(35.9° C to 37° C)

Precautions for Glass Thermometers

A small wad of cotton should be placed at the bottom of the thermometer container to prevent breaking or chipping of the thermometer.

If a thermometer breaks in your mouth, do the following:

- Try not to swallow.
- Spit out whatever you can.
- Rinse your mouth with water and spit several times.
- Examine your mouth for glass bits or cuts.
- Report the accident to a medical person at once; mercury is a poison.
- Eat some bread if you have swallowed glass. Bread collects the glass bits and lessens the chances of injury.

BREAST SELF-EXAMINATION

How to Examine Your Breasts
(This is a must for women of all ages.)

1. **In the shower:**
   Examine your breasts during bath or shower; hands glide easier over wet skin. Fingers flat, move gently over every part of each breast. Use right hand to examine left breast, left hand for right breast. Check for any lump, hard knot or thickening.

2. **Before a mirror:**
   Inspect your breasts with arms at your sides. Next, raise your arms high overhead. Look for any changes in contour of each breast, a swelling, dimpling of skin or changes in the nipple.

   Then, rest palms on hips and press down firmly to flex your chest muscles. Left and right breast will not exactly match—few women's breasts do.

   Regular inspection shows what is normal for you and will give you confidence in your examination.

3. **Lying down:**
   To examine your right breast, put a pillow or folded towel under your right shoulder. Place right hand behind your head—this distributes

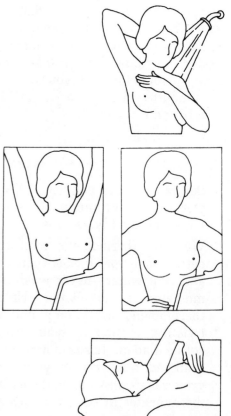

breast tissue more evenly on the chest. With left hand, fingers flat, press gently in small circular motions around an imaginary clock face. Begin at outermost top of your right breast for 12 o'clock, then move to 1 o'clock, and so on around the circle back to 12. A ridge of firm tissue in the lower curve of each breast is normal. Then move in an inch, toward the nipple, keep circling to examine *every part of your breast*, including nipple. This requires at least three more circles. Now slowly repeat procedure on your left breast with a pillow under your left shoulder and left hand behind head. Notice how your breast structure feels.

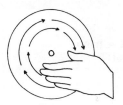

Finally, squeeze the nipple of each breast gently between thumb and index finger. Any discharge, clear or bloody, should be reported to your doctor immediately.

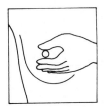

Why You Should Examine Your Breasts Monthly

Most breast cancers are first discovered by women themselves. Since breast cancers found early and treated promptly have excellent chances for cure, learning how to examine your breasts properly can help save your life. Use the simple 3-step breast self-examination (BSE) procedure shown above.

For the Best Time to Examine Your Breasts:

Follow the same procedure once a month about a week after your period, when breasts are usually not tender or swollen. After menopause, check breasts on the first day of each month. After hysterectomy, check your doctor or clinic for an appropriate time of the month. Doing BSE will give you monthly peace of mind and seeing your doctor once a year will reassure you there is nothing wrong.

What You Should Do If You Find a Lump or Thickening

If a lump or dimple or discharge is discovered during BSE, it is important to see your doctor as soon as possible. Don't be frightened. Most breast lumps or changes are not cancer, but only your doctor can make the diagnosis.

On the following lines post the dates of your breast self-examination.

_____ _____
_____ _____
_____ _____
_____ _____
_____ _____

Reprinted with the permission of the American Cancer Society.

Self-Change Charts

Self-Change Plan

Self-Change Goal	Specific Behavioral Change	Self-Observation

Patterns that Aid or Hinder Self-Change Efforts	Skills and Tasks Required for Self-Change	Plan Summary

Self-Observation

Behavior:

Date	Situation (Briefly describe where you were and whom you were with.)	Thoughts and Feelings in This Situation (Briefly describe how you were feeling and what you were thinking.)	Actions (Describe how you responded to the situation.)

REFERENCES

American Red Cross. *Temperature, Pulse, and Respiration.* Washington, D.C., 1984.

Belloc, N. B., and Breslow, L. "The Relation of Physical Health Status and Health Practices." *Preventive Medicine* 1 (August 1972): 409–421. Also see "Relationship of Health Practices and Mortality." *Preventive Medicine* 2 (1973): 67–81.

Berland, Theodore. *Fitness for Life: Exercises for People Over 50.* Washington, D.C.: AARP; Glenview, Ill.: Scott, Foresman & Co., 1985. (An AARP Book).

Brooks, D. N. "Use of Post-aural Aids by National Health Service Patients." *British Journal of Audiology* 15 (1981): 79.

Butler, R. N.; Gertman, J. S.; Oberlander, D. L.; and Schlinder, L. "Self-Care, Self-Help and the Elderly." *International Journal of Aging and Human Development* 10 (1979–80): 95–119.

Christakis, G., and Miridjanian, A. "Diets, Drugs and Their Interrelationships." *Journal of the American Dietetic Association,* 52 (1968): 21.

Fuchs, V. *Who Shall Live?* New York: Basic Books, 1974.

Giglio, R. V.; Spears, B. W., and Edy, N. B. *Personal Life Plan.* Amherst, Mass.: Self-published, 1977.

Gray, G. M. "Drugs, Malnutrition, and Carbohydrate Absorption." *American Journal of Clinical Nutrition* 26 (1973): 121.

Kannel, W. B., et al. "Vascular Disease of the Brain—Epidemiology Aspects. The Framingham Study." *American Journal of Public Health* 55 (1965): 9.

Kemper, D. W. "Self-Care Education: Impact on HMO Costs." *Medical Care* 20 (July 1982): 710–718.

Leslie, D. K., and McLure, J. W. *Exercises for the Elderly.* Iowa City: University of Iowa Press, 1975.

Mossey, J. M., and Shapiro, E. "Self-rated Health: a Predictor of Mortality Among the Elderly." *American Journal of Public Health* 72 (August 1982): 800–808.

Nocerino, J. T.; Pringl, W. B.; and Shenert, K. W., M. D. *Health Activation for Senior Citizens.* Vienna, Virginia: Health Activation Network, 1977.

Pell, S., and Fayerweather, W. E. "Trends in the Incidence of Myocardial Infarction and in Associated Mortality and Morbidity in a Large Employed Population, 1957–1983." *New England Journal of Medicine* 312 (April 18, 1985): 1005–1011.

Recommended Dietary Allowances. 9th ed. Washington, D.C.: National Academy of Sciences, 1980.

Roe, D. A. *Drug-Induced Nutritional Deficiencies.* Westport, Connecticut: The AVI Publishing Company, 1976.

Sagov, S. E., M. D. *The Active Patient's Guide to Better Medical Care,* New York: David McKay Company, 1976.

Taylor, F. "How to Talk to Your Doctor About Yourself." *FDA Consumer* (October 1979). U.S. Department of Health, Education, and Welfare, HEW Publication No. (FDA) 80–1070.

———. "How to Talk to Your Doctor About Yourself." *FDA Consumer* (September 1984): 681–684.

Trocchio, Julie. *Home Care for the Elderly.* Boston: CBI Publishing Company, 1981.

U.S. Department of Health, Education, and Welfare. *A Guide to Medical Self-Care and Self-Help Groups for the Elderly.* (November 1979). NIH Publication No. 80–1687.

U.S. Department of Health and Human Services. *Exercise and Your Heart* (1981). National Heart, Lung and Blood Institute, National Institutes of Health, NIH Publication No. 81–1677.

Vickery, D. M., et al. "Effect of a Self-Care Education Program on Medical Visits." *Journal of the American Medical Association,* 250 (December 1983): 2952–2956.

Zapka, J., and Averill, B. W. "Self-Care for Colds: A Cost-effective Alternative to Upper Respiratory Infection Management." *American Journal of Public Health* 69 (1979): 814.

INDEX

ABOUT THE AUTHORS

Eugene C. Nelson, D.Sc., is executive director of the Dartmouth Institute for Better Health and vice-chairman for community medicine at Dartmouth Medical School, Hanover, New Hampshire. A leading innovator in promoting self-care for good health, Professor Nelson is an originator of Dartmouth's medical self-care education program for older adults begun in 1977. He is working also with the Rand Corporation on evaluating community health programs and has written many professional articles on primary-care research and patient education. He received his doctor of science degree from the Harvard School of Public Health.

Ellen Roberts, M.P.H., is an instructor in the Department of Community and Family Medicine at Dartmouth Medical School. She has been coordinator of self-care programs at the Dartmouth Institute for Better Health and directed the educational program for the medical self-care project for older adults. Among other writings, she contributed to the book *Wellness and Health Promotion for the Elderly* (1985). She was a Peace Corps volunteer in Central America and received her master's degree in public health from the University of North Carolina.

Jeannette J. Simmons, D.Sc., is a clinical professor in the Department of Community and Family Medicine at Dartmouth Medical School. She is the author of *Making Health Education Work* for the American Public Health Association and a contributor to the book *Wellness and Health Promotion for the Elderly* (1985) and has written extensively on community health topics for professional journals. She served in a number of overseas assignments for the World Health Organization and is a former chair of the board of directors, National Center for Health Education. She received her doctor of science degree from the Harvard School of Public Health.

William A. Tisdale, M.D., is a director of the Gerontology Unit and professor of medicine at the University of Vermont College of Medicine. He has taught at the Dartmouth, Yale, and Harvard medical schools and has written many professional articles on internal medicine and the elderly. He was a contributor to a national plan for research on aging for the National Institute on Aging. In addition to his teaching and research in Vermont, he provides primary care for geriatric patients and serves as a consultant. He received his medical doctor degree with honors from Harvard Medical School.